Alarming Sleep Secrets

Alarming Sleep Secrets

YOUR DOCTOR IS MAKING AN ASS OUT OF YOU

Elizabeth Shannon

PUBLICATION NOTICE
This book is published by Ingram Spark. It is also available electronically through Kindle.

ISBN-13: 978-0-6485584-2-2
ISBN-10: 0-6485584-2-8

About the Author

Elizabeth Shannon is a sleep evangelist, researcher, educator, and outlying industry expert. She was introduced to brain wave technologies and meditation in 1978 at pioneering personal development seminars. This interest continued outside of her professional work at KPMG, Kellogg's and the NAB – as peak performance was not discussed in workplaces at the time.

After marrying a grazier and moving to a remote sheep property, her *Compatibility Blanket*™ bedding invention in 2000 saw a return to sleep research.

Elizabeth Shannon

Her *Sleep with the Experts* webinar program in 2009 was attended by insomniacs and health care professionals from all 5 continents, and lead to the *Sleep Mojo* book, which has been updated and incorporated into *Alarming Sleep Secrets*.

Shannon is a regular on the *Today Show*, featured on *9am with David and Kim*, Radio KPCC Southern California, 2UE, 3AW, 4BC, 6PR, ABC, the *Sydney Morning Herald, Herald-Sun, The Age*, the *Sunday Telegraph, HC Online* and numerous publications.

She makes no apology for not being a medical doctor or professor. This book highlights mismanagement, malpractice, conflicts of interest, professional negligence and corporate and government duty of care breaches.

"Qualified experts" created, represent, organise and actively support this fundamentally broken system that is costing many lives, and the lives of children.

Clearly an independent review is what's needed, starting with a Royal Commission.

Disclaimer

Elizabeth Shannon is not a medical professional. The information in this book has been prepared and/or obtained for general information, education, reference, and entertainment purposes only and is not intended to provide medical or psychological advice. The author of this book and owner of websites is not a doctor, psychologist or psychiatrist, and does not pretend to be.

The information is not intended in any way to be a substitute for advice or assessment from a medical or healthcare professional, nor should it be implied as such. It is the reader's responsibility to determine the validity, accuracy and applicability of all information provided.

Changing medical prescriptions and other interventions requires the supervision of exceptionally knowledgeable experts.

The information in this book is broadly available, in plain sight, on the internet, in books, and can be followed up by pursuing the references supplied.

By continuing to read this book you agree that you will not take any action without first confirming the information with a third party expert.

By purchasing this book you agreed to the Terms and Conditions and Disclaimers of the writer. For further information go to: http://www.sleeplessnomore.com/disclaimer/, http://www.sleeplessnomore.com/terms-of-service and http://www.sleeplessnomore.com/privacy-policy/.

Dedication

Dedicated to Henry.

Acknowledgements

Looking back it seems the varied parts of my life have all been leading up to this book, and I consider this my legacy.

It began with my father who constantly told me to 'never be afraid to ask a question', and my mother who had a stint in censorship during World War II.

Who knew that these would be the seeding traits that might lead to this book?

I was a maths and science sort of a girl at school, and after graduating in economics from the University of Sydney moved jobs and careers every few years because once I understood something I wanted to move on to something else. After learning very little at university (except how to party), getting a masters/PHD was never even tempting. That would have required staying in one discipline for far too long. B-o-r-i-n-g.

Acknowledging people by name is not what I will do here because the list would probably be a hundred or so people, from intelligent friends to radicals and even my restrictive catholic boarding school where I toed the line ... until one day when I decided not to. Funny how many of my most outspoken friends with leadership qualities were restricted and challenged at some point in their lives, and later decided to make their own rules.

Boarding school and control freaks have given me a heightened sense of looking at the world through power bases.

Who is telling who what to do and why?

In sleep and mental health, this is just about all you need to know. As you will find out.

I've had awesome bosses at most of the companies I've worked in, from fastidious to demanding to worldly-wise, and I've learned a lot from the dodgy ones too. See that... how can you thank someone for being dodgy – but I genuinely learned heaps from them.

And learned a lot about leadership from a small country community I lived in where their answer to my ideas and suggestions was usually no.

They did me more favours than I realized at the time.

I understand that many people are not going to listen to what I say in this book. And many will dismiss what I say because I'm not a professor.

Making excuses for my lack of PHD is not going to happen, I know plenty of intellectuals who I regard as thick, limited and boring. Some should be in jail because they actually know the facts, got too dirty, and are working in their own self interest. And yes, in this field.

I'm writing this book for people who want to listen to a new perspective. And especially for people who have been touched by mental health and/or sleeping problems – and are finding it difficult to find real solutions.

The doctors and intellectuals are clearly failing.

Why else would we have so many millions on prescription drugs?

It seems that people no longer want to do any work towards finding a solution to their underlying problems – they have bought the marketing that "popping a pill" actually works.

Unfortunately you'll learn in this book that popping a pill can be the start of the escalation of your problem. Not the solution.

I'm writing for YOU, if you want to get the *quick and easy solution* by reading this book. Or at least the quick and easy *understanding* of this complex environment.

I've included all the expert references, from real evidence-based medicine, so that you can double check the information by yourself, in your own time.

And added enough information so that you can see the lies and harmful information that is being promoted to you, in the name of profits and business models – not your health and mental health.

So here's to the awesome people and friends I have known in school, university and college, accounting, KPMG, the NAB, Kellogg's, DEC, consulting, art, motivation, internet marketing, the media, presenters and speakers, personal development, alternative health, retail, hospitality, mentors, agriculture and horticulture, Landcare, community groups, charities, clients, experts and randoms.

If by some miracle this book gets any real traction they'll be doing a "Chapter 5" on me for sure, so I'll tell you now I'm no saint, not qualified to be writing this (ahem..) and yes, I did inhale.

My question to them is why does this book need to come from me, the outlier? Who, in 1.5 million people employed in Health Care and Social Assistance in Australia, is doing any clinical governance? And where are the brainy types when we need them to lead and disrupt?

Cheers to the leaders you will learn about in this book. It has taken me a very long time to isolate this small group of outspoken, amazingly competent world leaders in the mental health and evidence space that have the courage to speak out, and take the heat from powerful organisations who prefer you did not know the truth.

These experts are the ones leading peer global organisations, publishing quality papers in the British Medical Journal, reviewing clinical trials, appearing in court cases and exposing frauds.

People like Professor Peter Gøtzsche, Robert Whitaker, Professor David Healy and Professor Jon Jureidini.

Most of the truth tellers are overseas, and they're thinly spread.

That is what this book really offers.

Links to *their* knowledge, *their* research and *their* courage.

Don't miss this opportunity to learn from them.

Once you get it, there will be no turning back.

It might make you angry, or sad, or both. But it is worth the effort.

Thanks to my sister Margaret, who has supported me in writing this book in many ways, and quietly believes in what I do in spite of my blunt, over the top attitude and annoying focus.

Thank you to many friends who support me in myriad ways over many years. Many I don't see any more, but I remember you all. Some helped me grow up, some pushed me along, all of them were accepting, and others were wicked and funny.

They keep me sane and give me the confidence to stick it up the system through this book.

Yes I'm old-school, that's what happens when you've lived a life and watched things develop over decades. If you think I'm having a senior moment, I can assure you that this book is not one of them.

By the way, if you haven't noticed – I'm not an author or editor and I don't want to hear complaints from the grammar police. I was taught how to speak and write properly, I just choose not to.

I do however apologise for my bluntness. This book cannot be written in a politically correct way by me – look for someone else who might be doing that. Yes, I use the word 'nuts', and worse, as part of my effort to get a jarring feeling when you read it. It needs to be noticed. We need to be noticing when people go a bit nuts, before they get worse and get really nuts. It can happen when they're reacting to something they saw that deeply disturbed them, being abused, feeling lonely, if they're not coping, going through puberty ruggedly, "bored to tears", getting divorced or moving house.

Many of us have lived straitjacket-lives, looking totally sane.

I'm also using the word nuts as a "trend stopper". In my opinion the pendulum has swung too far towards labelling people with the politically correct 'mental health issues' of ADHD, OCD, PTSD, WHATEVER, instead of having a proper friendly and supportive conversation and listening to their story. Really listening. Then waiting for more. Most people actually know what's going on that is disturbing them: it's just not that easy to talk about it. So they internalise it, and squash it down some more, instead of letting out a "bit of nuts" and releasing the pressure.

Once labelled, it's all too easy to *not* engage. Then we get a bigger problem.

I'm pretty sure everyone has feral times in their lives when they are acting out and doing weird stuff, to deal with pain that they are suffering at that particular time. I also think that in order to make major changes in our lives we need to go to the extreme to unhook ourselves from the hum drum that looks like normality, but will probably kill us – certainly our spirit. We all have passion and we all have spirit – sometimes it comes out in emotions and expressions that look normal, other times they do not. It's called having a life. And thank goodness we are different.

There's a great quote in Paulo Coelho's book *Veronica Decides to Die:* "I should have been madder. But, as doubtless happens with most people, she had found this out too late."

Be a great friend to people if you can – and especially when they're feeling dodgy or acting out.

Wishing you love, happiness, passion, courage and fulfilment.

And healing, if that's what you're here for.

Love and peace

Elizabeth

Table of Contents

Part One: The Lights Are Out And No-One's Home.

CHAPTER 1

Introduction

The intention of this book is to simplify the scientific and medical research around sleep and mental health and provide you with real solutions to these challenges.

For every so-called-expert that is promoting a particular solution to these problems there appears to be another that is disagreeing.

Some of the discussions in this field are heated, and some are downright aggressive.

Some of the solutions are deadly.

Either way, the problems of insomnia, depression, anxiety and PTSD, etc. are increasing.

And the result for you and me is confusing.

Here is the situation:

- 1 in 6 Australians (or 16.6 percent) are taking antidepressants[1]. (If you think America is weird and backward, we have exactly the same figures),
- Over 35 million psycho scripts are being written annually in Australia[2],
- If you present to your doctor with insomnia you will be prescribed in 95.2 percent of cases[3], medications which will never solve the underlying problems that present as the symptom of insomnia,
- The 2013-14 BEACH study showed that patients present to their doctors with the following health concerns: 16 % depression, 12 % anxiety, 3.9 % Insomnia, 2.2 % sleep apnea; and 2.3 % dementia[4],

- Approximately 95 percent of the Medical Benefits Scheme's listed items are not evidence based[5],
- I can find *no study* into what percentage of the Pharmaceutical Benefits Scheme is evidence based;
- Total government expenditure on the Pharmaceutical Benefits Scheme increased by 19.5 percent, in one year, between 2014-15 and 2015-2016[6],
- Health Care and Social Assistance is now Australia's largest employing industry, with 1,523,000 workers or 13 percent of the Australian work force[7]. (Is that a good thing, or an indication of our incompetence?)
- Antidepressants double the suicide rate in children[8],
- In April 2017 GlaxoSmithKline was ordered to pay $ 3 million over the suicide death of Stewart Dolin who was taking antidepressants and jumped in front of a train[9], and
- About 30 percent of Australian women take the contraceptive pill which is associated with increased rates of depression and higher than average antidepressant use (particularly in adolescents).

What's more, we are being told that there are many more people in Australia with mental health problems, that the problem is understated, and that we should see our doctor about it.

Really?

Let's stop for a minute and actually consider the situation.

We need to look behind the marketing, power plays, significant amount of publicity and news stories surrounding mental health.

It's time to learn the truth.

It's time to simplify the confusion.

And it's time for the facts to be revealed in everyday language so that we can understand what's actually going on in the sleep and mental health industries.

What if I told you that what is being marketed and prescribed as evidence-based best practice is often misleading and even fraudulent?

It is costing lives and adversely affecting the health of millions of Australians, including children as young as infants.

The systems are entrenched, and complicated – but once you understand the forces at play it becomes very simple.

Very, very simple.

Recently I explained to a friend that my book would provide the 'everyman's/everywoman's version' of medical research, so that YOU, the potential patient, parent or mental health sufferer can understand what is going on – without doing a doctorate/PHD.

And that's not to put you down.

Or me either.

Part of the problem is that everyone's arguing (even screaming) about evidence-based medicine, but no-one is explaining what "evidence based medicine" actually means, and how it affects you and your life.

I know many people who have worked in the medical profession all their lives, and they don't get it either.

Yes, you read that correctly.

And I've met many professionals and experts who knock the peak bodies that are endeavouring to ascertain the truth.

Because it doesn't suit their agendas.

Sleep and mental health seem to be the biggest game in town.

And they're telling us that most mental health problems are largely undiagnosed.

So does that mean that 50 percent of the population is nuts? 60 percent?

Here are some of the **Alarming Sleep Secrets** revealed and developed in this book:

- Antidepressants don't work and have serious side effects including increased suicide, violence and *akathisia/akathesia* (the new word you **should** know about, fast).
- Doctors are failing at clinical governance, continuing to prescribe dubious drugs when other evidence-based obvious solutions such as talk therapies are being largely ignored.
- How the drug companies define the word "addiction" to suit their commercial aims – deceiving patients and doctors.
- Why clinical trials can be biased, deceptive and fatally flawed, and how the drug companies retain the raw information to avoid scrutiny.

- How Australian doctors prescribe in 95.2 percent of cases when patients present with insomnia, drugs that the Therapeutic Goods Administration unsuccessfully attempted to reclassify from Schedule 4 to Schedule 8 in 2012.
- The shocking misinformation being promoted by leading mental health charities, institutions and do-gooders.
- The side effects of sleeping pills and antidepressants – important when you know that 35 million psycho drugs are being prescribed every year.
- Why drugging the symptoms of insomnia, anxiety and mental health issues makes the problems worse. By overriding these most valuable early warning symptoms for health and happiness, solutions are delayed and sometimes become impossible to resolve.
- Why the present mismanagement of insomnia and mental health problems is costing Australians billions of dollars a year – money we cannot afford to keep spending. The *Wasted* documentary by Four Corners showed that approximately 95 percent of the subsidized Medical Benefits Scheme is not evidence based. There is yet to be a similar study on the Pharmaceutical Benefits Scheme. Wonder why?
- Health Care and Social Assistance is now Australia's largest employing industry, employing 13 percent of workers. Have we backed ourselves into a corner, where cleaning up our health industry would cause a national recession? Is that worth dying for?
- The power and money games that are so entrenched that you pay – with your money, your sanity and sometimes with your life.
- Why the pussy-footing around doctors' responsibilities?
- What is a mental health problem and what is not? For example social anxiety disorder (being shy, or introverted?) is classified as a mental health condition, but bonking your horse is fine. Apparently. Who knew?
- The Australian media tolerates medical and pharmaceutical advertising direct to the public when most other developed countries do not allow it. Mainstream media advertising income has become more and more challenged as social media and the internet reach their target audiences more efficiently. Expect to see more and more

advertisements telling you that you have a physical or mental health problem (if that's possible!). And expect to see the continuing death of independent reviews of medical evidence by journalists. Don't wait till the major movie stars advertise xyz drug before you wake up. You know it's happening with vitamins and supplements. And you've watched journalists' careers being compromised as they speak out.

- ASX listed companies in the health industry have a primary motivation of profit, not your health. They include the drug companies, government providers, medical practice administrators, medical services companies, medical training, medical appliances, medical diagnoses, etc. Accept that as a given and a continuum. It's laughable to expect the stock market to change anytime soon as shareholders expect ever increasing dividends and stock price increases. Fines for fraudulent misrepresentation of information, encouraging off-label prescribing, and being sued for the occasional death are just business costs. Successful cases are rare, the risk is low, the payout immaterial. That's it. Move on.
- Our super funds invest in these companies, so we are all complicit.
- The next advertising frontier is Google rankings, other search facilities and social media. With one in twenty Google searches now related to health, algorithms are changing. What an opportunity! E.g. Google is working with the Mayo Clinic as the apparently peak-evidence-base in the world[10]. That won't be my 'doctor Google': I'll be googling a bit deeper, thanks. I will be searching, searching. It just makes it harder for Joe Blow, who won't bother, and they know that.

What you'll discover in this book:

- How the medical system works, both mainstream/allopathic and complementary so you can work your way through the system to survive.
- Get your argument straight for all the 'conspiracy theorist' nay-sayers you will encounter, who don't have a clue and have their heads in the sand. But want to take the mickey out of you every time.

- Akathisia... a potentially deadly side effect of antidepressants. Learn the word "akathisia" and how to pronounce it. It's the new new word that needs to slip off your tongue in any discussion about mental health and how some drugs are not looking after sufferers. Say it after me: A-ka-these-e-a. And for the purists, phonetically it looks like this: /æ.kə.ˈθɪ.si.ə/.
- What 'evidence based medicine' actually means. The part played by randomised controlled trials (RCTs) and meta-analyses.
- How RCTs sometimes mis-translate down the system to your prescription.
- Proof that your doctors and psychiatrists are not advising using evidence-based-medicine in the areas of sleep and mental health.
- Don't wait for the federal or state health ministers to wake up. They are going down another path, and have been for a long time.
- Stop the confusion, and know the facts.
- Learn what you can do to find your solutions.
- Discover easy, practical solutions.
- Get back your life.

There are some serious problems, and they are affecting every one of you reading this – because the problem is now very common – or more precisely *marketed* to be very common.

Whether it's you, an immediate family member, a friend or "all of the above" that have been affected with sleep and mental health issues.

If you're anything like me, this book is going to make you angry, or worse.

I first took notice of brain wave patterns when I was learning to meditate in 1978, and I was unaware at the time where that curiosity and discipline would lead in my life.

My sleep research began in earnest about 2000, and it was a life changing experience. I was always interested in natural solutions to sleep, as I learned early (or knew instinctively) that insomnia was a symptom of something else. An underlying problem.

I probably started off a bit alternative, with an interest in herbal solutions. As the years went on I found myself more and more interested in the "maths and science" of it all. For years now I've been most interested in peak research bodies and the real evidence base.

And combining that with my very practical understanding of sleep, stress, relationships, reluctance to change, personal development, children and families, nutrition and food, and life in general.

There is always a reason why we can't sleep. And it can be easy or hard to find out that reason.

For some people they just can't switch off at night because they are pro-actively doing work related things right up to bedtime and simply have very bad lifestyle habits that need to change.

For others, resolving the problem is much more complicated. Mental health issues are connected to anxiety and other problems that might prevent someone from sleeping well throughout the night. Resolving mental health issues requires understanding personal problems, which can be complicated, even painful. We often have to discover exactly what set off anxiety, for example, that built up over time – and may have been triggered by a seemingly insignificant, misinterpreted event, even in early childhood.

So addressing the problems early is a great idea. And it reinforces the responsibility of parents that the way we nurture and support our children and families is vital – for now and later throughout their whole lives.

"Nipping things in the bud", that old-school saying, is actually a great idea if you can, when it comes to sleep and mental health issues.

Another complication is if you, the parent, were subjected to abuse or neglect or abandonment in your youth – and don't really understand or feel the problem 'from outside'.

Many behavioural problems are generational and familial. As kids we consider our circumstances as 'normal' – and absorb it all subconsciously - which can be good or bad. Or good *and* bad: as there are many traits we pick up.

Mental health problems can result from remembered, or forgotten, childhood abuse, feelings of abandonment, other significant problems such as having fought in a war or working in traumatic jobs.

One of the most important things is that we recognise the problem, talk about it openly, and get help from someone who will actually help us.

You'll read more about that in Part Three of this book, where we discuss and discover the underlying reasons why we can't sleep.

Insomnia does not always relate to mental health problems. But it often does. For example when people are stressed, anxious, grieving or traumatised in any way.

Or more basically, if your teenage child isn't getting enough sleep and they start being really feral. You know ... that one?

Mental health problems and sleeping problems go hand in hand. Without good sleep, the mental health problems get worse. It only takes one bad night's sleep to understand that. But it's a fact that alludes many so-called-experts.

Sleeping problems are the ultimate early warning signal of mental health problems, in my opinion.

Sleeping problems are also a great early warning signal of general health problems and lifestyle challenges too.

That's why I'm banging on so much about sleep. Duh.

For now, though, it is important to give you the background information on the sleep and mental health story from an industry perspective.

The big picture on it. So you'll totally 'get it'.

Natural Solutions, Non-Drug Interventions, Talk Therapies

Years into my research I read the book *Anatomy of an Epidemic, Magic Bullets, Psychiatric Drugs, and the Astonishing Rise of Mental Illness in America* by Robert Whitaker.

The book totally messed with me. I found it very disturbing. I kept putting the book down thinking 'this can't possibly be true' and also because I couldn't cope with the consequences of it being true.

I can remember thinking 'this guy is just dramatising', or 'he's got an axe to grind', and 'he's a conspiracy theorist'. All of that while my gut kept saying his background was very sound, that his research looked exemplary, that he seemed like an honest guy.

Basically I did not *want* to believe that the book was true. Because if it was, the world was a nastier place, and the problems with mental health and sleep just got a whole lot uglier than I had previously thought.

But I agreed with his research and understanding of how to deal with mental health issues. That people need to be listened to, and that there is always more to the story of psychotic incidences and the inability to cope as 'normal' human beings.

And who, after all, is calling who, "normal".

And doesn't everyone in their lives have some nutty stages? When they have to cope with serious distress such as deciding to leave their profession, divorce their partners, or as the aftermath of traumatic and/or emotionally damaging incidences, when they are under enormous pressure at work, or having to deal with really bad news?

And if you try to avoid life and its ups and downs sooner or later the Mac Truck will come to mess up your carefully orchestrated avoidances.

After integrating the extent of the systemic problems the challenge to fix the problems became enormous.

Reading that book was a major turning point that I didn't realise at the time.

This book is part of my contribution to the same cause of making sleep and mental health sane.

And I'm pitching it to "intelligent Joe Blow", hopefully not bogging you down in too much research.

But at the same time, including enough hard core research that if you want to go and check what I'm saying, you can verify the information for yourself, today and now.

And protect myself from "Chapter 5 incidences". You'll find out about them as you read.

Not Anti-Drug and not Anti-Doctor

I am not anti-drug or anti-medical-profession, nor am I against allopathic medicine, and I don't have an axe to grind.

What I will say is that if the rest of the medical and health systems are as crap at looking after their patients as they are at looking after insomniacs and people with mental health issues, then there is very little hope for our system at all.

I often go looking for good news stories to balance out the rubbish that I find in sleep/mental health that I have got to know intimately over the last 33 years.

And often when I go looking it gets worse. Like the night I watched the Four Corners *Wasted* television program[11], where it was revealed that of about 5700 listed items on Australia's Medical Benefits Scheme (MBS) only about 5 percent are REALLY evidence based!

No wonder we can't afford our medical system and medical insurances.

And I wonder why it takes people like me, from outside the medical profession, to feel the need to write books on the failings of the medical and mental health systems.

If an untrained person can see all this, why is there complete silence – just about – from the medical professionals?

Are they dumber than we think? Corrupted? Afraid? Confused? Given no alternatives?

All of the above?

Has the system reached the point of no return?

My 'axe to grind' if I have one, is that it is ME that is compelled to write this book.

Not one of the 1.5 million Health Care and Social Assistance professionals employed in Australia that observe this system every single day.

Or that it takes a Four Corners "Wasted" program for the truth to be exposed in the medical profession. And then, afterwards, basically no changes are happening.

Argh.

There are people dying every day, and continuing with their mental and physical health problems because of the gross inadequacies in the system.

Which means it is only going to get worse without a paradigm shift in the way we do things.

Children suiciding.

Parents killing their children and then themselves.

How do we possibly ignore this?

Open Your Mind and Prepare to be Shocked

Lies, manipulation, culpable behaviour, outdated regulations, and 'evidence-based' myths.

I could fill this book with shocking stories of parents' finding their children after they had committed suicide, and parents who have killed their children and then themselves.

But I find it too disturbing to think about. And even worse to write about.

Aren't we traumatised enough?

The stories provide no help to the sufferers. There is no comfort for them.

Instead I hope to prevent it happening by exposing the problem for what it is.

This is not a pretty read, but for your health and the health of your loved ones and families it is worth reading this book.

So Far Behind

I'm Australian, but the research for this book is internationally relevant.

For example, our drug approval agency in Australia is the Therapeutic Goods Administration (TGA), but references are also made to the US Food and Drug Administration (FDA). Each country obviously has their own equivalents. UK readers will think of the Medicines and Healthcare Products Regulatory Agency (MHRA), etc.

The research is mainly from overseas. Australia is embarrassingly behind.

What you will learn in this book is not limited to the sleep industry, insomnia, and mental health issues.

Systemic and Institutional

I can see the same patterns repeating themselves across the health industry, medical profession, doctors, corporations, registered training organisations (RTOs), nurses, schools and university education bodies, leading health institutes, research centres and foundations.

It's systemic and institutionalised – and it's very serious.

It's costing Australians billion of dollars a year in ineffectual medical treatments, drugs, addictions, rehab clinics, road accidents – even suicidal ideation, suicides and homicides.

It's costing lives, our children's lives.

And it's costing businesses, and the economy. Big time.

But no-one is talking about it.

If this book gets any traction I'll be getting some serious flack from the industry, drug companies, medical professionals and everyone who doesn't want you to know this stuff... all the people and organisations that are profiting from your inability to sleep and resultant mental health and performance issues.

Don't shoot the messenger. I've got very little to gain from this book. I'm just compelled to write it.

Most of it has been told before, by more impressive people than me.

It's not new news.

That's the irony – all this information is in *plain sight*.

But the message and the antiquated systems aren't being "seen" by enough people and children.

That's the frustrating and really ugly fact.

Question: What is the similarity between cigarettes and lack of sleep?

Answer: Cigarettes were proven to be addictive and damaging to our health in old-timers-time, and still they are readily available in Australia, with the government making billions out of their sale. The companies producing the cigarettes still persist in selling us a product they know damages our health.

The government subsidises medical and psychological practices which are not evidence based.

What's more, the medical system continues, with no leadership being shown to change what is wrong.

Highly Qualified People are Sustaining this Broken System

The system is being run by "qualified" people.

And the system is fundamentally broken.

The only conclusion that anyone can make is that the qualifications are fundamentally compromised. Common sense tells us that.

BUT, thankfully I've found a very few good people.

They are both qualified and courageous, and they have common sense too.

Listen to them, and follow them.

After reading this book, when you approach your medical professional, don't mention me, that won't work.

Clearly.

Instead, quote your personal research from the world experts that I have led you to – and let them deal with the quality information sources.

If and when your medical professional argues against Cochrane, Professor Peter Gøtzsche, the British Medical Journal's publication of *Restoring Study 329* (September 2015), the warning labels on the medicine packs, and the $ 3 million suicide payout given in the Dolin vs. GSK case in April 2017 then you can form your own opinion about the quality of your health care.

There are obviously many cases where antidepressants did not lead to suicide. And there are many people who swear that their medications saved their lives, and help them.

People say that as soon as they start coming off their medications they feel bad again – and that that justifies them continuing... not knowing about the withdrawal effects of the medications – and that the tapering stage is seen by many experts as the most dangerous stage.

Others swear black and blue that their medications are working.

I'm directing you to the best people I have found internationally.

The responsibility is yours. Always has been, always will be.

The responsibility is not your doctor's, or your psychiatrist's, or your health care professional's – but yours alone. Only you get to feel the rewards of your own good health care, and only you get to feel the pain of bad health care.

I think this book should be compulsory reading.

If you don't read it for you, then read it for your children, friends' children, grandchildren, workmates, friends and associates.

Doctors Have Responsibility

I'm not anti-doctor, but dangerous drugs would have no power if they were not prescribed by doctors, and if patients did not trust the doctors who are prescribing.

The drug companies will continue to maximise their profits, they are listed on the stock markets and that is their aim. Don't live in fairyland and expect that to change.

Hold your doctor accountable.

Look up information from the sources I have supplied in this book. Check out the research in the Cochrane Library.

Demand your doctor explain the side effects of the medications they are prescribing to you, and the withdrawal effects. All drugs have side effects. Ensure that they know.

I find it interesting that only this month (May 2017) I'm noticing damage control advertisements being aired on television to elevate the image of doctors in Australia.

Doctors are the linchpin.

The pressure is building from both sides.

Patients should demand transparency and full disclosure. Why are questions not being asked about the enormous amounts of prescriptions being written each week by Australian doctors for sleep and mental health problems when the evidence supports other solutions?

Doctors have to take full responsibility. They are the ones that are trained at universities to advise patients. They are the ones that supposedly know more than the general public about what is good for us. They are apparently the elite brains in our society. They are the ones prescribing the drugs.

To distract from the main game, they're trying to make it about alternative medicine, anti-vaxxers and conspiracy theories.

We know better.

The problem is main stream.

The general population is growing a brain.

Things are beginning to blow.

Let's not pretend to be surprised.

You need to know where to stand and how to protect yourself.

A Few Good Men and Women

I've kept the message straight forward by featuring only a few world leaders in the field.

I'm into clarity.

I do not want to muddy the waters through argy bargy.

The system loves confusion.

You'll get a very clear picture from the few good people I feature and if you want to argue the point after that, tell someone who cares.

I'm getting on with my next project.

CHAPTER 2

History of a Problem

We sleep for about a third of our lives, or we should sleep for about a third of our lives.

Obviously as babies and children, we slept a lot longer than a third of the time.

But for many it is easier said than done.

And because of the sleeping problems that people have endured for centuries there have been a range of so-called-solutions and real solutions put forward.

"Symptom" versus "Underlying Problem"

You will see as a repeating chant throughout this book that "insomnia is a symptom of something else".

It is important to very clearly understand the difference between a "symptom" and the actual problem.

We'll call the problem the "underlying problem".

Why is this so important?

Because the health/medical industry and medical solutions are often pitched to "cure" the symptom, not the underlying problem.

Which is no solution at all.

If you graze your leg against a very sharp object and end up with a bleeding gash in your leg, the *symptom* is a bleeding gash in your leg. The *underlying problem* is that you grazed your leg against a sharp object. There is no benefit in stitching, binding and/or applying pressure to the gash in your leg if you do not learn that you should not graze your leg against very sharp objects in the future. That that action leads to the adverse 'symptom' of a bleeding gash in your leg.

Actually, the bandaging solves the problem of the *symptom*. The leg gash symptom will probably heal. That's the "quick and easy fix".

But unless you have learned that you should avoid grazing your body against sharp objects in the future, you have not addressed the underlying problem.

And the problem will present itself again, because we missed the point.

Please don't think I'm being derogatory here, but this book will demonstrate just how far this ludicrous basic concept is being used in the sleep and mental health industry.

And exactly why health management in some disciplines is getting worse over time, not better, costing Australia and other countries a fortune.

Getting back to 'insomnia' being a symptom of something else: here are a few *underlying problems* that present as the *symptom of insomnia*:

- A general lifestyle issue, such as lack of exercise, which might mean that at the end of the day our bodies are not tired, because they have done very little physical work;
- An underlying mental health issue that caused anxiety, which means that when we go to bed we are thinking and worrying about a myriad different things, and unable to relax;
- The side effect of medications, recreational drugs, alcohol, food allergies and intolerances; or
- Circadian rhythm disruption from jetlag or shift work.

This book will demonstrate that the solutions being presented by the health and mental health industries generally are only dealing with the symptoms.

That's where the money is.

And over time, the industries have strengthened their broken systems to include best medical practice guidelines, government policy, media advertising, clinical trials, published medical reports, prescribing guidelines, drug approval procedures, government instrumentalities, clinical governance procedures, prescribing guidelines, research facilities, lobby groups, publicly listed companies, international conferences, remuneration schemes, even charitable organisations and university departments.

And you are part of the problem, because you are generally looking for the 'quick and easy fix'.

It is more difficult to investigate the underlying problem that causes insomnia and mental health problems, it takes longer than popping a pill or sleeping overnight at a sleep clinic, and it might require discipline and lifestyle changes – but if we really address the underlying problem, we will find the solution.

And that solution will likely be final and long term.

But that's not where the medical industries are focused.

In the area of sleep, fatigue and mental health, we will find that the allopathic medical model is severely lacking, even culpable.

Alternatively talk therapies, psychotherapy, counselling, exercise, relaxation techniques, meditation (and the like) can be beneficial. And there is real evidence to support them.

Curing the Symptom

So if people can't sleep, let's *force* them to sleep! Let's deal with the symptom.

In the beginning were chloral hydrate, paraldehyde, then barbiturates used as sedatives, ethylchlorvynol, carbromal, glutethimide, methyprylon and methaqualome.

It was benzodiazepines, commonly known as sleeping pills, that have stayed with us since the 1950s.

The "discovery" of benzodiazepines has been attributed to Hoffman-La Roche's chemist Leo Sternbach in the 1950s, who conducted experiments with rats, looking for compounds that would make animals less aggressive and numb to pain. In these experiments, under the influence of the chlordiazepoxide, rats would press a lever to eat, even though they knew that the food would be accompanied by an electric shock.[1]

The public did not hear about these animal tests, but an article published in the *Science News Letter* explained that if you took a tranquilliser "you might still feel scared when you see a car speeding toward you, but the fear would not make you run."[2]

The first benzodiazepine, chlordiazepoxide was brought to market in 1960, selling as Librium[3].

Early sedatives included meprobamate (sold as Miltown), chlordiazepoxide (selling as Librium) and Valium.

The dependence-producing properties of sedatives and tranquillizers has been a problem since the earliest chemicals, and continue with the benzodiazepines. See chapter 9.

Thalidomide was first brought to market in 1957 as a hypnotic sleeping pill by Chemie Grunenthal, under the name "Contergan" – the only non-barbiturate sedative known at the time. "Clinical trials" were conducted, and they advertised their product as "completely safe" for everyone, including mother and child, "even during pregnancy," as its developers "could not find a dose high enough to kill a rat." By 1960, thalidomide was marketed in 46 countries, with sales nearly matching those of aspirin.

In a post-war era when sleeplessness was prevalent,
thalidomide was marketed to a world hooked
on tranquilizers and sleeping pills.
At the time, one out of seven Americans took them regularly. [4]

It was also claimed to cure anxiety, insomnia, gastritis and tension. Later it was used off-label for nausea and morning sickness in pregnant women. Throughout the world about 10,000 cases were reported of babies being born with malformed limbs, only 40% of them survived.

Thalidomide changed the way drug approvals were made in the United States, with more rigorous approval processes being introduced by the US Food and Drug Administration (FDA).

You will learn more in the next few chapters, how clinical trials turned out to be a marketing and business bonanza for the drug companies, and did NOT clean up the industry OR guarantee proven health and mortality benefits.

Off label prescribing of drugs is still very much alive today! There are multi-million dollar law suits and fines to prove it. Incidents and cases are so common that I'm convinced the drug companies consider it is just a 'cost of doing business'.

And the sad part is, through all the banter that everything is getting better – we have come full circle.

The latest information I'm reading now is that anti-depressants are again associated with compromised babies and neurodevelopmental delay, with a new link to autism.

And the most common drugs that are being taken by pregnant women are antidepressants[6].

Hard to believe!

We have come full circle now...

Have we learned nothing?

60 years, men on the moon, Hubble telescope, the internet, Cochrane, neuroscience, CERN, and we still can't guarantee that drugs do no harm before they are marketed.

So much for randomised clinical trials (RCTs), the FDA, the TGA, clinical governance, doctors' due diligence, drug company checks and measures and full and honest disclosure of drug side-effects.

Thankfully we are bright enough to see that there is more in play than making the world healthier.

The responsibility for you and me is to ensure that we know where to get the right information.

This book uncovers the games at play.

CHAPTER 3

Keeping Us in the Dark with "Evidence Based Medicine"

The means to protect ourselves from a recurrence of the thalidomide disaster have been our undoing. Product patents gave an incentive to pharmaceutical companies to produce blockbuster drugs — drugs that were so valuable to a company and its survival that the incentives to breach regulations and hide any safety data that might be inconvenient for the company are so huge that entire trials are hidden, that almost all trials are ghost-written to ensure the data looks right, and no one, not even the FDA, has access to the data.[1]

Every entrepreneur is taught "out of a problem comes opportunity", and the Thalidomide story was no exception.

As it turns out the challenges and costs associated with having to conduct proper scientific trials became the cornerstone of the greatest commercial opportunity for the drug and medical equipment companies.

Then Came Patents

With a patent taken out for particular drugs, you are protected for 8 years. You can keep your clinical information secret as commercial in confidence information and as protection for your shareholders and charge the price the market will absorb without the threat of a generic version of the drug being made.

It will also be prudent to prove the efficacy of your patented new drug against similar or competing drugs on the market, thereby proving your competitive and professional advantage – and create a marketing opportunity to the medical professionals.

Then Came Professional Negligence/Exposure and Insurance

Once a drug is proven to be evidence-based through published clinical trial information in world leading journals, and passed by the FDA/TGA it becomes 'best practice' and recommended as the latest advanced solution for the particular health or mental health problem being addressed.

What's more, if the medical professionals chose to go outside these new established guidelines they leave themselves exposed to professional negligence law suits.

The insurance industry benefits from this, by taking on these risks from the doctors through professional negligence insurance.

That's the Slam Dunk

Not only do we recommend these drugs for certain patients, but they are approved by the FDA/TGA.

The drugs are now "evidence-based" and they become *best practice*. Doctors and medical professionals have a duty of care to follow best practice and evidence-based medicine. Doctors can be seen to be professionally negligent if they do not consider prescribing, and they risk being professionally sidelined if they rock the boat.

This FDA approval process was strengthened in the 1960s. The present system has had about 50 years to be polished and fully entrenched.

Clinical trials, FDA/TGA approval, patents, best practice guidelines, clinical governance, professional negligence and insurance.

They all go hand in hand.

You can see how this all developed, can't you?

Taking a Closer Look at Clinical Trials and How Evidence is Established

Recently I found an awesome and simple video explanation of evidence based medicine and the establishment of clinical efficacy[2] given by Dr David Healy, who you will see featured a number of times in this book.

Here is the link if you want to go there immediately. https://vimeo.com/59145379

The video is of Dr David Healy presenting the hypothetical case to make alcohol an approved antidepressant.

He presents the case using clinically accepted principles and the processes by which drugs become approved by the FDA/TGA and other approving bodies.

It's a great insight into what the approval process looks like, and it's shocking.

So here are the steps taken in order to get your drug or substance approved as an antidepressant, on to the market and into mainstream and subsidized use (as explained by Dr David Healy):

A. First establish that you have just 'invented' the substance and it is capable of being patented. (Otherwise there's no money in it, so why bother?)

B. Run a trial for 6 weeks, comparing your substance to another (in this case alcohol to Ribena drink, say). You don't have to show that you have saved lives, or got people back to work – the outcome measure is done using "rating scales".

C. The rating scales might include questions such as "do you feel less anxious?" and "are you getting better sleep?"

D. Only one out of 5 trials has to be positive to get a drug approved, or say 2 out of 10 trials.

E. Report the results of say 2, successful trial(s) in 100 different publications, which look like there were 100 different positive trails showing that it is very positive and works well. It is common for companies that do the trials to publish 50 different articles per trial, and they do not give an indication that they are dealing with just the one trial.

F. In the reports, alcohol might be only marginally better than the placebo, but we can include all the benefits of the alcohol and discount the placebo controllant totally. Accentuate the positive.

G. In extreme situations if a number of clinical trials do not perform well, we might use data from positive results in another country. By combining the information from the trials we can produce a positive result overall for alcohol. For the approval bodies such as the

FDA and MHRA, even if it looks strange, they still so ahead and give licensing approval based on the overall studies. Another way to do this is to attribute *all positive outcomes* to the drug/alcohol – even if, for example, the patient was to feel better in a week naturally.

H. Other companies and organisations are then able to bring their own, different forms of the product to the market.

I. What happens then, if you are not getting much better from just one product, is that multiple prescriptions can be made of the various different product versions, or brands. The product is now assumed to work, *proven to work*, and been approved: so if you are not getting better then different options should be investigated. E.g. it is not uncommon for medical practitioners and psychiatrists to meet people who are on 5 antidepressants from the same class, 5 antihypertensives, etc.

J. If the publications and trials are deemed satisfactory, The National Institute for Health and Care Excellence (NICE in England, or the national equivalent in your country) will *endorse* this drug as the number one solution that the medical profession should be using.

K. Then comes the cost-benefit proof that if the National Health Service (NHS or your country's equivalent/PBS, etc) spends money on this drug, then the country will be financially better off by using it in the long run. If we provide the product for free, or at a subsidized amount, it will be very beneficial, and save the country money.

L. You will be told, on the basis of 6 week trials, that you should be taking alcohol for life.

Here are some more problems outlined by Dr David Healy:

- Since the trials are for 6-8 weeks it is uncommon for significant side effects to turn up in that brief time span (explained for the alcohol example). So the reporting of side effects is limited to a very short window of time. *Actually* in the SSRI trials there were double the number of suicidal acts and violent acts also.
- It is only required to report a side effect if it affects 10 percent or more of the people in the trial.

- The results of the trials have been extrapolated to include the benefits to pregnant women.
- If the patient tries to withdraw or stop their medications and suffers from withdrawal symptoms, they will be told that it is caused by the illness that is being treated (not the withdrawal symptoms of coming off the alcohol/drugs). Which supports and reinforces the idea that you should be taking the alcohol/drugs for the rest of your life.
- If we do find adverse side effects caused by the alcohol/drugs there are thousands of studies to trawl and many writers who will come up with evidence that supports the premise that the illness causes (or "is") the side effects, not the drugs/alcohol. In this case that depression causes liver dysfunctions.
- The fact that the drugs are available by prescription only reduces the perceived risk of the drugs, and perhaps increases the length of time that the drug is taken for. He uses amphetamines as an example, showing that on the street they are regarded as calamitous, but when approved for prescription, pressure begins to be put on the medical professionals because not prescribing them is seen to be a problem. Because they are now being endorsed as the number one solution to the problem – not as ineffective or even dangerous - it has become "your duty to treat".

Also shown on the presentation screens, but not in this video are:

Stockholm Syndrome

After a bank raid in Sweden in 1973, it was recognized that isolation, a threat to life, and the kindness of captors can lead to Stockholm Syndrome. According to Dr David Healy, Stockholm Syndrome is exactly what prescription-only arrangements impose on patients and doctors.

In this comfortable, confidential environment that exists between the doctor and the patient, often outside influences are ignored, and doctors may not fastidiously tell patients about the side effects of the medications they are prescribing, nor follow up patients who are newly prescribed to ensure that they report any adverse side effects of medications, etc. And if the patient finds their condition worsening, it is very difficult for them to have the discussion that perhaps what the doctor had recommended was making them worse.

I'm a pretty confident and outspoken person, yet I have often found it difficult to broach topics with my doctor – and any attempts to present another point or suggest another avenue have resulted in a strained relationship. Not only for that day, but often permanently.

The other issue at play is the fact that you, as the patient, often want to condense your conversation to the absolute minimum, because it is the 'norm' to have a 10 minute or so consult. Only twice did I have doctors that actually asked general, friendly questions (when I lived in a country town and knew them) that might result in an holistic view of my health at the time. And of course they got a far better response. In fact when I lost weight my doctor was shocked that I had actually done what he had suggested I do – I think he said I was the first one ever. I attribute that to his open, friendly and negotiable approach.

But, as a general rule, I hate going to the doctor just like the next person. And minimizing the conversation always seems to be advantageous. To what? Certainly not to my best outcomes.

But we've got used to it. We have been 'trained' that way.

I think doctors get so used to 'being the expert' that they do not think they ever aren't. Even friends I have seem to think their opinion on marketing and bulldozers (whatever) is superior simply because they're doctors and they spent years at medical school.

Tell me you haven't encountered this?

Healy persists by saying that no medical school on the planet offers training on how to handle Stockholm Syndrome, how medical practitioners induce Stockholm Syndrome, and what they can do about it.

None.

"It is the reason doctors fail to recognize that adverse events happen to their patients even though these are now the fourth leading cause of death and how they rarely intervene to save their patients."[3]

Legal Exposure

Because treatment with the particular drugs is now regarded as best practice and endorsed by government health authorities, doctors and practitioners now leave themselves exposed to being sued if they do not prescribe. They can also be seen to be professionally negligent, and/or ostracized by their colleagues, their professional bodies and government authorities.

> *"Clinical trials were introduced as the eye of a needle*
> *through which the financial camel, that is*
> *the pharmaceutical industry,*
> *would have to squeeze if it wanted to get drugs*
> *on the market and make money.*
> *These trials would establish if drugs worked*
> *and would lead to a clear recognition of their hazards.*
> *But we have been led badly astray.*
> *The most extraordinary symbol of just how badly lies in the*
> *fact that the one drug that had been through a controlled*
> *trial before it was supposed to be marketed in which it had*
> *been shown to be safe and effective was ... thalidomide.*
> *This is the system on which we now depend*
> *to avoid future drug disasters."*[4]

How are you feeling about 'evidence-based' medicine, clinical trials, professional journals, and the approval processes for drugs right now?

Selling Sickness

Let's also keep in mind that in order to prescribe a drug, the doctor needs to see an illness, and name that illness.

Over time it has been documented by a number of the experts cited in this book, that the 'line of disease' (my words) has moved closer and closer to the normal situation, and in some cases is totally out of hand.

e.g. Listed in the *Diagnostic and Statistical Manual of Mental Disorders*, which is a list of all currently recognized mental health disorders, published by the American Psychiatric Association (APA), bereavement is defined as a depressive disorder if it has lasted for more than the following period of time:

1980: In Psychiatric Disorder List DSM-111: 2 years (to grieve is fine).

1994: In Psychiatric Disorder DSM-IV: 2 months (to grieve is fine).
2013: In Psychiatric Disorder DSM-V: 2 weeks (to grieve is fine).[5]

They're kidding, right?

Since when are we given only 2 weeks to grieve a loved one before we are considered to have a mental illness? That's insane. I know people who grieve for longer over a pet.

Looking at this trend, dive for cover before the next exciting update of DSM-VI is released! Especially if a compulsory new adverse 'best practice' is implemented by then.

I'm not listening to any grief diagnosis that any psychiatrist gives me. Now if you're real, you're mad.

Talk about the pot calling the kettle black!

The same trend is happening across a lot of health and mental health issues, and a great book to read about moving the "line of disease" is *Selling Sickness* by Ray Moynihan and Alan Castels.[6]

CHAPTER 4

Cochrane: Who are They and Why do They Exist?

Most people who talk to me about "evidence based medicine" have no idea about Cochrane, what it is, or what it does. Or they dismiss it.

Some even laugh about it!

I admit it took me a while to learn about it. (Unfortunately Cochrane are really crap at marketing. But that is not what they are good at.)

I'd heard about it, but I had never really GOT it.

It's time everyone understood Cochrane and what they do.

In 1992, the distinguished British health services researcher, Iain Geoffrey Chalmers was appointed director of the UK Cochrane Centre, leading to the development of the international Cochrane Collaboration, now known as Cochrane.

The Cochrane Collaboration conducts the world's most thorough independent analysis of healthcare research, and publishes the results to assist health care professionals, decision makers and patients.

They are the ultimate peer reviewing body for healthcare.

The Cochrane Collaboration is a network of more than 31,000 researchers from over 120 countries, working to evaluate the effectiveness of health care practices.

In 1993, Peter Gøtzsche co-founded The Cochrane Collaboration (the gold standard for the review of medical research data) and The Nordic Cochrane Centre, where he is Managing Director. In 2010 he became professor of Clinical Research Design and Analysis at the University of Copenhagen. He has published more than 70 papers in "the big five" (BMJ,

Lancet, JAMA, Annals of Internal Medicine and New England Journal of Medicine) and his scientific works have been cited over 15,000 times.

In lay persons terms Cochrane prepare, maintain and disseminate systematic reviews of the effects of health care.

This can include reviewing all the clinical trials on a particular topic or drug, the selection methodologies, randomization, reporting, blinding, placebo comparisons, vested interests etc. They scrutinize trials in detail to find flaws in them that are not obvious, in an effort to find the truth and efficacy around a particular health care system or drug.

They do meta-analysis (combining figures of multiple studies) and longer term population reviews to watch results over time, to see, for example whether mammography and early detection of breast cancer actually leads to longer lives of the women involved. (The answer is no, by the way. See Peter Gøtzsche's book *Mammography Screening, Truth, Lies and Controversy.* So much for Australia's BS television ads.)

The reason Cochrane exists is basically they don't believe everything they're being told. And they attempt to get to the truth with rigorous investigation.

*There are **more than 31,000 researchers and medical professionals** around the world that not only have a similar opinion about "what we are being told" but are prepared to spend time and effort to do this investigative work in the name of truth and better health outcomes.*

Well, that's a relief!

Clinical Trials

Clinical trials of one sort or another have been happening for many years, but the first published randomized clinical trial (RCT) in medicine is attributed to Austin Hill in his study entitled "Streptomycin treatment of tuberculosis" and 1948.

The idea of a randomized trial is to reduce bias in the clinical trial. Such things as randomly selecting the participants who are included in the study, and not telling them if they are being given a placebo instead of the trial drug help in researching the responses and collecting the data. Ultimately it is hoped that RCTs lead to more reliable, scientific conclusions as to the efficacy and safety of a particular drug or intervention being trailed.

And hopefully they ascertain the truth.

They are still considered the gold standard in medical research.

As honest people we generally assume that the people doing the trials are also honest. Especially if there are lives, addictions and serious side effects to take into account.

This is not the case. When billions of dollars can be made from a successfully marketed drug, by companies listed on the stock markets, whose main aim is to make money for their shareholders – the waters can, and have, got muddy.

Most people just regard a "clinical trial" as the ultimate proof.

But they don't understand that clinical trials can be unreliable, falsified, compromised, hidden, unregistered, not conducted correctly, not randomly selected, and a myriad of other issues.

And most people don't follow Cochrane.

Bias in Clinical Trials

According to Forbes Magazine industry sponsors 90% of published clinical trials[1].

What's more, industry sponsored trials are four times more likely to produce positive results than independently run experiments[2].

So here are *some* of the ways that clinical trials can be biased, or how the 'books can be cooked':

- Subjects not randomly selected. E.g. you select people for an antidepressant trial that are unlikely to ever be depressed, and perhaps aren't typical of the sort of person who will be taking the medications, thereby biasing the trial towards positive results for the drugs.
- The placebo group is not an unbiased placebo group.
- "Breaking the blind". In double blind placebo trials, the people in the trials sometimes figure out exactly which group they are in, because the trial did not properly hide whether patients were in the active or the placebo group. This distorts the reliability of the data as the 'active' patients are positively biased in their feedback generally. The results of the trial are compromised.
- Trials that do not include enough people: therefore not rendering a statistically valid 'population sample'.

- Reports do not correctly and clearly show how many people taking a drug (for example) left the trial because they felt no better and couldn't be bothered continuing the trial. Or the reasons are not shown correctly.
- Limitations placed on the reporting and the trial parameters. E.g. in some trials adverse events are only reported for 1 day or 1 week after taking a drug. This may be very misleading, especially if it takes a while for the drug to accumulate in the system, for addictions to begin, etc.
- The trial is held for a limited amount of time.
- The results of the trials are not fully reported, and/or the wording of incidents is not clear e.g. "hospitalization" instead of "suicide", etc.
- Ghost writers are engaged to write the results of the study, who previously had very little to do with the study, but are experts at jumping through the TGA/FDA hoops.
- Lies. It does happen and there are court cases that prove it.

And there's more:

- RCTs generally do not take into account the long term changes that a participant encounters. They are time-limited. Sometimes with an agenda.
- RCTs do not generally test the effects of coming off the drug - the withdrawal and tapering effects. (One of the agendas...)
- RCTs are not meta analyses, and do not study large population samples against one another. Nor over long periods of time.
- RCTs can be, and are, publishing in respected medical journals, even though the results are flawed.
- The raw data from RCTs does not have to be shown or revealed. The raw data of clinical trials remains the property of the entity that funded the trial. Some raw data has been revealed *only after successful litigation against a company for misleading the public*, where the judge directed the company to make the raw data available in his final judgement. This was the start of the ground-breaking *Restoring Study 329* which features prominently in Chapter 10.

- All clinical trials are not registered (there is current action to change this, but I'm not sure it will be successful, nor how it will be policed).
- The results of unfavourable clinical trials are generally not reported. And the study does not get published. Revealing all trials, even if unsuccessful, would help others who might benefit from the failed trial – and help eliminate duplication. Results are certainly not published as failed trials (and I'm not sure the publishers would even accept them.) Yes, I know this is complicated in private industry/ listed companies, but if governments really cared about the population's health they would act more decisively to deliver tested solutions. After all, we are paying for the fake solutions.
- There are very few, if no, procedures for independent third parties to review the raw data of clinical trials against the results, and what is published in medical journals.

Prescription Drugs – The Third Leading Cause of Death

All this, and the fact that according to Peter Gøtzsche's research "Our prescription drugs are the third leading cause of death after heart disease and cancer in the United States and Europe."[3]

You might be interested in Professor Peter Gøtzsche's other comments:

- "My studies in this area lead me to a very uncomfortable conclusion: Our citizens would be far better off if we removed all the psychotropic drugs from the market, as doctors are unable to handle them. It is inescapable that their availability creates more harm than good."
- "The hypothesis about serotonin is stone dead. The good studies that have been made could not see that depressed patients were different from normal patients. What these drugs do is .. they do not correct a chemical imbalance, that's another lie psychiatrists love .. that you have a chemical imbalance, like a diabetic that lacks insulin, so now we are going to correct your chemical imbalance ... it's a lie, they are creating a chemical imbalance and it is exactly for this reason that it's difficult for patients to stop after two or three months ... because there is now an imbalance".

- "We are doing, more or less, exactly the opposite to what we should be doing." "These drugs are dangerous."
- "Most depressed patients recover by themselves, so why not wait and see, some weeks, then many of them would never get an anti-depressant, and then they would have no problems stopping the drug."
- "We know that these drugs increase the risk of suicide, in young people, up to the age of 40, according to FDA data ... and we don't really know what they do above the age of 40 because the drug companies have cheated so enormously in their randomised trials, so, in the worst case these drugs might increase the rate of suicide in all age groups."[4]

So next time someone questions you about why you would be such a fool to question accepted medical practice, ask them *why Cochrane exists.*

They will either have no clue about Cochrane (which hopefully will get them off your back), or they know about Cochrane and you will elevate the conversation to something more meaningful.

Culling The Clinical Trials and Randomised Control Trials

Here is a very rough diagram I drew up for a talk I presented for school children to help them understand what evidence-based actually means.

Hidden from the Masses

As a normal member of society, not having the time to do all this research, you have no way to know that this is happening. Your health could be adversely affected by not knowing the facts. You need to have the courage to tell your doctor that you do not want to take a particular drug or undergo a particular operation or intervention.

And risk the not unusual responses of "are you a doctor?", "I didn't go to medical school for nothing", etc.

It must be the country girl in me, 'cos I can sure see the bullshit.

(No, I haven't tried that response.)

You'll see in this book that your life could depend on your courage to argue the point.

And your courage to say no.

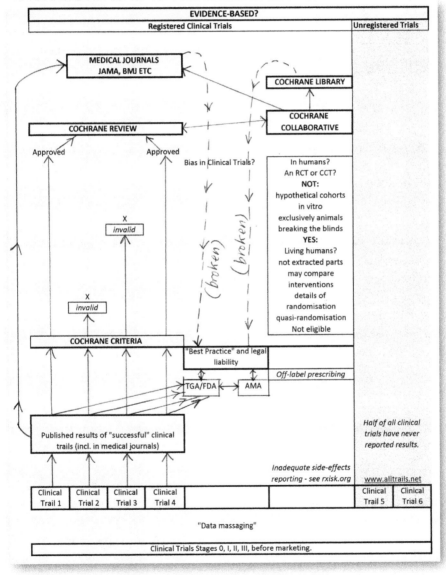

What Does "Evidence-Based" Really Mean?

CHAPTER 5

"Promote a Dickhead" and other Marketing and Public Relations Strategies.

At this point the system is pretty well established. If you disagree with the way that health care is being run in Australia, or you have the audacity to question what is supposedly 'evidence based medicine' *you* will be the one with the problem, *certainly not* our best-in-the-world medical practices.

And if an argument looks like it's growing legs (e.g. it's appearing on social media and picking up some significant traffic), then 'the power base' start pulling in the big guns to make sure that any dissenting view is squashed.

(FYI the prescribing patterns of *doctors* are being monitored by drug companies. The American Medical Association (also 'AMA') has sold doctors' demographic data to the pharmaceutical industry continuously since the 1940s, and the information sharing includes individual patient information – without showing the patient's actual name. The American Medical Association sells individual doctor's identifiers to health information organisations (HIOs). Further information can be accessed from *Prescription Tracking and Public Health*[1].)

This chapter talks about techniques that can and are being used to ensure that any free thinking that might disagree with the status quo is quashed. Hopefully they work so well that others fear speaking up in a similar manner, forever.

A great book to read that gives some insight into marketing, public relations and spin is *The Father of Spin, Edward L. Bernays and the Birth of Public Relations*, by Larry Tye.

You won't have to get too far into the book to get the gist of it, but here are over 100 methods and techniques to manipulate public opinion (and/or individuals) on any topic or product, and I'm compiling this list at page 70! Conduct opinion research to support your mission; assemble a distinguished front group; enlist or create public charities or causes to promote your idea or product; launch a product at an established and respected place; use education as the means to promote; use inventive slants on stories; change names; colour spreads in the media; trademarks, brands and slogans; stunts; gimmicks; public visibility; sensationalize; sexualize; design products to match current trends and publicity; featured articles in respected journals, publications, blogs, radio and television; press releases; visits to editors and publishers; coined phrases; create a crisis; solve a crisis; fire imagination; create heroes; testimonials; celebrity endorsements and testimonials; associate with other artists and successful people and concepts; plant propaganda; boost morale; organize, promote and report on rallies; make the news; hustle; promote fear; free giveaways; moving the free line; salesmanship; big promises; limited offers; limited time opportunities; luxury; discredit opposing research and views; crystallize public opinion; enlist experts; pay experts to agree with your product and solutions; conduct and report on opinion polls; cherry pick research results; create new fashion and other trends; latest findings; expert opinions from organisations such as health bodies; lie; cheat; bribe officials; engineer your product as the solution to another (hopefully related) problem; surveys; create trends; make claims; assume the adoption of a trend or product and forward think new trends; coverage through created controversy; discredit the competition; take the high ground; create a sub-issue; repetition; community group support; long-range programs; market to a new market; public events; rallies, protests and demonstrations; appeal to and align with traditional values; institutionalize; extend the marketplace; alignment with the churches; calendar driven events; international day of the "given aim"; scarcity; staging; history making coverage; "page one" news; media captions and slogans; product launches and demonstrations; academic and scholarly articles; media advertising; anonymous backing and secretive sponsors; move expert and/or created opinion down the line to press, then public opinion; dramatic appeals; charity involvement and donations to charity; address the shortcomings and promote the solutions; secrecy; duplicity; payments; stonewalling; refusing to comment; fight the enemy; competing publicity companies; jokes and humour; hire detectives; hire the competition; colour and branding colours; use emotions; align with environmental, health and other movements; publish and promote from different sources; billboards; psychoanalysis, psychological studies and slants; side-promotions and counter pitches; cover up the negatives; editorial persuasion; circuitous appeals; medical opinion; involve competitors without them knowing; create a void; simplification; new ways of behaving; big think; letter-writing campaigns (would now include online petitions); alliances; deception; charge more; make it exclusive and hard to get; lobby groups; make it an everyday need; influence and intervene in government policy; persuade government to fund; overt acts; collaborate against a common enemy; appeal to pocket book issues; movies; product placement; study groups; fear and safety issues; co-opt the enemy; scientific evidence including published clinical trials; identify the market; institutionalize and traditionalize; targeted lists and mailings; fight dirty; credentialize; bad publicity can be good; sensationalize; letters of tribute; memorabilia; commemorative stamps; association with national leaders; live and risky demonstrations; super-advertising and align with national celebrations.

By the way, if you don't understand some of these, you are the target market.

And yes, these are *conspiracies*. And because of your ignorance and/or apathy you are shark bait.

Capturing the minds of the public doesn't stop there either.

Wars have been started to promote ideas and commerce, and continue to this day. We know that, why pretend.

So let's admit it: if you aren't aware of what's going on, or at least attempting to know, then you are part of the *manipulated class*.

You are part of someone else's solution, not your own. And at the sticky end the price you pay can be your life, or the lives of your loved ones.

I'm going to expand on six deceptions that I know are being used in the medical industry, for those of you who might not be totally clear at this point.

Strategy 1: Clinical Trial Publications.

Previously covered. You're all over that one now, right?

They're not included in the long list above, but they should be.

Strategy 2: "Promote a Dickhead".

This is one of my favourites, and I see it reasonably often but not a lot.

It works like this: if there is a real truth that is getting some traction, and you really don't want people to be listening and taking notice of the discussion, then find a dickhead who is talking about it.

A real dickhead.

Someone who no-one wants to be associated with. You know ... maybe ugly, overweight, untidy, preferably looking a bit extreme, feral, perhaps a 'hippy', talks weird, unqualified in the traditional sense, extreme, flat-earther, unfriendly, aggressive – and "all of the above" to win the jackpot.

Then, when counter discussions are being made for that point of view in the media or social media – promote this person to the nth degree. Make them the spokesperson. They will generally be pleased, because they are helping get the good message out, but they might not realise they are being stooged.

Manipulated because what they have to say is probably going to be discounted by the masses because they don't look and/or behave like they have a clue. And they're generally not 'media trained' to handle the curly questions that they will *surely* be asked. (And if all else fails, just edit the grabs.)

They will do a marvellous job of discrediting the truth, because the general public have no idea what is happening.

Also this person will be called on to 'give a balanced view' sometimes when the media is required to present the "for and against" arguments, without bias.

Well, nice try, but it is biased after all.

And if you're the one organising this PR stunt, you might even suggest this person as a possible person to interview to represent the opposing view. And you might even suggest some questions that might be asked, or design your media release to lead the questions in a particular direction.

Lamb to the slaughter.

OK, you've got this haven't you?

Can you remember seeing one of these cases?

I've got one person in mind here, and thanks to her courage I woke up about a particular issue – AND realised why they chose her as the spokesperson. I haven't seen her lately in the media, and thankfully the discussion has gone way beyond "you have to be old, untidy and crazy to believe that", with support for her argument coming from all over the place.

Keep an eye out for this one, because it's a pretty hot strategy. Maybe you can use this technique in a good way.

And beware of organisations asking you to endorse their products, especially if you are a handsome/beautiful celebrity and/or expert in your field. One shonky endorsement and you have ruined your chance of being taken seriously. I'm amazed at how little research established experts and celebrities do before they endorse products, or agree to a board appointment for organisations that might be included in future royal commissions, etc. Or maybe they're not as smart as they appear, or they like the remuneration more than their reputation/contribution.

Strategy 3: The Media's "Balanced Argument".

This is a new one I've just come across.

If the media is on to a really big story and they are looking for only the top people (there are generally only a very few of these), you can sometimes shut down a story simply by not being available to give your opinion.

It doesn't always happen that way, if the media has the fortitude to say "we contacted xyz person, but they declined to be interviewed", but in some cases, where the producers are not strong (or inclined), the story may just not be aired because the piece did not represent both sides.

And a one sided argument might leave the television company/broadcaster open to be sued.

This is a good technique to use if you know the other person being interviewed will totally discredit your argument or position, especially if you are in the wrong. And it has been used successfully by a few shonky experts.

Strategy 4: Call Out "Conspiracy Nutjobs".

If you're not a conspiracy theorist on at least some issues, you are just plain dull.

There, I've said it.

Strategy 5: "Encourage" The Start of a Community/ Charitable Institution/Foundation/National Organisation, That You Know will Indirectly Benefit Your Product or Services Through The Back Door.

I'm not going to expand on this by listing the suspect organisations that many smart people watch.

I'm not completely stupid.

But I will ask you to start thinking about what sorts of organisations you might support if you wanted to promote your product, through the back door, while appearing to "save the world".

And getting a hellova lot of, *often free*, publicity because the idea is so marvellous.

And involving key public figures in the organisation.

Not you or your organisation. Other people, duh.

And if it is a charity or foundation there will be definite opportunities to make donations. Even tax deductible ones. Nice.

Come on!

This one is subtle, because it never shapes up like this initially. It will be all about a "great mission".

And sacred because of that.

Tell me, you know this one.

Strategy 6: Go Hard on "Evidence-Based" Discussion – Even if It Isn't.

- This has the same effect as confusion, as it totally shuts down the conversation for most. Only the brave will continue.
- There must be one in a thousand (or even less) who actually knows how to look up clinical trials, and double blind placebo trials. And about one in a thousand of those (?) that can recognise any bias in clinical trials, and which trials pass muster. (FYI, you can be trained by Cochrane on how to discern relevant clinical trials, without having a doctorate. It's not even that hard, so why aren't all medical practitioners put through this training?)

- Speak the words 'evidence-based' and don't be intimidated. Don't squirm.
- They're going to believe anything you say, because they don't want to look stupid.
- And who has ever heard of Cochrane or The Cochrane Collaborative?

Here's my redress for these types:

Go hard on 'evidence based' back. Ask them to *cite the exact reference, publication, study or trial they are talking about.* You want the details, because you're going to look it up. The name of the authors, the title of the paper, the date it was published and where.

Works like salt on snails for the shonkies. And there are plenty of them.

The legitimate people will honour you with a full answer, and generally a full discussion. They have found a kindred spirit.

Then, if they honoured you with the answer, write it down and look it up in Cochrane, Google, the BMJ, JAMA, wherever. It will take 5 minutes to find if they've given you valid information. (Yes, you can "Doctor Google".)

Other Strategies

Other strategies include confusion (because who knows what evidence-based really means?), Astroturfing, 100 government departments (and you can't complain effectively to any of them, they're all toothless tigers and ditherers, and they're all in the middle of a "full scoping investigation to fix the problem ... that will be open for public discussion in a year, and we encourage you to put a full report in" – so we can ignore it after you have spent a week giving your best opinions for free)...

Establish the peer body yourself, run annual conferences (charge high prices), lie, cheat, lobby, bribe...

There are hundreds of them, you understand.

If they ever get a Royal Commission happening, restrict the terms of reference so the real stuff doesn't come out, and then don't act on the recommendations that cost a fortune to make.

Too frustrating to continue...

The ultimate strategy is to make something 'quick and easy' and to market it as such.

That's the extent of people's commitment to most things. Unfortunately.

Just wise up if you aren't already, and continue to be intelligent and disruptive.

The world needs you. Big time.

CHAPTER 6

The Trojan Horse. Lessons from Ancient Greece.

I fell in love with Greece when I travelled there years ago, and was captivated by the myths and stories – some of which turned out not to be myths at all.

A teacher at school tried to persuade me to do ancient history, but I hated reading.

Unbeknown to me, I had reading dyslexia, but no-one suspected because I was bright (particularly in maths and science). I didn't see jumbled letters or numbers, which is a usually the problem with dyslexics. I just never read anything if I could avoid it – certainly never read any of my English novels cover to cover. I used to feel like falling asleep and had to read things over and over and over – which didn't help me remember anyway. I just thought those books must be boring. Many were.

My eyes were opened when an alternative healer fixed my problem when I was about 28 years old, well after graduating from university. I have now read thousands of books and articles.

I started to respect the work of alternative and natural healers a lot more because of that particular incident that seemed to "unlock my brain" to remember what I was reading, and to enjoy it. (And this week I noticed that Jamie Oliver, Britain's most published non-fiction writer, was a reading dyslexic too.)

You'll notice this book is not full of long-winded paragraphs. I've kept the content pretty 'conversational' for this exact reason. And because I know that if you're tired or stressed, you don't want to read a whole lot of boring stuff. Ever.

The Trojan Horse

The *Trojan Horse* story can be sourced back to Virgil's *Aeneid*, and Homer's *Odyssey*, and is variously thought to have actually happened in the 12th, 13th or 14th century BC.

It was the controversial figure Heinrich Schliemann (1822 – 1890) who envisioned as a child that he would find the city of Troy, thereby proving that it was not a myth, but rather a fact. He is attributed to discovering Mycenae and Troy in conjunction with English archaeologist Frank Calvert in the late 19th Century.

According to the varied Trojan Horse stories a war raged between the Greeks and the Trojans for many years.

Under the leadership of Epeios the Greeks built a very large wooden horse, fashioned after the emblem of the city Troy.

The horse was so large that it could house Greek warriors inside.

The plan was to convince the Trojans that the Greeks had retreated from the war, and returned to their boats... that the Trojan horse was either left as a gift for the Trojans or as an offering to the gods.

The ultimate intention of the Greeks was to persuade the Trojans to bring the horse inside the protective and powerful walls of the city, where the soldiers would escape to fight and conquer the Trojans.

A pity Brad Pitt wasn't around then, it might have saved a hell of a lot of woodworking.

The Trojan priest Laocoon guesses the plot and his warning is apparently the beginning of the saying "beware of Greeks bearing gifts". His warnings are ignored.

The Trojan Horse is indeed brought inside the walls of the city, and the horse led to the downfall of the city of Troy.

What's The Trojan Horse Got to Do with Modern Medicine?

Power games are always being fought, and modern medicine is no different.

Imagine the health industry as the powerful and protected fortress that is Troy. Troy is the power base, the rule maker, the strength and fortification, the government subsidies, the tax and money collector, the home for intellectuals and educators, the political centre with foreign connections, the patron, the enforcers...

Troy is the castle: physically, philosophically and financially.

Anyone who wants to rule has to conquer the castle. That's how the battle goes.

Now imagine the drug companies as the Greeks.

They want to infiltrate the establishment, with the power and wealth that comes with it.

Medicines and drugs haven't had that much of an impressive history really considering the amount of resources, universities, research and funding that has gone into the industry over decades. A lot has developed since the original snake oil salesmen, but most of the improvement in life span for many years was attributed to lower death rates during birth, general hygiene, education and dealing with infectious diseases.

A strange thing happened with Thalidomide.

Thalidomide first entered the market in Germany in 1957 as an over-the-counter sedative that was marketed as "completely safe for everyone including mother and child". It was the only non-barbiturate sedative known at the time and by 1960 was marketed in 46 countries, with sales nearly matching those of aspirin.

The "clinical trials" of Thalidomide involved distributing more than two and a half million tablets of thalidomide to approximately 20,000 patients across the United States alone, at least 207 women were pregnant. More than one thousand physicians participated in these trials, but few tracked their patients after dispensing the drug.[1]

In 1961 Australian Dr. William McBride noticed that the drug seemed to be related to the birth defect phocomelia. Phocomelia means 'seal limb'. Babies were born with limbs that looked like flippers, or hands or feet were attached close to the trunk, or the limbs were grossly underdeveloped or absent. (Dr McBride had been prescribing Thalidomide off-label to his pregnant patients as a morning sickness remedy.)

The makers of the drug ignored various reports, but took the drug off the market in Germany after a newspaper reported 161 babies were born with these shocking birth defects.

Other countries noticed the same problem, and by March 1962 the drug was banned in most countries that it had been available.

Frances Kelsey, the head of the FDA in America had refused formal FDA approval of the drug because of the lack of proper reporting, follow up and evidence.

This event brought about a major overhauling of the system of drug approvals in the US, requiring drug manufacturers to prove that their drugs were both safe and effective before they could be approved.

It was a step just down the track that was to have far more reaching effects.

With the implementation of Randomised Control Trials (RCTs) to prove both efficacy and safety, a number of conditions developed:

- RCTs became regarded as the gold standard of evidence based medicine,
- RCT results were published in leading medical journals around the world,
- The cost of RCTs made them the domain of large companies who could afford to conduct them,
- The raw data from RCTs did not have to be revealed or documented in detail – therefore prohibiting review from interested third parties,
- RCTs formed the basis for best practice models and professional treatment standards, and
- RCTs underpinned professional negligence exposure.

The formation of Australia's *Therapeutic Goods Administration* came a long way down the track.

Unfortunately there was more than a bit of dithering in the Australian government when Sir Earle Page introduced the *National Health Bill* and the *Therapeutic Substances Bill* to parliament in 1953. His comment that "I regret to state that at present there is evidence that drugs are being supplied that do not conform to the requisite standards and, so, are incapable of carrying out the job which the medical profession believes that they will carry out. It would be criminal to allow such a state of affairs to exist and continue merely through lack of appropriate action."[2]

Australia's Therapeutic Goods Administration (TGA) was finally founded in 1989.

Seems we still haven't got Sir Earle Page's message from 1953.

The criminal behaviour continues.

Heck, it's only been 64 years.

From a business and financial perspective here's what can and does happen, sometimes:

- A clinical trial is performed by a university or respected institution that has been the recipient of a donation from a company whose drug or intervention is being trialled. Interestingly in Australia I see significant moves towards *increased* commercial sponsorship of universities, and the research they are doing. In my opinion it is not enough that a university, for example, declared donations in its financial reports – as these declarations rarely show the name of the donor specifically linked to a university department or study. That would be stupid, right?
- A clinical trial is performed, but because the results were not favourable the trial results are never printed and never published. Even though that information and trial being unsuccessful could be highly beneficial to medical progress.
- There is no requirement for all clinical trials to be registered at the time the trial is being established. There are people agitating for this to happen, but it has not happened yet.
- Professors, directors, doctors, PHD students and masters' degree students can be employed and/or remunerated by private enterprise and work for universities, including taking part in trials. Conflicts of interest are often curly and very often completely ignored. There are many cases published where doctors, for example, are later found to have received special speaking and consulting fees from drug companies who they have favourably advantaged. This includes foundations and charitable organisations who list donations in the fine print, but do not declare that these donating companies may have influenced their opinions and policies. Of course they need medical experts on the board: but who do they choose?
- Off-label prescribing. Drug companies have been found guilty of marketing to doctors in areas where the drug has not been proven to be beneficial. They have been sued because they have mislead

doctors as to the efficacy of a drug in a different market – e.g. marketing to adolescents, when the drug is only approved for adults, etc.

- Drug companies patent the drugs - strengthening secrecy and limiting investigations.
- I won't go on, you get the drift. Now they are moving into schools. Get 'em young and train them. Yikes!

The Trojan Horse is the Randomised Control Trial (RCT).

RCTs are now inside the castle walls and have taken power.

They are the establishment.

You've seen how RCTs can be unregistered, biased and untruthful?

How has it been going since 1948 and the beginning of published RCTs?

The main killers of heart disease and cancer remain the main killers today in spite of the enormous resources being thrown at the 'cure'.

There is increasing interest in evidence-based medicine, but an evidence base isn't easy to prove, and we can't tell the difference between the good RCTs and the bad.

There remains increasing discussion about the processes that are in place today that are flawed.

The Greek conqueror is "Randomus Clinicallus Trialus" and no one dares question his truth and power.

Except the people who know, of course.

And that includes you now.

The Trojan Horse Led to the Downfall of Troy.

Here's a great quote from Professor David Healy:

"More than 90% of all clinical trials are now run by private companies, which organize ethical approval through other private companies and outsource the trials to parts of the world where oversight is minimal. The results, sometimes stemming from patients who don't exist, are fed back to the parent companies coded in a manner that often causes problems to vanish. Those trials and their results that suit company marketing agendas are then written up by ghostwriters and published in the leading medical journals — even though the editors know what is happening and the lives they are putting at risk by publishing these articles."[3]

And another from Professor Peter Gøtzsche, co-founder of the Cochrane Collaborative from his book *Deadly Medicines and Organised Crime, How Big Pharma has Corrupted Healthcare* (2013):

"Drugs are now the third leading cause of death after heart disease and cancer."[4]

Throwing the Baby out with the Bathwater.

Our confidence in the health and medical fields is at a very low ebb.

Understandably.

People no longer know who to believe, so they are throwing the baby out with the bathwater.

The medical, drug and health industries have no one to blame but themselves.

They have proven to be incapable of clinical governance for so long now that the public are taking matters into their own hands.

Is it any surprise?

And we know why vested interests are telling us not to "Doctor Google", gagging nurses and doctors and naysayers who speak out.

The time has arrived for major changes to occur in health around the world. Because it is such a huge industry, and the ramifications are so complicated, they're trying to put a lid on it.

We need a very strong health ombudsman, a powerful consumer watchdog and effective health and mental health ministers who have the tenacity and capability to look at our broken system and save the Australian economy billions by implementing radical change.

The consumer revolt is well underway. The corruption evidence is on the internet for everyone to see. We just need more people to know how to access it.

By the way, we haven't trusted what Google pops up on the first page for ages, and less now since the latest algorithm changes.

We know we have to Google the *right people*, the *right groups*, the right *research libraries*, the *right leaders*.

And there's the Trans Pacific Partnership (TPP)!

I wonder why the contents are so secret?

Let's just say it's not only about exporting primary produce created by our wholesome, hard working farmers ... duh.

A flock of Trojan horses? Giddy up.

Slam Dunk

Create the ultimate construction, filled with danger, and wheel it into the castle – initially fight like hell.

Then infiltrate the establishment, make the rules to suit yourself, become the fortress.

Ultimately create the **standards of care** that everyone in a country must follow, or be penalized.

RCTs do more than miss the long term injuries a drug might do us. They get used to build standards of care to which doctors are obliged to adhere.

Anyone who figures it might not be wise to add a sixth drug into the mix a person is on, or that thinks that maybe adolescent crises are not something that need medicating, will find themselves up against these standards of care facing managers who ask "Who are you to go against the Standard of Care? Sorry we have to let you go."[5]

The drug companies are now omnipotent:

- They are the holders of the key: the RCT,
- They have commercial permission to hide the raw data and the detailed results of the trials,
- They dictate "World Best Practice", the "Gold Standard", the "Standards of Care",
- They refuse to supply government and doctors with the raw data,
- They promote off-label prescribing,
- They sponsor and donate to community help groups that serve their agendas,
- They withhold information from governments,
- They know the names of the professors, researchers and doctors who are "favourable to persuasion",
- They lobby and incentivize,

- They encourage the careers of their preferred medical professionals,
- They influence, nominate, and promote their preferred key influencers,
- They're listed on the stock market, so their KPI is increased profits for their shareholders,
- They have huge budgets and advertise in the media,
- They influence government policy, standards of care and professional negligence exposures,
- Their products are subsidized by governments (you, actually),
- They support *doctors*, and support *their* systems (they need them, big time). *Their* respectability, *their* standing in the community, *their* patients' trust, *their* direct link to the market, *their* strong lobby groups, *their* trust in what they are told. Hmmm, getting nervous? This is where the pressure is centred. Watch this space.

Where do we fit in here?

Well, we're becoming a bit untidy really.

However, they do need consumers/customers.

And they need consumers to keep saying 'yes' to their doctors.

Otherwise the castle falls.

Throw Out RCTs?

No way...

The RCTs **that have integrity** play a very important part, along with meta-analyses.

But "the game" has to be cleaned up substantially.

We need:

- All clinical trials to be registered before they begin,
- RCT registration should clearly state the aims of the trial and the methodologies being used,
- The raw data and results should be supplied to the participants of clinical trials, with full disclosure of their placebo or other status given at the completion, for their review, as part of the trial,

- A health ombudsman that overseas clinical trial participant practices, and
- A health ombudsman that has the power to review the raw data of all RCTs, in every case where government funding/taxpayer money is being used to subsidize the drug and/or medical intervention.

It is no longer acceptable that "commercial-in-confidence" excuses are used by medical companies who are motivated and legislated to make profits, and/or listed on the stock markets – *who derive financial and other benefits from taxpayer funds.*

Taxpayers should no longer be required to subsidise these companies' products through the PBS and MBS when we do not have adequate proof that their products even work, let alone do no harm.

This system has proved to be fatally flawed.

Vaccines and the National Childhood Vaccine Injury Act (NCVIA)

Before I leave this topic of RCTs I will mention the great amount of vitriol on social media aimed at people who question the status quo in medicine. Especially vaccines. By now I hope you will be questioning most things, whether they are procedures, medications, appliances, operations, vaccines, or anything else.

Actually, when I learned about the US government passing the 1986 National Childhood Vaccine Injury Act (NCVIA) and establishing the National Vaccine Injury Compensation Program (VICP) I became more curious as to what was happening there.

If vaccines were so incredibly safe, why did the liability and compensation for harm get moved to the government (*us...*) from the vaccine manufacturers?

No wonder there is a new wave of vaccines being introduced. From a commercial perspective why wouldn't you move to a "no responsibility" business model?

It's a no brainer.

Ka Ching!

The problem used to be that vaccines were administered through a needle, and a painful prick … which is obviously a marketing impediment.

Not surprisingly there are a few options emerging for needle-free "injections" of vaccines, such as putting the vaccine in a sugar pill (who would complain about having that?), or patches on your skin, nano patches, injector devices with a high pressure spray, etc[6].

Notice: we have had a not-so-subtle redefinition of "vaccine".

Now that we have moved the liability, let's call tablets, patches and sprays all *vaccines.*

Keep an eye out for this, because this is the ultimate get out of jail free card.

But I'm getting side tracked, the best is yet to come.

(By the way, Cochrane looks at vaccines too, so we're in good company. Don't give your brain away yet.)

CHAPTER 7

You are the Perfect Market. Ouch!

I know the content of this book is hard to digest and integrate, but it's not going to get any easier in this chapter.

The problem is this: if you aren't sleeping properly, feeling anxious, stressed, depressed and/or any number of issues that readers of this book will have – it affects your ability to *think straight*.

One of the ways to find solutions to problems is the ability to "take yourself away" from a particular problem, mentally (sometimes physically too) – and review it logically and intuitively until you can make sense of the problem, and hopefully find a solution.

Because of the situation you find yourself in, your ability to think straight is impaired, clouded or compromised depending on how much your insomnia and mental problems are affecting you.

I'm now talking to YOU.

No way you would have bought this book and read this far if you genuinely didn't want to solve your problem(s).

And good on you for doing that.

But...

Most of the underlying problems that manifest as sleep disorders, anxiety, depression, OCD, phobias and other sleep and mental health problems are complex, and need to be thought about in detail. Often they need to be discussed with competent people, in order to get to the bottom of them, and to eventually find a way out to feeling well rested, happy, healthy, relaxed and ideally even getting back your previous sense of humour and fun.

The solution to your problems does NOT come through "popping a pill".

It just doesn't make sense.

When you're tired, anxious, stressed and/or depressed you're not in the mood to be doing hours of research and arguing the point with doctors.

Hmmm, read that again.

Pills may look like an easy answer, but they never are with psychological or sleeping problems, according to my research.

In fact, they can make the problem worse.

A whole lot worse in some cases.

No organ of the body is affected by lack of sleep more than the brain.

Specific brain functions that are affected by lack of sleep are problem solving, decision making ability, memory, the ability to focus, verbal reasoning, strategic thinking, mental flexibility, task switching, attention span, response initiation, planning, working memory, cognitive processes – thinking properly.

They're called the executive functions of the brain.

I'm not saying you are the perfect market without good reasons.

And I understand why you might be tempted to hope that a pill will fix the problems. (Don't we all...)

We are not in a position to be taking bad advice.

Arguing the point when we feel and think like rubbish is not what generally happens. Right?

We have to actually work through our problems and talk about them to find solutions.

We have to kiss a few psychological demons before we find the answers.

Some of you are already on medications.

So here is what Professor Gavin Andrews of NSW University says about benzodiazepine use:

"Chronic benzo use …. produces stupid people."[1]

I can see your "backs up" right now.

But I'm on your side, and I want you to start thinking the right way to help you get yourself out of your fix.

We need our full faculties to know when we are being mislead, lied to and brushed off.

Unfortunately the overtired, stressed and depressed are not firing on all cylinders.

But you *are* totally capable of getting through this.

CHAPTER 8

Sick and Tired of Medical Evidence Jet Lag?

I met a woman at a party the other day that told me that the Australian Government started talking about an airport at Badgery's Creek in the 1960s. I found it hard to believe, so I checked it out. She was right: apparently it was first proposed as a potential site in 1969, and the Hawke Government named it as their preferred site in 1986[1].

Wow.

How slow are we?

Or should I ask, how slow is the Government? And how slow is legislation?

And how much lack of vision do our leaders have?

All that translates into our country, Australia, being as thick and two short planks. Have you noticed? And I'm not being political, both 'sides' are crap, and the others too, apparently...

If we had gone ahead with an international airport at Badgery's Creek in the 1970s, for good or for bad, how far ahead would we be today? How much cheaper would the land have been, how far more advanced would the airport transit transport be? Would we have at least solved some of our snarling road problems in Sydney?

I won't go on.

But let's look at the sleep and mental health industries.

Is this any different?

I first heard about different brain wave patterns and the connection between thought and health in the 1970s and I wasn't even trying. Just going to personal development courses. Yeah, OK, maybe slightly ahead of the curve there...

Now they're calling it "neuroscience", when it has been talked about in personal development and alternative health circles for decades.

And "Cognitive Behavioural Therapy" (CBT) is the new, very unsexy name for positive thinking. Epic fail there... You couldn't get a better name for a natural therapy doomed to fail. Yep, very tempting to hit the instant pill solution rather than engage in some "Cognitive Behavioural Therapy".

WTF is that about?

Yes, it works. Duh. Think about what you're thinking about, and if you're thinking about too much crap, change your thoughts.

Or at least make some effort about it.

Duh, again.

This is CBT and neuroscience.

Wow.

Then there's that very ugly word "napping".

Napping was apparently proven to be beneficial to performance by NASA in the late 1960s, and they're still researching it because of its benefits[2].

But when I talk to leading organisations in Australia, the mere mention of the word sends executives spare!

Most organisations tell me I'm encouraging their employees to "fall asleep on the job". (They are anyway, but they mustn't be noticing.)

In America it's a bit more encouraging.

35 percent of Americans say their workplace permits napping during breaks at work, and 16 percent say their employer provides a place for them to nap.

Organisations have encouraged napping since 1969 and now include the most progressive companies like Google, Cisco, P&G, BUPA, BMA, Virgin Active Health Clubs, iSelect Insurance, Yarde Metals, The New York Times, Huffington Post, NASA, Nike and Deloitte.

One N.A.S.A. study found an increase in their pilot's productivity up 34% from a 26 minute nap[3].

These are just a few examples of Medical Evidence Jet Lag.

Medical Evidence Jet Lag

Defined as that sick-and-tired feeling caused by a 40-year-lead-time between the evidence being in and arriving at the destination called "having-a-medical-clue"!

The time lag between evidence and policy uptake.

40-50 years is a hellova long time not to have your feet on the ground.

Smoking was first introduced to Australia by Indonesians in the 1700s before the first fleet arrived. Last century cigarettes were marketed as healthy, proven to be carcinogenic, and they are still freely and legally available in Australia.

Medical evidence jet lag. We've got it bad.

Only some people are well informed.

And only the well informed reap the physical and mental health benefits.

Don't wait until the government and policy makers catch up.

We'll be dead by then.

Part Two: Deadly Sins: Brain Damage, Addiction, Suicide, Homicide, Lies, Manipulation, Fraud And Avarice.

CHAPTER 9
Sleeping Pills: 34 Dark Secrets

Y ou now know about the Cochrane Collaborative, and you know it was co-founded by Professor Peter Gøtzsche, so let's see what he says about sleeping pills (benzodiazepines) and antidepressants (SSRIs):

"People I know, psychiatrists, have weaned off very many people from benzodiazepines and antidepressant drugs: all of them tell me it is far less to stop heroin in a street junkie than to get people off benzodiazepines and SSRIs. These are terrible drugs that we should use very, very little. So, we should focus on psychotherapy…"[1]

If you present to your doctor in Australia with insomnia you will be prescribed in 95.2 percent of the cases[2], so it's important to know about the medications you are being prescribed.

Often you will be prescribed a benzodiazepine or sleeping pill.

However you may be prescribed an anti-depressant or SSRI alternatively, or additionally - depending on your doctor.

Your research should go beyond just sleeping pills.

Information on anti-depressants/SSRIs is in Chapter 10.

The source of statements made here have been stated in each case so that you can do further research to make up your own mind independently.

Additionally, there are a number of medications being prescribed that effect sleep and mood. They include medications that:

- Have the side effect or withdrawal symptom of insomnia or other sleep disorder.
- Have the side effect of anxiety, restless sleep, depression, panic etc. Included in this group might be immunomodifiers, some cholesterol reducing medications, the pill, anxiety medications themselves, drugs to treat MS, carcinoma, some interferon drugs and HIV drugs.
- Those that can effect sleep for some people include psychotropics, antidepressants, stimulants, cardiovascular drugs, bronchodilators, decongestants, flu and cold medications, central nervous system stimulants, diuretics, steroids, respiratory medications, antihypertensives, some slimming tablets and diet pills, hormones and painkillers.
- Medications, in combination, have some adverse effects. If you are taking more than one medication it is not enough to look at the documentation on the individual medications/drug names because the effect of combining drugs will not be shown. This of course includes the combinations of drugs and alcohol and recreational drugs, and in some cases even food items etc.
- Medications have side effects that bring on or increase stress levels. They might include medications that cause sexual dysfunction, decreased libido, cause headaches, cause diarrhoea, bring about overheating and/or sweating, bring on nausea, are linked with depression, are addictive, cause weight loss or gain, or are associated with pain.

Freely Available and Legal

Commonly used substances that effect sleep and mood include alcohol, nicotine, caffeine and "energy" drinks containing stimulants.

Freely Available, Not Legal

Freely available substances that effect sleep and mood are amphetamines, cocaine, ecstasy, crystal meth, ketamine, etc.

Natural Sleep Aids

Natural sleep aids are beyond the scope of this book. Please note that just because it is 'natural' doesn't mean that it works, that it is valid, or that it does not have side-effects. Some herbal agents adversely affect sleep, and some interact adversely with medications.

Even some 'normal foods' affect the efficacy of some medications, and/ or your sleep patterns. Generally they should be shown on the labels and the documentation supporting the prescriptions, but that is not guaranteed, as you will see.

Food Additives, Chemicals, Colourings

The over 50 food additives, chemicals and colourings that affect sleep are talked about in Part 3, Chapter 27.

Here are the 34 Dark Secrets of Benzodiazepines/Sleeping Pills:

It is important to note that much of this information is not contained on the Australian National Prescribing Service's website, and certainly not in detail, with the appropriate references.

This list has been hard to come by, and compiled by me over about 15 years.

1. **Sleeping Pills will never address the underlying problem that lies beneath the sleep disorder.**
   Insomnia is always a symptom of something else.

   Insomnia itself is not the problem, its existence shows us that there is a problem – but doesn't actually reveal what the underlying problem is.

   The only way to cure insomnia is to cure the underlying problem that is causing insomnia.

2. **Sleeping pills mask the symptom(s) of insomnia and sleep disorders.**
   This means that it is more difficult to diagnose what the underlying problem(s) is(are).

By taking sleeping pills you are generally delaying the solution. If you become addicted to sleeping pills that delay can increase and become more complicated.

3. **Sleeping Pills are addictive.**
Benzodiazepines are addictive to highly addictive. "Addictive" means that over time you need more of them to get a similar result and/or when you stop taking them you have withdrawal symptoms which can include rebound insomnia and even more serious withdrawal effects such as suicidal ideation. (There's more about the definition of addiction in Chapter 10.)

One benzodiazepine, Xanax, previously prescribed for anxiety (and now moved to Schedule 8) has been described as "more addictive and harder to kick than heroin"[3].

The Australian National Prescribing Service recommends that doctors who prescribe sleeping pills discuss a stopping plan for the hypnotic medicine *at the time of the initial prescription*[4].

Because of their addictive qualities sleeping pills can become part of the problem, not the solution.

4. **One of the side effects when you try to come off sleeping pills is rebound insomnia.**
When you come off them you can get rebound insomnia, which makes you think that the pills were "working", and you need to go back on them – when it is just the 'rebound insomnia' side effect that is presenting. A very commonly overlooked aspect of benzodiazepines.

5. **Sleeping pills have a variety of symptoms and side-effects. They include:**
   ▪ Grogginess in the morning
   ▪ Headache
   ▪ Pain in the limbs, back and neck, teeth and jaw[40]
   ▪ Stiffness in the limbs, back and jaw[41]
   ▪ Paresthesia/paraesthesiae (stabbing pins and needles in the limbs and face)[42]
   ▪ Dizziness[43]
   ▪ Tinnitus[44]
   ▪ Hypersensitivity to sound, light, touch and taste[45]
   ▪ Muscle pain and twitches[46]

- Tremor[47]
- Fits and seizures[48]
- Drowsiness
- Nausea
- Myalgia
- Dyspepsia
- Hallucinations[51]
- Anxiety[49]
- Disorientation
- Drugged feeling
- Fatigue
- Lethargy
- Poor memory and concentration[53]
- Peculiar or bitter taste
- Dry mouth
- Changes in certain hormone levels, including testosterone and prolactin[5]. These changes could lead to sexual side effects, including decreased libido, milk-like nipple discharge, fertility problems
- Nausea
- Vomiting
- Abdominal pain, diarrhoea and constipation[52]
- Blurred vision
- Insomnia and nightmares[54]
- Agoraphobia and other phobias[55]
- Panic attacks and palpitations[56].

6. **Sleeping Pills have a half life.**
The length of time of the half life is variable between different benzodiazepine medications, varies between individuals and varies with age. Figures for half lives have been shown as 2 hours to 200 hours.[6]

The half life of a medication is the time it takes for *half* of the active components of the drug to go out of your system.

This means that, in a half life of 24 hour example, half of the active components in the drug are still in the body in 24 hours' time.

The expression 'half life' means that the dissipation of the active ingredients does not follow a straight line but a curve. (It's the shape of a reverse exponential curve, for the mathematicians.)

This also means that for the other 50% of the ingredients to leave the body totally takes *much more* than twice the length of the initial half life period of time.

In other words, if a sleeping pill has a half-life of 18 hours (for example), it is not eliminated totally from the body in 36 hours (2 x 18 hour periods). Instead the elimination is gradual, only eliminating half of what is left over the next 18 hours, then half of that residual again in the next 18 hours, etc. So, if you were to take another tablet in 24 hours (say, the next night), you would be dealing with the residual of the first tablet still in your system the next night, as well as the full strength of the tablet you just took. You can see how problems might accumulate if you have adverse reactions to any medication.

Most people do NOT understand the idea of a half-life. When you were prescribed your medication, did your doctor explain about half lives?

7. **The sleeping pills with a short half life aren't necessarily any better than the ones with a long half-life.**

If you investigate the information from one sleeping pill to another you will notice that some of the warnings that relate to the short half life medications can be stronger than those attached to the longer half life medications.

Don't believe that improvements have necessarily been made with the newer sleeping pills with shorter half lives.

8. **Stilnox, which has a shorter half-life, was the most complained about medication to the Australian Medicines Event Line run by the National Prescribing Service and Brisbane's Mater Hospital between September 2007 and February 2009.**

A quote from that article: "The figures come as a study linking Stilnox with sleeping behaviour was published in the Australia and New Zealand Journal of Psychiatry last month. The study, which examined 66 sleepwalkers being treated at a psychiatric clinic, found their abnormal behaviour was associated with the regular use of Stilnox. The pill was also linked to eating during sleep, with sleep walkers more likely to be overweight or obese."[7]

Of 1669 calls, 196 (or 12%) related to this one sleeping pill, Stilnox. (670% more calls than the second on the list!)[7]

9. **"Sleeping tablets usually make sleep problems worse, not better, in the long term."[8]**

10. **In spite of the National Prescribing Service recommending people investigate all possible avenues before using sleeping pills, the actual prescribing behaviour of medical practitioners in Australia shows a wide variance from those recommendations.**
Here is what is ACTUALLY happening in Australia:

- For new cases of insomnia being reported 81.7 percent were prescribed medications.
- Generally 95.2 percent were prescribed medications.
- Coupled with lower than normal rates of advice, higher prescribing rates (normally 54.5%), considerably lower referral rates and significantly lower pathology tests[9].

11. **Viewed as a group, sleeping pills will reduce the time it takes to fall asleep by 12.8 minutes compared with fake pills[10].**

12. **Viewed as a group, sleeping pills increase your sleep time by 11.4 minutes[11].**

13. **Sleeping pills have been blamed for some bizarre behaviours.**
The following weird and bizarre behaviours (parasomnias) have been connected to the use of sleeping pills.

- Sleepwalking,
- Sleep-eating and cooking,
- Making phone calls,
- Having sex while not fully awake,
- Behaving abnormally,
- Driving while asleep – see 20 below[12].

Often, people do not remember these events.

In March 2007 in Sydney it was reported that an Australian federal health watchdog was to review the safety of a certain sleeping pill following the death of a man who had, allegedly, fallen to his death from his 12th floor unit after having taken Stilnox[13].

There are other court cases sighting unusual and uncommon activities being undertaken by people under the influence of sleeping pills, where they have done illegal acts, but claim not to have remembered them.

14. **Some sleeping pills are associated with increased risk of depression[50].**

"Data for 5535 patients randomized to a hypnotic and for 2318 randomized to placebo were compiled. The incidence of depression was 2.0% among participants randomized to hypnotics as compared to 0.9% among those randomized in parallel to placebo (p < 0.002)."

"Modern hypnotics were associated with an increased incidence of depression in data released by the FDA. This suggests that when there is a risk of depression, hypnotics may be contra-indicated."[14]

As an aside, if 0.9% (less than 1 percent) is the figure for the 2,318 placebo group for depression, do you wonder why 16.6 percent of Aussies (and Americans) are taking antidepressants? Because I sure do.

15. **Sleeping pills have been associated with a four-fold risk of death and increased rates of cancer for people taking large amounts per year.**

Receiving hypnotic prescriptions was associated with greater than threefold increased hazards of death even when prescribed less than 18 pills per year[15].

16. **Some sleeping pills can change your perception of your sleep, for perceived benefits.**

"Most sleeping pills work on the same brain receptors as drugs to treat anxiety. By reducing anxiety, the pills may make people worry less about not going to sleep. So they feel better."[16]

17. **Most sleep medications affect people's memories.**

"Another theory about the discrepancy between measured sleep and perceived sleep involves a condition called anterograde amnesia. While under the influence of most sleep medications, people have trouble forming memories. When they wake up, they may simply forget they had trouble sleeping[17]."

Excuse me for being a little more cynical about that one!

18. **Patients are demanding them of doctors.**
Doctors are concerned that patients are demanding they prescribe sleeping pills, and indicate that if they do not prescribe them, they will seek out prescriptions from other sources.
Are you one of these patients?

19. **Because they are addictive, sleeping pills have withdrawal symptoms.**
The reported withdrawal symptoms include:
- Suicide[57],
- "Persistent withdrawal syndrome", which means that you can have withdrawal symptoms that last for years, even permanent damage where you do not recover from the symptom[58],
- anxiety,
- unusual dreams,
- sweating,
- shakiness,
- fatigue,
- rebound insomnia,
- unusual depressed or anxious mood,
- stomach cramps,
- vomiting,
- sweating,
- fatigue, and/or
- irritability.

Please note that not all these withdrawal symptoms relate to each different sleeping pill variety, the symptoms are randomly selected from a range of reports on sleeping pill withdrawal symptoms.

20. **Sleeping pills have been linked to sleep driving, impaired driving, sleep walking and other dangerous behaviours[67,68].**
One sleeping pill, Ambien (US brand name, Stilnox is the Australian brand name), ranks among the top 10 drugs found in the bloodstreams of impaired drivers, according to some US state toxicology labs.

In Washington state there were 78 arrested in 2005 for impaired driving, an increase of 40 percent from 2004.

Mixing these drugs with alcohol has very adverse effects:

"The behaviour can include driving in the wrong direction or slamming into light poles or parked vehicles, as well as seeming oblivious to the arresting officers, according to a presentation last month at a meeting of forensic scientists".[18]

"People get up, they take their car keys and they go drive. As you might imagine, that might be potentially dangerous to the patient and others as well".[19]

These bizarre occurrences have become so common, the American Academy of Forensic Sciences held a presentation on the odd effects of Ambien impairment on the body[20].

Zolpidem/Stilnox now has a black box warning in Australia because of its association with sleep walking, sleep driving and bizarre behaviours. The warning includes a caution with other central nervous system depressant drugs: that they should not be taken with alcohol, and its use should be limited to maximum four weeks under close medical supervision.[65]

21. **Sleeping pills are respiratory depressants and can exacerbate sleep apnea and related illnesses.[21]**

Sleeping pills should not be used if you have sleep apnea.

Sleeping pills, like alcohol, might prevent the necessary momentary arousals necessary to resume breathing in sleep apnea sufferers.

Although they are not as bad as barbiturates in depressing respiration, this observation should be considered important for some.

And the observation is particularly relevant when benzodiazepines are mixed with other drugs and substances.[60]

22. **Sleeping pills have been associated with increased fall and fracture rates in elderly people[22].**

Please refer to the information on falls in older people (over 65 years of age) in Chapter 10 on the side effects of antidepressants.

23. **Sleeping pills may help you fall asleep, but will not help you get all the way to stage 5 sleep.**

Stage 5 sleep is described by the National Prescribing Service as the rapid eye movement sleep (REM sleep) that occurs just before waking up at the end of a normal and beneficial night's sleep.

"To feel fully rested, you need to spend a lot of time in Stage 5. This stage is also known as REM sleep and it's where dreaming and deep sleep occur." [23]

I have a slightly different idea about what is regarded as 'deep sleep': it is not the REM part of the sleep, but the slower brain wave patterned parts of the sleep cycles. However, we agree that the value of REM sleep, especially the part before waking up, is huge. We have seen REM sleep associated with problem solving (very important for people suffering from anxiety and depression issues).

Waking up out of REM sleep at the end of a 'normal' night's sleep is also very beneficial because it generally means there is no 'sleep inertia' – that groggy feeling that you get when you wake up from slow wave sleep and feel disoriented and half asleep for a little while. REM sleep usually occurs and typifies the lighter phases of sleep.

What might have been meant by referring to this Stage 5 as "deep sleep", is that it takes all night to get there – you just can't 'click into' the elongated REM sleep stage at the end of a good night's sleep without cycling through the brain wave patterns of a normal night's sleep beforehand.

The benefits of this last stage of sleep include dreaming, the welding of the brain's learning network or potentiation, memory improvement, the sharpening of spatial abilities and perception, and the brainpower to execute complex tasks. REM also has a role in emotional memories and helps uncouple associations that are no longer productive[24].

We know that waking up too early has been associated with feelings of depression and grief. There is some question as to "which causes which". i.e. Does the lack of the last stage of sleep (Stage 5) cause the psychological difficulties of depression and grief, or vice verse – the psychological problems changing the sleep pattern to bring on early awakening?

What happens with some sleeping pills (SSRIs and some antidepressants) is that they prolong the time spent in Slow Wave Sleep (SWS) therefore inhibiting the time spent in REM at the end of the night[25].

24. While some sleeping pills prolong the time in slow wave sleep and reduce the time spent in REM (see 23 above), other sleeping pills (such as benzodiazepines) inhibit the time spent in SWS

and cause sleepers to have lighter sleep generally – or sleep spent in the higher brain wave patterns – such as REM[26].

SWS is associated with healing your body; bone and muscle growth; tissue restoration; protein synthesis; carbohydrate and fat metabolism (including cholesterol); decreasing stress, anxiety and the susceptibility to illness; the production of milk in new mothers, etc. Meanwhile our brains and the firing rate of neurons drops dramatically, and other activities that look like pruning mental deadwood and clearing your mind are carried out, and declarative memory is strengthened. Stage 3 and 4 are both regarded as SWS.

25. Completed Suicide.

The association between benzodiazepine use and attempted suicide is especially high for non-antidepressant users, for the young, and for males[27].

There have been 2158 reported cases of completed suicide for Zolpidem users alone, recorded by the Rxisk.org website[28].

"You can be suicidal on a benzodiazepine alone."[59]

26. Significant Lowering of Minimum Oxygen Levels.

Benzodiazepines significantly lowered minimum oxygen levels during the night when compared with placebo[29].

27. In 2012 the Therapeutic Goods Administration announced that it was considering a proposal to reclassify all benzodiazepines from Schedule 4 to Schedule 8, making them controlled drugs and effectively prohibiting most GPs from being able to prescribe them without specific authority.[30]

(See the Poisons Schedule, Appendix 5.)

Seventy public pre-meeting submissions were received; among them was an unfavourable submission from the Australian Medical Association (AMA), stating that the rescheduling "would have added significantly to the administrative burden on GPs and hospital staff".

The AMA said "while benzodiazepines were at risk of abuse, there were currently a range of controls in place, including electronic tracking of dispensing, patient and medical practitioner education, audits of prescribing, and prosecutions."[31]

Interestingly the AMA sees those checks and balances as working, given we now know that you will be prescribed in 95.2 percent of cases – see item 10 above. Other research I have conducted indicates that those controls were not in place at the time at all, and probably not even now, more than 3 years later.

The end result of this initiative was that the Alprazolam class of benzodiazepines was moved to schedule 8, but the other benzodiazepines remain at Schedule 4 in Australia.

According to Wikipedia, Alprazolam was the 12th most prescribed drug in the US in 2010, and remains in Schedule 4 in that country[34].

It is undisputed that Alprazolam/Xanax is highly addictive, and no doubt one of the reasons it was moved to Schedule 8 in Australia.

"…the pills they pop like Smarties are more addictive and harder to kick than heroin.[35]"

The Advisory Committee on Medicine's Scheduling (ACMS), and its members can be found on the Australian Government, Department of Health, Therapeutic Goods Administration website, here: https://www.tga.gov.au/committee/advisory-committee-medicines-scheduling-acms (Accessed November 18, 2016.)

28. Akathisia is a frequent and common adverse effect of treatment with antipsychotic (neuroleptic) drugs, including benzodiazepines, and in the withdrawal or tapering phase of use[32].

According to Wikipedia, the term 'akathisia' was coined by the Czech neuropsychiatrist Ladislav Haskovec (1866–1944), who described the phenomenon in 1901.

Akathisia predisposes suicide and homicide in some users[33]. See point 25 above.

29. Congenital Abnormalities/birth defects.

One study suggested higher risk of oral cleft, the floppy infant syndrome, dependence in babies, or marked neonatal withdrawal symptoms when using benzodiazepines during pregnancy[36].

An increased risk of congenital malformations in humans has been suggested with use of some benzodiazepines. Withdrawal syndrome has been described in neonates whose mothers took benzodiazepines during pregnancy. Withdrawal symptoms such as intrauterine growth retardation, tremors, irritability, hypertonicity, diarrhoea/vomiting, and vigorous sucking have been described. Floppy infant syndrome, which presents as hypotonia, lethargy, and sucking difficulties, has also been reported with the use of certain benzodiazepines, such as diazepam or lorazepam[37].

Benzodiazepines are in "FDA Pregnancy Category D" which recommends against their use during pregnancy.

30. Overdose deaths and poisonings using benzodiazepines.

The Victorian Drug Overdose Register showed that Diazepam (which is a benzodiazepine) was the drug that caused or contributed to the highest number of overdose deaths in 2014 (the year before the findings were brought down)[38].

According to the Drug Poisonings in England, NHS 2014 list there were 15,385 poisonings attributed to benzodiazepines, the next on the poisonings list was heroin (2,450) following by cocaine (2,306) poisonings.

There were 374 deaths in England and Wales in 2014 (an increase of 8 percent on the previous year and the largest since recording began). Benzodiazepine death numbers lagged death by heroin and morphine (952) and methadone (394).[61]

31. Doctor Shopping of Benzodiazepines

There are inadequate checks and balances to ensure that addicted benzodiazepine users do not and cannot 'doctor shop' to ensure supply of these drugs they want.

The inquest into the deaths of Christopher Salib, Nathan Attard and Shamsad Akhtar by the State Coroner's Court of New South Wales recommended a raft of measures in June 2015, including that benzodiazepines be moved to schedule 8 of the Poisons Schedule, that the state develop an online real time registration and monitoring system of all schedule 8 prescriptions, imposing a restriction on general practitioners to look into prescription histories before prescribing, continued education to pharmacists on prescription shopping and drug dependence case studies, clinical guidelines be developed around prescribing these drugs, the Royal Australian College of General Practitioners develop a clinical governance framework for schedule 8 medicines and that they pursue collaboration with the National Coronial Information System (NCIS) and database to share information on deaths linked to prescription medication, that general practitioners attend a unit of skills training related to opioids and benzodiazepines, all medical prescribers to be registered under the Prescription Shopping Program, and to establish local forums for multidisciplinary professionals to discuss pharmaceutical shopping, etc[39]. (See other detailed recommendations in the reference.)

32. Genetic Predisposition for more Severe Adverse Reactions.
Some genetic types can render the medications toxic through an inability to metabolise the medications. These patients have a significantly higher risk of problems with these prescribed drugs because of their genetic metabolisms.[66]

This means increased risk of suicide, for example.

Please refer to chapter 10 for further discussion on this genetic predisposition and Cytochrome P450 – it is relevant to some sleeping pills and antidepressants and is an important new area of study.

Poor metabolisers, which include a higher percentage of Asian genotype, have, on average, a 4-fold higher exposure to the reference drug than homozygous extensive metabolisers (EMs). Heterozygous EMs have, on average, a 2-fold higher drug exposure than their homozygous EM counterparts.

33. 50 percent increased risk of Alzheimer's Disease.[63]

34. Difficulty Walking.
Professor Heather Ashton reported in the British Medical Journal in 1984 that "all patients complained of difficulty walking. This appeared to result from a combination of sensory disturbance, muscle weakness, pain and stiffness".[64]

Further notes:
I have not studied how many benzodiazepines are prescribed in hospitals, government institutions, mental institutions, detention centres, jails and the like, and how much therapy is given before those prescriptions are given. I suspect the figures would be higher in these cases.

Polypharmacy is another issue I have not addressed in this book. I certainly know of cases where not just one medication is being prescribed, but a number of medications together (even of similar type), which is ... yes, alarming.

Tell me, is this list enough?

"Sleeping Pills are a Bandaid Solution"?

I can't complete this chapter without putting in my opinion on this comment that I hear often. It really aggravates me!

Since when are bandaids addictive, cause serious side-effects, require medical supervision to take off, delay and/or impair healing the underlying problem, impair your memory and cognitive functions, cause you to do weird things overnight, increase suicidal ideation and cause permanent damage?

Wake up.

Why Natural?

Because **world's best research** recommends solving your sleep disorders and psychological problems in non-drug ways – through human engagement, talk therapies, psychotherapy, counselling, etc.

By now you should be convinced.

What are the natural solutions to sleeping better?

And how do you tailor your solutions to exactly your sleep problem?

Find the answers in Part Three: Sleep Mojo.

WARNING: if you didn't read my warnings earlier... DO NOT WITHDRAW WITHOUT PROPER MEDICAL SUPERVISION. Stopping sleep, anxiety, depression and other medications suddenly can be dangerous and/or difficult. In fact, the tapering stage is reputed to be the most dangerous stage. Please seek expert and specialized medical assistance to reduce or withdraw from any medications.

One example I have found of a withdrawal strategy (and *don't quote me*, this is just an indication... if you are on one medication only...) is to taper, *under expert supervision*, 5 – 10 percent of your medication over a 4 to 6 week period – depending on how well you are going. Then repeat the process for another 5 -10 percent, etc. It is a slow and exacting experience. E.g. One woman I spoke to said the 'lick' stage at the end of her long withdrawal strategy was the most difficult for her to give up!

I'd be asking a few curly questions of my doctor before I selected the right one to help you off your medications. See the references at the back of the book for support groups.

In a statement for the inaugural World Benzodiazepine Day on 11th July 2016, the British Medical Association said:

"Benzodiazepines can cause short and long term harm to patients when their prescription and withdrawal is not carefully managed. Not enough is known about the levels of dependence and withdrawal and the level of harm that is being caused. There is also too little research about the long term effects of these drugs."[62]

This was the first statement made by a significant medical body in 50 years that recognised the suffering from benzodiazepines and the lack of research into their use.

Another example of medical evidence jet lag.

My conclusion: you have to be a bonzo to use benzos. Steer clear of them.

CHAPTER 10

Antidepressants/SSRIs: Facts to Make You Mad and Sad.

After reading the sleeping pills/benzodiazepines list, you're probably thinking that they're pretty bad. And they are.

So brace yourself for the scarier list for antidepressants!

50 shades darker? The safeword is no.

There are a number of antidepressant drugs, and a few types of antidepressant drugs.

I'm not going to go into the detail of the types and uses of antidepressants in this book.

You will need to investigate further before taking any action on your medications, including reducing or stopping your medications – which should not be done without expert help, as mentioned in my disclaimers, etc.

Selective Serotonin Reuptake Inhibitors (SSRIs) are the most commonly prescribed anti-depressants.

This chapter is directed at antidepressants generally, including SSRIs. I'm not distinguishing between the different types, otherwise we'll all miss the point.

I'll start with my top 3 quotes from international leaders and truth tellers:

1. Peter Gøtzsche: Co-founder of the Cochrane Collaborative, the most respected medical watchdog in the world, author of *Deadly Medicines and Organised Crime*, and numerous papers published in major international medical journals.

"Our citizens would be far better off if we removed all the psychotropic drugs from the market, as doctors are unable to handle them. It is inescapable that their availability creates more harm than good[1]."

2. Peter Breggin: Renowned author and expert witness in major law suits in the USA:
"They're not really antipsychotic drugs, they're just lobotomising drugs."[2]

3. "Irving Kirsch, the Harvard University psychologist responsible for the most thorough analysis of the effectiveness of SSRIs, says that: 'In the future, there will come a point when the prescription of antidepressants that we currently use will be regarded the way we now regard blood-letting: how could doctors have done this?'" [3]

If you like YouTube videos I can recommend the following to you:

- *Mental Health: Overdiagnosed & Overmedicated.* Professor Peter Gøtzsche, 2015. 90 minutes long, and worth every minute of it. https://youtu.be/ZMhsPnoIdy4
- *Psychiatric Drugs Are More Dangerous than You Ever Imagined.* Peter Breggin MD. November 4, 2014. http://youtu.be/luKsQaj0hzs 9 minutes long.

Let's start with 2 most important facts about the marketed "chemical imbalance" that apparently relates to depression and the brains of depressed people:

Fact 1: Professor Peter Gøtzsche of the Cochrane Collaborative states that chemical imbalance is a hoax[4].
Fact 2: Antidepressant drugs *create* a chemical imbalance, which is why it is difficult stopping them[5].

The following information is revealed in *Mental Health: Overdiagnosed & Overmedicated*:

A. The FDA analysis says that antidepressants increase suicidal behaviours till age 40[6].

B. Children and adolescents have about double the risk of suicides if they take antidepressants compared to not taking antidepressants[7].

C. The FDA data is grossly unreliable. Gøtzsche's review of the FDA analysis showed 15 suicides, not 1 for a cited study, meaning that he found *15 times more suicides* than the FDA analysis, an error rate of 1,400 percent in the FDA's statistics[8]. That's a huge error, I'm sure you'll agree.

And it's important to note two major flaws identified in this study:

- Only 'events' occurring within 24 hours were included in the randomised trial. E.g. If a person committed suicide (an 'event') two or more days after the trial, that suicide event was not included in the statistics.

- People with akathisia/agitation (which predisposes them to suicide and homicide) were put on benzodiazepines[9].

D. Addiction is a side effect of antidepressants. Some people say they are harder to get off than heroine.

E. Sexual dysfunction is a side effect of antidepressants. Which includes decreased libido and yawning while having sex[10].

F. Permanent sexual dysfunction. If you weren't depressed before, you sure will be now.

G. An increased risk of committing suicide is a side effect of antidepressants.

H. Akathisia, increased violence and homicide are associated with antidepressant use.

Some of the side effects of antidepressants that I've shown in this chapter are the same, or related. I've specifically explained each, even when they overlap or repeat, for the purposes of clarity and full disclosure.

Suicide, for example is one side effect of anti-depressants. So is suicidal ideation (or thinking about suicide).

You might ask why I'm including both.

Except if you are the parent of a child that has just been prescribed anti-depressants and seems to be "getting lower" on the day or days following the commencement of the medication.

If I was a doctor, I would not be recommending antidepressants.

To my knowledge it is "off-label prescribing" to prescribe antidepressants to children in Australia at the time of writing (June 2017). After reading *Restoring Study 329* and Dolin vs. GSK you should be in a position to make your own decision, whether for children or adults.

In every case of prescribing an antidepressant (or withdrawal) the doctor or psychiatrist should **definitely** be recommending that you and your family and friends keep a VERY close eye on the patient during this phase (and others)... It is far too late after an actual suicide to learn about the increased risk of suicidal ideation and suicide.

Likewise with akathisia - agitation that can lead to suicide or homicide. Be very careful of any downgraded explanations and definitions of "akathisia". It took me a while in my research to "get it", as most explanations just list it as a minor irritation – but never as the torment that some sufferers experience that leads them to kill or take their own life (or both).

List of side effects have the habit, in my experience, of being underplayed. I hope this book clearly demonstrates this.

You have been warned.

And some of you, unfortunately, will be hearing this information first from me.

It's called professional negligence. And culpable behaviour. I can't see it any other way.

It's not only the drug companies who are at fault.

Drug companies would have no sales of their products if doctors and psychiatrists did not prescribe the medications. Doctors and psychiatrists already have a duty of care to engage in evidence-based medicine, and to conduct their clinical governance in a way that results in evidence-based medicine.

I'll let you gauge how well you think they are faring at the end of reading this chapter.

The ABCs of Clinical Governance

Getting your pharmaceutical information from drug companies and acting on that information is not clinical governance and never will be.

Similarly, getting your Continuing Professional Development (CPD) education, as outlined by the Medical Board of Australia[11], from drug companies' approved trainings is a practice fraught with conflict of interest challenges, and potential clinical governance issues.

Yet it is exactly what is happening, and part of the accepted continuing education of medical professionals in Australia.

Conflicts of interest go beyond approved continuing professional development courses run by pharmaceutical companies and into universities and research foundations, as covered in other chapters.

And there is growing interest in having private enterprise sponsor the schooling systems and what is being taught there.

Danger Will Robinson, Danger!

Here Is My "Mad And Sad" List Of Antidepressants' Side Effects And Ramifications:

1. **Increased Risk of Suicide, even Double the Risk of Suicide.**
   Reliable and recent studies including the *Restoring Study 329*, published in the British Medical Journal September 2016 showed serious adverse effects of antidepressant use, including suicide[12].

   If you would like to read more about this groundbreaking investigation into the drug company that was found to have committed consumer fraud, and fined $ 3 billion visit https://study329.org/.

   "Thousands of North American children and adolescents
   were seriously harmed by taking SSRIs
   like Paxil. Many died.[13]"
   "In November 2012 GSK pleaded guilty
   and agreed to pay $3 billion,
   the biggest fine in corporate history.
   The next year, the number of prescriptions for paroxetine in the United States increased by 3%."
   (Note that the original Study 329 has
   never been retracted by GSK)[14].

   In the conclusions of *Suicidality and Aggression during Antidepressant Treatment: Systematic Review and Meta-analyses Based on Clinical Study Reports* it states that "in children and adolescents the risk of suicidality and aggression doubled"[15,16].

2. **Increased risk of suicidal ideation (suicidal thoughts).**
Suicidal ideation in layman's terms is thinking about suicide, which include thinking about how you might commit suicide. It is a known side effect of anti-depressants.

It may or may not lead to suicide, but certainly it can be a precursor to suicide.

I have included it here so that parents, friends and professionals can watch out for the signs, and hopefully act accordingly with support and help.

It is obviously *not harmless*, and this warning needs to be taken very seriously.

3. **Akathisia**
Akathisia is a restlessness or agitation which can manifest as crying, pacing, burning sensations or an intense inner restlessness.

Akathisia is described by some, in its more extreme form, as an internal agitation so severe that people feel like they want to "jump out of their skin"[17]. It can result in self harm and in severe cases it can become so torturous that "death can be a welcome result".

Akathisia predisposes suicide and/or homicide in some people[18].

During a significant episode of akathisia (agitation) some people may commit suicide, or homicide[19].

Many professional bodies, drug side effects sheets and online information sources list "akathisia" as simply some "minor agitation" that occurs[20].

In fact I'm sure the first time I heard about it, the word was connected to restless legs syndrome - that agitated feeling you get in your legs when you can't sleep.

Well, I now know that under the influence of certain medications, including antidepressants, you can suffer akathisia in its full blown form – which can lead to fatalities.

4. **Increased risk of homicide.**
For some people antidepressants increase the risk of committing violent acts, including homicide[21,22].

This had been the source of much debate for a long time now, with increasing numbers of violent crimes being performed by people who are taking antidepressants, tapering off antidepressants, or changing their prescription dosages.

Important work has been done on the connection between genetics and a predisposition to violent acts such as homicide by researchers including Dr. Yolanda Lucire[23].

Some people have a greater predisposition to violent acts and adverse reactions, which is explained further in point 14 below: "Genetic Predisposition to More Severe Adverse Reactions".

Further information can be obtained from the www.Rxisk.org website containing stories and data related to SSRIs.

5. **Increased aggression.**
Discussed previously.

6. **Suicide and murder combined.** Sometimes murder is followed by suicide[24].

7. **Sexual dysfunction.**
"Close to 100 percent of people taking antidepressants experience some form of sexual side effects". Known as Post-SSRI Sexual Dysfunction (PSSD). "PSSD affects both men and women. It can happen after only a few days exposure to an antidepressant and can persist for months, years, or indefinitely. There is no known cure."[25]

Here are some of the sexual dysfunctions that have been reported to the www.rxisk.org website:

- Reduced erogenous (sexual) sensation in genitals
- Genital anesthesia
- Erectile dysfunction/decreased vaginal lubrication
- Delayed or inability to orgasm (anorgasmia)
- Pleasureless, weak or "muted" orgasms
- Decreased or loss of libido (sex drive)
- Reduced response to sexual stimuli
- Decreased or lack of nocturnal erections
- Premature ejaculation, and
- Soft glans syndrome

8. **Permanent Sexual Dysfunction.**
There is some evidence that some sexual dysfunction is permanent, even after coming off the drugs[26][27].

9. Yawning while having sex[28].
10. Increased interest in consuming alcohol[29][30].
11. Visual problems on SSRIs[31].
12. "Antidepressant use during the third trimester (of pregnancy) has been associated occasionally with a transient neonatal withdrawal-like syndrome characterized by jitteriness, self-limiting respiratory difficulties, and problems with feeding."[32] My insertion of the words "(of pregnancy)", for clarity.
13. Antipsychotics May Boost Respiratory Failure Risk in patients with Chronic Obstructive Pulmonary Disease (COPD)[33].

COPD are lung diseases that make it hard to breath, including emphysema and chronic bronchitis.

14. Genetic Predisposition to more Severe Adverse Reactions.

Antidepressants are commonly prescribed without having the patient undergo genetic testing to ensure that they are capable of metabolising the drugs without increased harms due to toxicity.

It is important to note that there are genetic indicators of increased problems for some people taking antipsychotic drugs, and/or benzodiazepines. There is testing available.

Some genetic types can render the medications toxic through an inability to metabolise the medications. These patients have a significantly higher risk of problems with these prescribed drugs because of their genetic metabolisms[34]. This means increased risk of suicide, for example.

The specific test that is recommended by some experts is a test for genetically-determined metabolism of Cytochrome P450, which contributes to toxicity.

Cytochrome P450 is related to forensic and legal medicine through akathisia-related violence and suicide.

There are more than 50 CYP450 enzymes: 6 of them metabolise 90 percent of drugs[35].

This test is still not routinely recommended, so you will have to find a suitable expert should you want to participate in this testing. If you are in Sydney start with the Blacktown Molecular Research Laboratory, part of the National Association of Testing Authorities[36].

Poor metabolisers, which include a higher percentage of Asian genotype, have, on average, a 4-fold higher exposure to the reference drug than homozygous extensive metabolisers (EMs). Heterozygous EMs have, on average, a 2-fold higher drug exposure than their homozygous EM counterparts.

For leading thinkers it is already regarded as professional negligence that this test to establish metabolic vulnerability is not routinely given before prescribing antipsychotics and some benzodiazepines.

Download the Cytochrome Factsheet published by the Blacktown Molecular Research Laboratory for more information, and a list of the drugs which are made more difficult to metabolise if you have this genetic trait[37]. Not only are the drugs more difficult to metabolise, they become toxic in the body.

This downloadable Cytochrome fact sheet lists CYP2C19 inhibitors, inducers and other important information.

Please refer to this information and list of drug groups, which includes antidepressants and benzodiazepine.

15. Chemical Imbalance in the Brain.

Here are some quotes from Peter Breggin's YouTube video *Psychiatric Drugs Are More Dangerous than You Ever Imagined*[38]:

▪ Antidepressant usage is "producing multiple bio-chemical imbalances in the brain that don't have any biochemical imbalances – until a prescriber puts you on the drug"[39].

▪ "None of these drugs are good for your brain", "all of these drugs are bad for your brain"[40].

This opinion that there is no evidence of chemical imbalances in the brain of a depressed person is also shared by Professor Peter Gøtzsche, and spoken about earlier in this chapter.

16. Lack of Easy Access to, and Disclosure of, the Side-Effects of Antidepressants/SSRIs, or misleading information from your medical professional.

This is possibly the worst problem of all. It is very easy for your doctor or psychiatrist to prescribe these medications, and just as easy for them to overlook telling you about the side effects and adverse reactions. And in a 10 minute or short consultation I know they are not giving you this list as I'm stating it here.

There could be more side-effects and adverse reactions than this.

Is your medical professional talking about this list of over 20 serious problems with antidepressants and antipsychotic medications? At the time of you being prescribed?

Looking at this list, it is my belief that if they aren't they are being grossly negligent.

And I also believe that other members of a person's family should be involved in these consultations so that intelligent observations and protective behaviours can accompany any use of these medications.

It is not just my opinion that until this industry is cleaned up these medications should not be prescribed in the ways that are being prescribed at the moment at all.

The medical profession has proved itself incapable of self governance and self control around the prescribing and diagnosis of sleep and mental health problems – and the situation is getting worse – proof that what is happening at the moment is not working.

It is not enough that the drug companies list side effects of drugs in patient instruction sheets and black box warnings that come with prescription medications, because patients rely on their doctors to ensure that what they are being prescribed is suitable for their individual case, ascertained during their private consultation.

The drug companies, in this action of listing potential side effects in patient instruction sheets, probably move legal liability and exposure away from themselves and on to both the prescribing doctor and/or the patient, who might or might not take any notice of the warnings in these documents. Another reason to be cautious if you are a patient or a doctor.

If you play the game, make sure you know the rules.

17. Addiction

Apparently this depends on your definition of "addiction".

Now watch carefully.

In the BBC Panorama interview *The Secrets of Seroxat* the interviewer Shelley Jofre asked Dr Alastair Benbow, Head of European Clinical Psychiatry, GlaxoSmithKline: "if people can't stop taking a drug when they want to stop taking it, they're addicted aren't they?" Benbow answered "No, that's not correct."[41]

He explained that "addiction is characterised by a number of different criteria which includes craving, which increases the dose of drug to get the same effect and a number of other features, and these are not exhibited by Seroxat"[42].

Jofre continued by saying the *Oxford Dictionary* says "addiction is having a compulsion to take a drug the stopping of which produces withdrawal symptoms", to which Benbow replied " If you use that limited description of addictive, then most prescription medicines could be defined as addictive"[43].

I'll leave you to make your own conclusions on this topic.

(Note: Seroxat, Paxil and Aropax are the brandnames in the UK, USA and Australia respectively. The manufacturer of these drugs is GlaxoSmithKline).

18. Lack of Easy Access to, and Disclosure of, the Side-Effects of Antidepressants/SSRIs, or misleading information from national and other charities, respected organisations, tax deductible and other foundations, research facilities, institutes and universities, etc.

Let's revisit chapter 5 for a minute, and the marketing strategies used by corporations in the health industry to push their agendas including drugs.

I could list a stream of foundations, institutions, charities, research facilities and universities here that are not promoting evidence-based medicine, but I won't. I'm pretty confident that by the end of the book you'll be able to have a look at them yourself.

So let's have a look at one, as an example.

Beyond Blue.

Ouch!

Yes, we are going there. I don't care who's on the board, and I don't care how respected this organisation is, we are going to look at some facts.

Beyond Blue has an awesome reputation in Australia for helping mental health sufferers, so of course I went there to see what they say about antidepressants, and what their policy is around antidepressants.

And I downloaded their Antidepression Medication Factsheet, dated December 2014 from their website.

Tell me what you think of the following statements made in this downloadable Factsheet in December 2014:

A. **"No deaths from suicide have been reported in any clinical trials"**[44] on the first page of the *Antidepression Medication Factsheet BL/0125 02/15*

Thankfully in January or February 2017 the story had changed. (As I write this in February 2017 I thought I'd check if any change had happened...)

Now the *Antidepressant Medication Factsheet BL/0125 12/16* (reviewed and updated in December 2016) states the following:

- "There is concern that a small percentage of young people up to the age of 24 years taking Selective Serotonin Reuptake Inhibitors (SSRIs) for the treatment of depression may experience an increase in suicidal thoughts and behaviour. Research shows the risk to be roughly 4 per cent compared to 2 per cent for those taking a placebo (dummy pill)."[45]

- "A young person will require close medical supervision and monitoring in the early stages of treatment if an antidepressant is prescribed."[46]

- "The Therapeutic Goods Administration (Australia's regulatory agency for medical drugs) and manufacturers of antidepressants do not recommend antidepressant use for depression in young people under the age of 18. There are, however, no government (i.e. Pharmaceutical Benefits Scheme) restrictions placed on the prescription of antidepressants and doctors are not prevented from prescribing them if they feel they are needed."[47]

That's a pretty strong turn about, that took Beyond Blue until 2017 to change their factsheet!

And on a scale of 1 to 10 how do you like Beyond Blue quoting the TGA's stance on antidepressants for young people - and then immediately supplying a get-out-clause (see the last dot point)?

And for those wondering about the
4 per cent and 2 per cent figures above,
in layman's terms it means
that antidepressants double the risk of suicide and suicidal thoughts.

It's August 2017 now, and I'm still wondering exactly what sort of publicity they are going to be doing to announce this change of information on their website.

And I wonder how many children died relying on the information contained on the Beyond Blue website prior to this most recent update of the *Antidepressant Factsheet*?

B.   "People often want to stop taking antidepressants quickly because they are concerned they are addictive. This may be because they confuse them with sedatives, a group of medications that are used to help a person feel relaxed and, in some cases, fall/stay asleep. Sedatives are designed to be used only for a short time. If used for long periods of time, sedatives may cause withdrawal insomnia and anxiety and be needed in higher doses in order for them to have the same effect. Sedatives may be craved and become addictive. **This is not the case with antidepressants.**"[48] (Author's bolding emphasis)

This statement did not change on the *Antidepressant Medication Factsheet* at the end of December 2016, from their previously published stance in December 2014.

I'd like to know where this research comes from.

Beyond Blue is not the only organisation or website with misleading information. Be aware.

19. **Autistic children born of mothers who take antidepressants while they are pregnant[49][50].**

Antidepressants are the most commonly prescribed medications to pregnant women.

One in six babies in America is born to a mother who has taken antidepressants while pregnant[51]. This is basically the same percentage of pregnant women taking antidepressants and the general population – which indicates to me that there is an attitude that "just because you're pregnant doesn't mean you should behave any differently than if you weren't".

And just because your *patient* is pregnant doesn't mean you shouldn't prescribe an antidepressant!

You've got to be kidding, right?

The risk of birth defects can persist for months or perhaps longer after stopping an antidepressant[52].

Other problems that have been documented around pregnancy include preterm births, increased risk of miscarriage, babies having trouble breathing, Persistent Pulmonary Hypertension of the Newborn (PPHN), and neonatal seizures[53].

So now let's have a look at this statement from the Beyond Blue Perinatal Mental Health National Action Plan 2008-2010:

"Antidepressants in pregnancy are as effective and necessary as for any other depressive episode, as evidenced by the rate of relapse in pregnant women discontinuing medication prior to conception"[54].

An interesting medical justification. And a *more than* confusing statement, given what we now know.

20. Increased risk of falls in older people, followed by death for one in 28 of them.

"For every 28 elderly people treated for 1 year with an SSRI, there was one additional death, compared to no treatment." Or for 100 people, you will have 3 deaths in a year[55].

In the over 65 years group, Peter Gøtzsche states that over half a million people die each year in the US and UK because of psychiatric drugs.[65]

21. Adverse effects on general health outcomes and mood disorders.

A study conducted by the World Health Organisation in fifteen cities around the world to assess the value of screening for depression did not support the view that failure to recognize depression has serious adverse consequences.

In fact, contrary to the study's expected results, of the 740 people identified as depressed in the study it was the 484 who weren't exposed to psychotropic medications (whether diagnosed or not) that had the best outcomes. "The group that suffered most from "continued depression" were the patients treated with an antidepressant."[56]

22. **Adverse outcomes for people diagnosed and treated for major depression in the areas of "Cessation of Role Function" and "Became Incapacitated".**
"A US National Institute of Mental Health (NIMH) investigation showed that at the end of six years the treated patients were much more likely to have stopped functioning in their usual societal roles (approximately 32% "Cessation of Role Function" in the treated group, compared with about 9% in the untreated group). And the treated group were much more likely to have become incapacitated (about 8% in the treated group compared with about 1-2 percent in the untreated group)."[57]

"In the United States, the percentage of working-age Americans who said in health surveys that they were disabled by depression tripled during the 1990s."[58]

23. **Shortened Life Span**[59]

24. **Tardive Dyskinesia**[60]
Wikipedia explains tardive dyskinesia (TD) as a difficult to treat and often incurable neurological disorder resulting in involuntary, repetitive body movements. "Tardive" means that they have a slow or belated onset, and can be the result of long term (usually at least 3 months duration) or high dose use of antipsychotic drugs.

25. **"Virtually wreck the part of the brain called the basal ganglia"**[61]
Other Side Effects?
There are other side effects of antidepressants, but I think I've covered enough.

I could spend years doing more research into this, but if you haven't got the message by now, my time will have been wasted anyway.

I'll list some other potential problems here, for my research-oriented readers, if *you* want to see if any of these have legs or not: increased breast and ovarian cancer risk, weight gain even after ceasing medication, increased risk of stroke, bladder and urinary problems, gender dysmorphia, self harm, mental turmoil, mammoplasia (growing breasts), galactorrhea (milky nipple discharge), personality drained away, huge weight gain, brain cell damage, weakened bones, insomnia, becoming introverted, head shocks, feeling terrible, increased risk of dementia, increased apathy, impaired memory, increased blood pressure, increased heart disease, etc.

Here is a page you can refer to for some of the sources/research, if you are interested. https://ssristories.org/antidepressants-risks-with-20-reasons-to-be-concerned-mythsandrisksinfo-com/

I'll leave the final comment here to US psychiatrist Peter Breggin, author of *Toxic Psychiatry* and prominent critic of SSRIs since their introduction:

> "They are causing a huge amount of misery, loss of quality of life, loss of love life,"
> "These drugs are devastating to people."[62]

Be Especially Careful During the Taper Phase

The most severe adverse affects occur in the taper phase. An area of study not well publicised[63].

And don't believe it when your doctor (or others...) says that heightened problems are a sign that the medications are working.

There are significant and dangerous *side effects* experienced during withdrawal.

That's why I don't recommend changing your medications at all without competent and expert help. These people aren't so easy to find. In fact, Professor Gøtzsche says that we do not have the facilities in the world to deal with everyone coming off these drugs.

It is a real problem, and will become more real as the truth becomes better known.

It's a Fake Epidemic!

Given the extensive research you have just been shown let's have a look at what the Australian Government tells us is "world's-best-practice" and a "gold standard health system".

Who cares what political persuasion you come from, left or right – this system has been set up for generations now. This level of ignorance, misinformation and deception didn't happen overnight, it has taken multiple governments, legislation, medical training programs, drug information sheets, best practice guidelines, clinical governance oversights and apathetic medical professionals to get us to the present mess we are in.

A lot of silence really. Don't you agree?

From people who are meant to be looking after our health and health budgets.

And WE are all individually paying for it, whether or not we take antidepressants and sleeping pills.

We pay by subsidising these medications through the PBS (Pharmaceutical Benefits Scheme), we pay in insurance fees (Medicare and private health insurance), we pay in MBS servicing (listed medical procedures subsidised by the government), we pay in emergency call outs and deaths, we pay in road accidents for people not paying attention or who are drugged to the eyeballs, we pay in medical consultation fees with doctors not recommending evidence-based solutions, we pay because we do not have effective preventative medical training, we pay because incorrect diagnoses and procedures often result in putting off the correct medical actions, we pay in complications that arise later when the actual underlying issues are found (if they are found), we pay the salaries of medical professionals who are not doing their job, we pay through the deaths and sickness of our family and friends, we pay through a dumbed-down society where people's minds are dulled and unproductive .... I won't go on.

But I could....

On and on...

And the government says we can't afford a better health system.

Let's clean up this broken system first, and then see what we can and can't afford.

What we can't afford is bad medical advice, procedures and training that are *not* evidence-based.

And this book only covers sleep and the antidepressants in mental health.

We know from the Four Corners *Wasted* program that 95 percent of the MBS is not evidence based. It means that 95% of the MBS funding is wasted, and that doesn't count any damage that is being done by tests and procedures that should not occur.

Here are some figures on how many people are affected: that's how I *know* this book should be read by everyone:

The following data were taken from the Australian Government, Australian Institute of Health and Welfare, Mental Health Services in Australia website, relevant at August 2017. (The figures for the previous year 2015-16 are stated in brackets, I have updated them just before going to print.)

- There were 36.0 (35.3) million prescriptions for mental health-related medications dispensed (subsidised and under co-payment) in 2015–16. This equates to an average of 9.0 prescriptions per patient.[66]
- There were a total of 24.2 million prescriptions for subsidised mental health-related medications in 2015–16, which was 67.2% or nearly 7 in 10 of the total number of mental health-related prescriptions.[67]
- 87.6% of the mental health-related prescriptions (subsidised and under co-payment) were provided by GPs, with 8.0% being pre-scribed by psychiatrists and 4.4% by non-psychiatrist specialists.[68]
- Antidepressant medications accounted for 68.7% (67.8%) of total mental health-related (subsidised and under co-payment) prescriptions.[69]
- Females, those aged 65 and over and those people living in *inner regional* areas had the highest mental health-related prescription and patient rates.[70]

The 36 million prescriptions (35.3 million) for mental health-related medications is equivalent to 1503.9 mental health-related prescriptions per 1,000 population. These prescriptions were provided to 4.0 (3.9) million patients, which equates to 167.6 patients per 1,000 population (or 16.7% (16.6%). Combining these data, there were an average of 9.0 prescriptions per patient in 2015–16.[71]

Yes, I'll repeat that: There were 36.0 million prescriptions for mental health related medications in 2015-16, provided to 4.0 million patients or **16.7 percent of the Australian population.**

So the figures of 1 in 6 people being on psychiatric drugs in Australia exactly matches the figures for the US.

Political Correctness Gone Mad

When I was a kid we would call people 'nutty' who were obviously not coping or 'unusual'. In my small country town in the Hunter Valley there were a few. Roamers, disengaged, emotionally disturbed, looking stressed...

People in the community were generally aware of them and looked out for them (in good and bad ways – generally good).

Now they would say that the person had a mental health problem, which is probably correct.

But now there are 1 in 6 people in the community who are apparently 'nutty', and we are told that it's the tip of the iceberg!

You've got to be joking.

Think about that for a moment.

Let's go old-school for a moment – **no** apologies for those who don't want to listen to old-school talk, or want to jump on me for my non-PC languaging. Bear with me.

In your mind line up your partner and all your friends and family and pick out 1 in 6 that you think has a "mental health problem".

Did you find one in six of them?

Really?

Because I sure can't. Tempted as I am for some I know...

I can see anxious friends, I can see stressed friends, I can see friends who are having major challenges in their lives, I can see friends who are a little eccentric at different times (generally when they are in major life changing stages, such as divorce or job struggles), and I can see people who are stressed over their 900K mortgages, or 4 kids and high powered jobs, or because they get no exercise... etc.

I can also see friends who are emotional. Thank goodness for that, I like people who feel and express themselves freely – they are my true friends.

But I don't see these problems as mental health issues. I see this as 'feeling the pain', which is often a precursor (and motivator) to finding a solution and taking appropriate action to solve the problem(s).

If you don't feel pain, you don't know something is wrong, and you don't make any effort to change.

My group of friends pay more attention when we find someone who's about to "lose it". (Yes another non-PC 'old-school' technical term.)

Then we *really* start paying attention, because there are signs that the problem(s) are escalating beyond being able to cope in their usual ways. And we might start to "force" a conversation in an attempt to address the issue, in a non-judgemental and supportive way, etc.

There are people in my sphere who drink too much and take recreational drugs. These habits do indicate underlying emotional and life issues that need to be addressed. Sure. And they are addictions.

But I wouldn't be giving them antidepressants to add to the cocktail. And I wouldn't be telling them not to feel the pain. You wish it was possible, but it isn't.

Emotions are what make us human, and expressing ourselves is what is important to stay sane. It's when you are trying to suppress your emotions that things get very wobbly. Or you haven't got anyone to talk to.

And I can bet that people who do not have good friends have a higher percentage of emotional problems, because of the lack of support and honesty that good friends honour you with. Like when you tell them about some ugly incident that happened in your life (and we all have them), and they allow you to talk about it in a non-judgemental way. Or they share that a similar thing happened to them – and both of you now have a deeper friendship and understanding. You might even make some black joke and laugh about it together. Or someone might suggest someone else to talk to. Or put it into some sort of perspective.

And it's such a relief to get it off your chest.

"Talk therapy". Yes it is valid. I'm glad I'm a girl – 'cos we do a lot of it.

Friends are right up there as "greatest mental health solutions". Just don't tell them that... haha.

Prescription drugs appear to calm people down, reduce their feelings, make it harder to express themselves, and reduce their motivation.

Or they can hype people up, and make them very restless, agitated and destructive.

And now you know they can be fatal.

Prescription and recreational drugs do not address the underlying issues. And none of them *solve* the underlying issues.

It is exactly the same with benzodiazepines.

What you need is a solution to your problems. Covering up the problem is never the solution.

Now getting back to your line up of partner, friends and family members....

Now I want you to pick out people who you would call 'nuts' in the old-school days.

Is this confronting?

Or not! Because I can't see one (out of a lot) that I would call 'nuts' in pre-politically-correct terms.

So maybe we shouldn't be politically correct.

Maybe we need to go back to that nasty word 'nuts' to see the extent of the problem that has been created.

I think we are being sold a lie by the drug companies and by the people who are following their rules, and influenced by them.

Admitting to being 'a bit OCD' is reasonably harmless (it probably ensures the gas really IS off...), and probably helpful.

But it's not harmless if you then take a cocktail of drugs to 'fix it'.

Wake up guys.

Does anyone else feel like Australia is "getting to dumbo" fast? Or is it just me? No wonder we can't seem to get much sense out of a lot of people!

Class Action

If you have had a child adversely affected by antidepressant drugs you can find out more about the Australian Antidepressant Class Action by referring to Tony Nikolic at Drayton Sher Lawyers. Email: Tony@draytonsherlawyers.com.au.

Or the Facebook Page: https://www.facebook.com/AustralianAntidepressantClassAction/

And you can help with donations to help fund the class action in Australia: https://www.gofundme.com/HelpOurAussieKids

CHAPTER 11

The Cost of Lack of Sleep and Mental Health to Australia

This chapter will focus on some of the costs to Australia as a nation, and individually.

For more information on the costs of lack of sleep and mental health issues to organisations, productivity, intellectual capital, profits and the economy, refer to Chapter 16 *What Has Sleep Got to Do with Fatigue* and Appendix 1 *Fatigue and Mental Health: Bedroom to Boardroom.*

Here are some of the alarming numbers:

- The cost of mental illness in 2016 was $ 207 billion – equivalent to about 12 percent of the economy's annual output.[1]
- This cost has climbed from $ 159.7 billion in 2005-06 to $ 203.1 billion last financial year. The drag on wellbeing caused by mental illness was $ 52 billion in the June quarter alone.[2]
- As a nation we spend about $ 155 billion a year on health. And about a third of that, $ 46 billion, each year is being squandered.[3]
- In 2007, people with a mental disorder in the previous 12 months were more likely to report their main source of income as government pensions and allowances than people without a 12-month disorder (26% and 22% respectively). For people with a psychotic disorder, the proportion was much higher—85% reported a government pension as their main source of income in 2010 (Morgan et al. 2011).[4]

- In 2013 almost one-third (31%) of people in receipt of the Disability Support Pension had a primary medical condition of 'psychological/ psychiatric' (DSS 2014).[5]
- 70 percent of people say they frequently don't get enough sleep, with 30 percent saying they don't get enough sleep every single night.[6]
- 20 percent of Australians admit to falling asleep at the wheel at least once[7]. In the USA a million people **each week** nod off and fall asleep on the nation's highways.[8]
- 1 in 6 Australians are taking antidepressants[9], with pressure for more mental health interventions.
- 35 million psycho scripts are written each year in Australia.[10] (Update: This year's figure, just released, is 36 million.)
- Police personnel, medical interns, emergency and ambulance personnel, the military, first responders, hospital shift-workers, and nurses are among the most at-risk personnel for mental health issues, accidents and errors. They have pressure from 3 angles: working in traumatic situations, dangerous shifts, and making life and death decisions. Now this *is* insane.
- Medical errors were recently revealed by John Hopkins University researchers as the third biggest cause of death in the US[11], which throws light on the urgent need for a thorough workplace overhaul of hospital procedures including shift work hours, sleep habits and night time working conditions. (Yes, I recognise that elsewhere in this book I reference Professor Peter Gøtzsche's research that indicates that pharmaceutical drugs are the third leading cause of death after heart disease and cancer.)
- Very little of the Medical Benefits Scheme (MBS) has evidence attached to it. Of the 5,769 services listed on the MBS about 269 are evidence-based. About 5,500 items do not have that evidence base.[12]

Who will similarly review the Pharmaceutical Benefits Scheme (PBS) and National Prescribing Service's (NPS's) evidence base? Will the Therapeutic Goods Administration, medical profession and health ministers leave that up to the media too? FFS.

I don't think the mental health figures include problem gamblers in Australia, but I don't want to give anyone ideas. And heck, 10 percent of all state revenue comes from gambling, with Victoria the most dependent at 13 percent of revenue.[13] Do we cost that in too?

Actuarial Help?

I wish I had continued with maths at university in order to do this chapter justice.

If you are an actuary and would be willing to help me with these figures, I'd love you to contact me. My contact details are at the back of the book.

No-one is calculating these costs correctly: they are underestimating the importance of this issue, and not including many connected factors.

Australia's Largest Employing Industry

Healthcare and Social Assistance is now Australia's largest employing industry, employing 13 percent of workers, and projected to grow another 16.4 percent in the next five years.[14]

From the sheep's back to mining, now health. Who'd a thought it?

Everyone's so proud of Australia being a 'service industry' country.

In cynical moments I think we're a country of baristas serving other baristas coffee ... sometimes with smashed ava.

But it's worse.

We are a country of health care professionals serving *sick and unhealthy* people.

That's the industry that's growing.

It's the biggest game in town.

What's not to love about that?

The Australian Bureau of Statistics (ABS) and the Mental Health Commission

According to the NSW Mental Health Commission about 1 in 2 people experience mental illness in their lifetime, 707 people died by suicide in

2012, 2.7 million workdays are lost each year because of mental health issues, and 54 percent of the NSW mental health budget is spent on inpatient care.[15]

The ABS 2007 National Survey of Mental Health and Wellbeing stated 3.2 million, or 20 percent of the adult population reported experiencing a mental health disorder in the last 12 months. Of these only one-third had accessed medical services to assist them manage their disorder.

The 2014 Fairfax Lateral Economics Index of Australia's Wellbeing Report

This report acknowledges in footnote 45 (page 56) that the quality or effectiveness of treatment is the preferred way to report on treatments, but that *sufficiently detailed data* was unable to be found.[16] (My italics.)

I think Robert Whitaker's book *Anatomy of an Epidemic: Magic Bullets, Psychiatric Drugs, and the Astonishing Rise of Mental Illness in America* provides that "**sufficiently detailed data**", if you're looking.

The book is listed in Recommended Reading and was a major motivator for me writing this book.

Things are not pretty.

Council of Australian Governments (COAG) National Healthcare Agreement

With what we know about how poorly mental health issues are addressed in Australia, I don't agree with how the COAG National Healthcare Agreement measures progress in addressing mental health issues.

COAG has two measures of progress, they are:

1. The proportion of the population receiving clinical mental health services, and
2. The proportion of people with mental illness who have a GP treatment plan.[17]

You're less than half way through this book, but tell me what you think about their criteria for "measures of progress"!

"Come To Jesus" Moments

Interestingly that same Australian Institute of Health and Welfare report[18] stated on page 2 that: "Mental disorders can vary in severity and be episodic or persistent in nature. Recent estimates suggest that 2–3% of Australians have a severe mental illness, as judged by diagnosis, intensity and duration of symptoms, and degree of disability caused (DoHA 2013). This group is not only confined to those with psychotic disorders, who represent only about one-third of those with severe mental disorders; it also includes people with severe and disabling forms of depression and anxiety. A further 4–6% of the population have a moderate mental disorder and 9–12% a have a mild disorder (DoHA 2013)".

These figures are significantly lower figures than the medication figures.

For example, if the above figures are correct, why are 16.6 percent of Australians taking antidepressants (or 1 in 6)?

Do you understand from the above figures why over 16 percent of Australians would be taking an antidepressant?

The 1 in 6 figure does not include any other psycho drugs – just *antidepressants*.

And why are there 35 million (36 million, 2017 updated figure) psycho scripts written in Australia yearly?

Costs to be Included in an Actuarial Computation

I won't bother revisiting the previous 2 chapters, but if anyone thinks that aggressive behaviour, cognitive impairment, suicidal ideation and sexual dysfunction (just 4 off those very long lists) doesn't affect the Australian economy, they're dreamin'.

Here are **some** of the costs that don't seem to be added into the figures I've seen:

- Chronic insomnia. The Lancet, 2012 revealed that sleep disorders contribute to 5.3% of strokes, 10.1% of depression, 4.3 % of motor vehicle accidents and 4.5% of workplace injuries.
- Social security payments and unemployment benefits payments made to people with a mental health problem who are incapable of working, working in jobs beneath their capability, cannot get a job, and/or are discriminated against at work.

- Work inefficiency and errors. Anyone who is taking a sleeping medication with a half life of say 20 hours, will have their work performance impaired for at least the next full day at work, possibly two. That's from one sleeping pill, once a year. (This is <u>not</u> a recommendation for short half life sleeping pills.)
- 1 in 5 motor accidents are fatigue related.
- Errors at work caused by fatigue – such as placing incorrect trades, incorrect financial information, bad strategic decisions, etc;
- Ineffectual grumpy and short tempered management, with the resultant lack of work productivity in their departments and organisations;
- Relationship problems, divorce, lack of self esteem, abuse;
- Domestic violence – medicated and not medicated;
- The cost of listing ineffectual drugs on the PBS, and the cost of those prescriptions to the patient (e.g. approximately 7 million benzodiazepine prescriptions written each year alone);
- The cost of medical conditions being overlooked, and worsening, because the root cause(s) of insomnia and mental health problems are being medicated, not investigated;
- The cost of not addressing the underlying problems that manifest as sleep and mental health disorders – many never uncovered, some uncovered too late;
- The cost of suicides, suicidal ideation and homicides;
- The cost of anguish, counselling, family and personal stresses, family disruption and shock when there are mental health episodes in households around Australia;
- The costs of medical appointments, medical examinations and counselling that are related to sleep and mental health problems;
- Polypharmacy and other pharmacological problems associated with the fact that the drugs do not work. They include multiple drugs, increased medications, testing and trialling medications, increased falls, renaming mental health problems, etc;
- The cost of emergency crews, phone counsellors, school counsellors, websites, chat rooms, forums, conferences that deal with sleep and mental health problems;

- The cost of the side effects of medications – short term, long term and permanent – including brain damage and permanent sexual dysfunction (refer to chapters 9 and 10);
- Hospitalization and incarceration costs associated with mental health episodes;
- Court room costs, coronial enquiries, jail costs, legal fees associated with medically induced and mentally induced crime;
- Loss of human rights associated with forced treatment in institutions, and/or against the wishes of the patient and/or their families/carers;
- Mistreatment of mental health patients by not engaging with them correctly to allow them to reveal underlying abuse problems, trauma, life stresses, family dysfunctions, parental pressures and the like;
- The cost of not looking beyond the obvious to such things as overexposure of young people to hours of violent video games that "desensitise" them to violence, sexual abuse, pornography and the like;
- The cost of not recognising that no-one really is desensitized – it always reveals itself somewhere. In the case of our military personnel it is no wonder that there are huge problems with PTSD and reactions to what they see, hear and experience in war zones and during training;
- The cost of carers and support groups;
- Funerals, wills, probate and other costs associated with every single unnecessary death;
- Opportunity cost of all psycho-pill taking Australian citizens' days spent in a dopey daze because they are sleepy, unmotivated, drugged, desensitised and distracted;
- Drug rehabilitation processes to get people off the addictive and sometimes dangerous medications, which many of them should not have been prescribed in the first place;
- The cost of the proven loss of drive, employment, self esteem, engagement, confidence and relationships caused when people are labelled as "bipolar", "depressed", "anxious", "ADHD", and the like;
- The accumulative effect of the sadness and shock of mentally ill people and their problems felt by families and loved ones who then find it harder to cope with life;

- Legal exposure and litigation costs associated with the known gap between proven, peer reviewed medical science and the practices of medical professionals and psychiatrists;
- The costs associated with medical information lag and denial. While we deny any of this is happening we are putting off ever finding valid and excellent solutions to these problems, and ruining the careers of people who are unrecognised leaders and who already hold solutions;
- Education costs, standards revisions and clinical governance reviews to match the health and mental health industry knowledge and practices with known scientific information;
- Federal and state law revisions to ensure that proven medical systems are legislated and enforced.

You get the idea.

Let's Talk about our Children

The Youth Beyond Blue website states that one in four young Australians currently has a mental health condition. 26.4 percent of Australians aged 16 to 24 currently have experienced a mental health disorder in the last 12 months. This figure includes young people with a substance use disorder. This is equivalent to 750,000 young people today.[19]

Off-Label Prescribing to Young People and Children In Australia

In spite of the fact that antidepressants are not approved for use for children under 18 years of age in Australia, there are 49,052 children under 17 taking antidepressants.

In other words, there have been **over 49,000 off-label prescriptions written** in Australia in relation to these drugs being prescribed for depression.[20]

It is illegal for drug companies to promote off-label prescribing, but not illegal for doctors to prescribe off-label. And observing their activity, apparently not illegal for foundations and charities to promote off-label prescribing.

1,459 of those children are aged 2-6.[21]

WTF!

Despite the known risks, warnings and regulations the TGA's Adverse Drug Reactions Database for antidepressants reveals that as of 31/10/16 there were:

- 94 completed suicides, a 118% increase since April 2011. Of these, 4 were aged 14 to 16.
- 848 reports for suicide attempts (311), suicidal ideation (511) and suicidal behaviour (26), a 46% increase since April 2011.[22]

Schizophrenia

Here are some figures shown on the Schizophrenia Institute's website:

- In Australia, approximately 1 in 100 people have or will develop schizophrenia during their lifetime and it is usually life-long.[23]
- Schizophrenia ranks among the top 10 causes of disability in developed countries worldwide. Onset is typically between the ages of 15 and 30.[24]
- It is a major cause of suicide – up to 50 percent of people with schizophrenia attempt suicide, 5 percent complete suicide. People with schizophrenia have 2.5 times the death rate of the general population, and life expectancy is reduced by up to 18 years.[25]
- In addition to the profound emotional cost to families, schizophrenia costs the Australian community approximately $2.6 billion per annum in both direct health costs and loss of productivity; 85 percent of sufferers receive welfare benefits.[26]

Unemployment and Economic Disadvantage

Australia has a shocking record for looking after the mentally ill.

For example, in a *One Plus One* interview with Deputy Commissioner of the NSW Health Commission, Fay Jackson, it was revealed that 10 percent of schizophrenics in Italy are unemployed, whereas 90 percent of schizophrenics in Australia are unemployed. Many people who have taken mental health medications for long periods of time die in their 50s, gain weight and are marginalised.[27]

Rehabilitation, Addiction, Withdrawal and Detoxification

Here is a very sobering prediction for the future when people wake up to the extent of this problem.

Professor Peter Gøtzsche stated in his *Mental Health: Overdiagnosed and Overmedicated* lecture in Australia that if everyone who is taking antidepressants were to move to taper off their medications the system would be incapable of dealing with the extent of the problem.[28]

With one in six Australians on antidepressants alone, and 36 million (35 last year) million psycho drug prescriptions being written it is important that you find out now which places are doing the best job.

And unfortunately "for some people, they never succeed" (in successfully getting off the drugs).[29]

If this was me, I'd be getting in early, ahead of the wave.

(Remembering the warning again: The tapering stage is sometimes the most dangerous.)

CHAPTER 12

Why a 10 Minute Quickie with Your Doctor is Never Enough

So you can see it now, the medical system is entrenched and inflexible. If you are a doctor, working in a medical practice, you are probably rather disillusioned with how the job has panned out.

After being the cream of the crop at school, working incredibly hard to get into medical school, then studying for years to get your medical degree, working ridiculous hours as an intern in hospitals, you end up being stuck in general practice seeing people all day with the common cold, emotional issues, the occasional fractures... and a lot of insurance claims and paperwork you would rather never do.

At lunch time you are being sold to by medical sales reps plugging the latest drugs, it is a continual challenge to keep up with the latest innovations, and to work out what *real improvements* are being made out of all the new products, drugs and procedures that are introduced.

The community thinks you are earning a fortune, but in actual fact, for the work you have put in, and what you do at work, the rewards are not that good.

They certainly aren't what you visualised when you chose to be a life saving doctor and community leader. And it isn't like the 1950's when doctors were respected above all other professionals, and patients believed what they were being told.

You are dealing with the following problems:

- Limited consultation time with each patient.
- Patients who want a quick fix, and aren't willing to make the life-style and other changes to make themselves better, such as losing

weight, drinking less alcohol, doing daily appropriate exercise, choosing more appropriate jobs and lifestyles, having more uplifting friends, etc.

- Patients who come to doctors demanding drugs.
- An endless stream of paperwork, including case reports, insurance documentation, test results and referrals.
- The fear of being sued if you make a mistake.
- Ignorant patients. Some of them argumentative.
- Team challenges working with other members of your practice.
- Increasing costs of running your business, including building maintenance, supply, staffing, etc.
- Profitability goals, especially when your practice is being administered by publicly listed medical companies.
- Often working in a medical practice, as part of a team, many operated by administrative companies that are listed on the stock exchange and motivated by profit and performance only.
- You find it difficult to research the correct solutions to the problems your patients have. There are too many different problems, too complicated solutions and too little time.
- Hearing only negative stories all day.
- High stress situations and emergencies that take a huge emotional toll on you and your family life.
- Increasing questions from patients for information on alternative therapies and supplements.
- Increasing scepticism from patients on the advice you are giving.
- Competition with Doctor Google.
- Increasing pressure from patients moving away from allopathic medicine.
- Activity based payments and income, even if you aren't convinced the 'activity' is warranted.
- Your prescription patterns being reviewed by drug companies.
- Your consulting behaviour being reviewed by associated medical listed companies.
- Continuing professional development, sometimes with conflict-of-interest pharmaceutical companies.
- Incentivised opinion making.
- Incentivised conferences.

- Incentivised behaviours.
- Universities with links to corporate interests.
- No time or incentives to review the real evidence.
- No time or incentives to do the best job.
- No time for thorough diagnoses in every case.

It's quite a list, and I'm sure there's more.

I probably don't have to go into further detail, but how, in the space of a short or even a long consultation, are doctors supposed to *really diagnose* the underlying problem(s) that are manifesting as insomnia, sleep disorders and mental health problems?

I have personally developed a *Sleep Diagnostic Questionnaire* with 200 questions on it, to establish underlying issues that present as sleep disorders and insomnia.

They are aimed at uncovering lifestyle problems, unresolved emotional issues, dietary issues, side effects of present medications, mental health issues, sleep patterns that indicate different diagnoses, age related sleep issues, food additives and colourings that effect sleep, the sleep environment, recreational drug and alcohol use, technology usage issues, light related solutions, sleep quality, circadian rhythm questions, work pressures, shift work and jetlag questions, relaxation scores, etc.

Sometimes the patient can't even remember what triggered their emotional problems in the first place, especially in cases of early childhood trauma.

Here is a sample of 10 questions taken from 200 in my *Sleep Diagnosis Questionnaire (Appendix 6)*:

- How long have you had a sleeping problem?
- Do you have difficulty falling asleep, staying asleep or waking too early in the morning?
- Are you, or have you ever been a shift worker?
- What stress are you feeling at the moment?
- Tell me about your job?
- What sort of family relationships do you have?
- Has someone died recently, lost your job, or any other shock?

- How long have you been overweight for?
- What bed coverings do you have on your bed in summer and winter?
- Tell me about your sleep environment and habits?

It would be difficult, if not impossible, to properly cover just these 10 questions in the time allocated for a short or long consultation with your doctor. And there are 190 more that could be relevant. And for those who are wondering, they are not asking them at sleep clinics either. They are focused on sleep apnea and snoring, with less than a handful of sleep clinics giving any sort of effective general sleep education. More on that later.

Where there are mental health issues, it is known that doctors and psychiatrists are not covering the basics well, and not covering them properly before medicating their patients[1].

What power do doctors have to fix the problems?

Very little it turns out, as the systems are set.

Moving outside the accepted medical model is professional suicide. There has been a lifetime invested in your career development, with many sacrifices already made.

There is far too much to lose.

Let's just stick with the present system.

Or not?

CHAPTER 13

Preventative Medicine. Why Bother When the Money is in the Illness?

" Follow the money trail" is a common saying to decipher what is going on around us.

The sleep and mental health industries are exactly that – industries.

If we were really solving our health and mental health issues in Australia, and Australia was so technologically advanced, the 'gold standard internationally', why is Healthcare and Social Assistance now Australia's largest employing industry, employing 13 percent of workers, with growth projections of 16.4 % in the next five years[1].

Who is celebrating that fact?

All I can say is that if the sleep and mental health industries are any indication of the gross negligence being displayed in all other health disciplines we are in a mighty pickle.

And I have absolutely no indication that what I have researched for this book could not be duplicated in many other aspects of the health industry in Australia and overseas.

It's time for some real leadership in health.

Where the hell are they?

1,523,000 people employed in the Healthcare and Social Assistance industry in Australia in November 2015[2] and it takes me, an economics graduate from the University of Sydney, to have the passion (and knackers) to write this book in an attempt to save people's lives through evidence-based medicine.

How's that for a laugh?

If it's so obvious to me, what the hell are you all doing?

Bring on the outliers, if that's what it takes.

Don't dare tell me I'm not qualified in health: it's very clear where quali-fications take you, and what a mess the 'experts' have created.

Why are people becoming more and more obese?

Why are 1 in 6 Australian's on antidepressant medication?

Why do the experts indicate that only one-third of mental health patients are actually being treated?

Patients are buying the BS, because so-and-so is a doctor, psychiatrist, or a professor.

Really.

Instead of using common sense, especially in the sleep and mental health areas, they are popping pills, going without sleep, eating rubbish, not exercising, and celebrating sleep machismo!

The most lame television ad I've seen recently is Victoria Alonso, Executive Producer of Marvel studios, claiming in a Microsoft Surface Pro 4 ad that "I know my superpower is to not ever sleep", working 14 hours a day, 7 days a week for decades...[3]

So that's a superpower now?

FFS!

The money is in the drugs, the sleep appliances, the overnight sleep clinic tests, the psychiatry sessions and the "quick fixes" that don't work.

And the most common 'solution' – drugs that impair and worsen the problems.

Brilliant.

The sicker the population is, the more money the health and medical professionals and staff make.

Wow, that's interesting.

Why would anyone want to change that?

CHAPTER 14

The Medical Profession Created their Own Terminal Case.

The Hippocratic Oath (Excerpt)

"I will follow that system of conduct and treatment which according to my ability and judgement I consider for the benefit of my patients and will abstain from whatever is deleterious and mischievous ... I will give no deadly drug."

So with all the evidence freely available and in plain sight, why are we pussy footing around doctors and psychiatrists?

And why are we pussy footing around their professional bodies, their professional development rules and their practices?

As a profession they are very silent.

How many doctors and psychiatrists have you seen publicly outing the system, calling for a royal commission, complaining about their professional standards, objecting to their professional development bodies, their dangerous long hours, etc?

Does the silence make you suspicious?

Many worry about the professional ramifications of speaking out, and some have already been subject to "adverse events" that seem to be designed to discourage certain behaviours.

With the situation as it is we should be seeing doctors and psychiatrists revolting against the system, with leaders challenging the Pharmaceutical Benefits Scheme (PBS), the National Prescribing Service (NPS), the Therapeutic Goods Administration (TGA/FDA/MHRA), the drug companies' off label marketing, the backhanders, the treatment of mentally ill patients, the AMA, the listed companies, the 10 minute consultation standard, etc.

But what we hear is silence.

What we see is drug advertising on television, the inappropriate power of drug companies, systemic drug solutions at the cost of patients, incorrect information in powerful charities, and doctors who appear not to even bother reading Cochrane reports or world's best practice publications.

They are blindly following the status quo, and have been for decades, at the detriment of our health and wellbeing.

Not what they promised with their Hippocratic Oath.

I remember taking a Cochrane report to my doctor questioning my blood pressure medication, given the fact that my blood pressure at the time was in the low range of concern, I had lost weight and I was taking the minimum amount of medication possible.

In spite of the Cochrane information, he still wanted me on the medications – his advice to me was simply that he would still recommend the medications.

No question about any adverse side effects I might be experiencing? Why my change in attitude? Any further information that may help in the decision?

None of that, just the implication that I had no idea.

Well doctors, sometimes we do have an idea.

The internet will allow any idiot (just about…) to look up the Cochrane reports, and reports coming out of the BMJ, NEJM, JAMA, Lancet, etc.

If the average Joe Blow wants to do some serious research on the internet they can come up with BETTER information than their doctor or psychiatrist is giving them.

It is possible.

Today.

The Cochrane Library information is freely available on the internet.

The top journals have been known to be corrupted and corruptible, I have to say that, depending on the editorial "attitude" at the time etc., but you are still going to get a much better picture in some areas than your "10 minute quickie" with your doctor.

And the other thing that we can do as average citizens is visit the https://www.rxisk.org website to see a list of side effects reported for most drugs.

The side effects listed on this website are generally not being talked about during your consultation, and many aren't even listed on the NPS website, or the product disclosure information.

The worst that can happen by doing your own research is that you have some quality questions to ask your doctor when you visit.

Another problem I have is that I can't find a list of general practitioners anywhere that respect Cochrane research. It would be an excellent market-ing idea, as many people now wish to *discuss* health solutions with their medical practitioner, including information they download from Cochrane – not just be 'told'.

Cochrane could set up a membership where the top doctors (i.e. those who don't mind Cochrane being discussed in a consult by their patients) can register so that patients like me can find the best doctors who aren't just aimlessly following "normal practices". It would be great to be respected for asking questions from Cochrane research (or BMJ/NEJM etc) in a consultation.

And I have very little doubt that these patients would be the ones to take ownership of their health issues, and want to do something good about them.

My guess is that these patients might actually lose weight or exercise – if you showed them they were REALLY evidence based, and discuss their best course of action.

Unnecessary drugs, X-rays and procedures cost a fortune - for us and the government. (Same thing, unfortunately.)

I would love to have one of those discussions without being seen as disruptive, even stupid!

"Cochrane Medical Practices", instead of the present groups of prac-tices that are listed on the stock exchanges and motivated by profit, would improve outcomes for the patients and reduce costs to the nation.

They could also hold evidence-based preventative health seminars that would become best practice guidelines instead of the present broken system.

Cochrane Reviewers

The Australian Government should encourage interested members of the public to become Cochrane-approved clinical trial reviewers to help the international system they have set up. I did not know that people like me could be trained to review clinical trials to ascertain if they can be included in higher review by the Cochrane experts – or culled as irrelevant or biased.

But we can.

That would be a contribution a lot of people would love to make. Especially, for example, older, retired, community minded, intelligent individuals, interested in research.

It could be established as a university subject available to a range of faculties, and would help eliminate the distorted information being promoted in the medical fields, during consultations and in the media.

Searching The Internet for Answers

Since the opening of the world wide web to the public in 1991 people have been able to find information themselves from various sources all over the globe.

The internet has enabled individuals to research health facts, research and conversations about their particular health conditions.

Provided they do not rely on what information has been "SEOd" and that they know the difference, they are in the position to become more informed than their doctor on specific health issues – if they have the time to research.

To explain to readers who don't understand: SEO (Search Engine Optimisation) allows individuals and organisations to advance their website to the top of the search engine results for particular words and phrases, not based on fact, but algorithms set by the search engine companies such as Google and Bing. These algorithms change from time to time, governed by Google and Bing, etc.

This means, generally, that until Cochrane, for example, spend money on SEO techniques (which they shouldn't have to), they will NOT turn up in a prominent position, if, for example you Google "high blood pressure". You are very likely, with searches like this, to come up with results that are unreliable (sometimes very unreliable) because they are "marketed answers", not evidence-based answers.

That's why you should search "Cochrane Library" then enter *blood pressure* in the Cochrane Library's search box – to get the results you are looking for. i.e. http://www.cochranelibrary.com/, then locate their own search box at the top right hand side of their home page.

At the very least you can search scholarly articles in Google, by going to scholar.google.com, which can be done in your country, such as https://scholar.google.com.au/. This is better than a normal Google search on a health term, but you will still be presented with publications of clinical trials etc that are not necessarily REALLY evidence-based, and can be just part of the 100 published articles of the 2 clinical trials that 'worked' for a drug company, for example, and spoken about in Chapter 3. Hence my reservation about how scholarly Google Scholar really is. But it is better than total dumbo Google searches and *believing* what you read in those results – especially if your life depends on it!

Doctors' and Psychiatrists' Responsibilities

But somehow, the doctors don't seem to be doing this! Or they sure aren't telling me when I go for my "10 minute quickie". Or "long consultation" of what, 20 minutes, to solve the full history of my mind and body's problems!

Here's what's happening:

The cat's out of the bag. As you're seeing very clearly. The MBS and PBS are fundamentally flawed, and real evidence is hard to find – including for the medical profession.

And there are forces which don't care, and are profiting splendidly by the overall confusion and bullshit.

- Doctors and psychiatrists are playing the game, which is increasingly set in stone, as you saw in Chapter 3.
- Individual doctors do not have time to research every single ailment and illness in Cochrane and reliable sources to help you, when they are really busy all day (and often overnight) with 10 minute consultations and emergency hospital visits, etc.
- Doctors do not want to be sued. However they continue with what everyone else is doing, and what they see is happening around them, and what is established as "best practice" by flawed systems (see chapter 3), and recommended by their drug representatives, and recommended at subsidized conferences, constrained by their

10-minutes-or-so consultations "encouraged" by their publicly-listed-profit-motivated-medical-practices company, etc.

- Our system that incentivises 'activity based' solutions is deeply flawed. Especially since it is coupled with majority MBS and PBS items which are *not evidence based*. Activity based incentives mean that you will be sent to have an x-ray occasionally, even if evidence shows that it is not really going to be part of your solution at all. This incentivises bad practice, and perpetuates incompetence.

What is the Result of Institutionalised Incompetence?

- You and I are waking up big-time.
- The average mum and dad and Joe-Blow-citizen can see the BS and want to do their own research.
- Most have no idea about **how** to research, but they're doing it anyway. Understandably: it's the first step you have to take to take back responsibility for your own health – and should be encouraged, of course.
- And no-one is bothering to tell us the REAL research – save a very few. You **now** know some of them as world class courageous and informed experts and heroes.
- Patients are becoming suspicious of what their doctors and psychiatrists are telling them. Understandably. And thankfully.
- People are throwing out the baby with the bathwater. E.g. because they read that a certain vaccine is linked to autism they no longer have any vaccines at all, even if they have not done proper research into individual vaccines at all.
- Some people might never do what their doctor tells them again.

There are a number of places to lay the blame, including with the patient, who generally goes to their doctor for a 'quick fix' – i.e. A pill to fix the problem today. Or a procedure that will take a day in hospital, for example.

Anything "quick and easy", which is a growing trend for everything. (Now I'm sounding like your mum, but it has to be said.)

They want the "snapchat" medical solution. Quick and dirty is fine.

BUT the blame also has to be taken by the doctors and psychiatrists.

Gone are the days when the public looked up to their doctor and believed everything they said.

I'll say it again, to the doctors and psychiatrists reading this: *Gone are the days when the public looked up to their doctor and believed everything they said.*

We don't care if you worked your butt off at school to get 99.99 in your HSC to get into med school at the best university, we don't care if you studied for 14 years to become a specialist in your profession, and if you have 15 letters after your name.

We just want REAL evidence-based solutions to our health and mental health problems, and we KNOW that you are *not* giving them to us.

The cat is out of the bag. Big-time.

And doctors and medical professionals only have themselves to blame.

It has been decades of misinformation on some illnesses and procedures. We want the industry cleaned up.

And we only want to pay for REAL evidence based solutions.

In all the political palaver about how much the health system is costing us, and how the government can't afford proper medical treatments – there is NO mention of the fact that most of the medical treatment and drugs have nothing to do with REAL evidence-based solutions.

And we know why, because none of us were born yesterday. Certainly no one reading this book.

We have a flawed, fraudulent, overly expensive, manipulative, harmful medical system, which is crippling the nation, and the doctors are saying nothing.

The doctors are saying nothing, the government is saying nothing, the hospitals are saying nothing, the TGA is powerless, the clinical governance experts are saying nothing.

It is the alarming truth.

And they still ask for our respect?

What is an emerging trend is that people who speak up are being professionally sidelined and rules are being strengthened to stop any medical professional rocking the boat.

We've watched this happening for ages, and no, that is *not* the solution. It doesn't matter if the boat gets rocked, it's sinking anyway.

Clear to most people now, not just the intellectuals and smart people.

In fact, its trending. That's why there is so much damage control happening.

We don't want to have our Medical Benefits Scheme's clinical governance done by the Four Corners *Wasted* program. (Why are they the only ones interested? And thank goodness they did.)

That's insane.

And I notice that even after this burning *Wasted* investigation, we have had a bit of chit-chat about knee arthroscopies but bugger all else.

Hello!

We ARE noticing.

What about the other over-5000 items on the MBS that are not evidence based?

And we aren't even mentioning the Pharmaceutical Benefits Scheme.

The medical profession has created its own terminal case.

Ironic and chronic.

I'm aware that it is people's livelihoods at stake, we did not create that situation, you did. The medical professionals, the hospitals, the universities, the "best practice guidelines", the activity based remunerations, the supporting industries and professionals, etc.

Just because it is a huge problem does not mean that we ignore it.

The people are speaking, and unfortunately it will probably get worse before it gets better.

My guess is the situation is at Stage 3, fast approaching Stage 4. Optimistically.

The Berlin wall seemed to fall overnight.

We're dying to see what solution you come up with.

Here are some more disturbing facts:

- Doctors have above average suicide rates. Male doctors 41 percent higher than the normal population, and female doctors have more than double the suicide rate of the normal population at 2.27 times.[1]
- "Antidepressants — now the most commonly prescribed drugs in pregnancy — even as the evidence accumulates that these drugs cause birth defects, double the rate of miscarriages, and cause mental handicap in children born to mothers who have been taking them."[2]

- Doctors appear to be unable to change their dangerous shift work patterns in hospitals.
- Their negligence in this area is causing costly health mistakes, errors, bad decision making in life and death situations, and death in some cases. The health system, the AMA, the hospital administration and clinical governance are all neglecting their duty of care to both the doctors and the patients.[3]

The silence is deafening.

Medical leadership is profoundly missing.

CHAPTER 15

Our Kids at School. Mental Health Care or the New Marketing Frontier?

"In Australia no antidepressant (including any SSRIs) is currently approved by the Therapeutic Goods Administration for the treatment of major depression in people aged less than 18 years"[1][2].

In spite of this fact, there is considerable argy bargy in a variety of places about the circumstances where you might consider it...

In other words, there are a number of places which openly discuss *off-label prescribing* of SSRIs to children less than 18 years old. (FYI It is illegal for drug companies to promote off-label prescribing, but not illegal for doctors to prescribe off-label.)

For example, here are some very confusing, contradictory and misleading statements on the *Headspace* website:

- "an association has recently been drawn between these declining rates of prescriptions and an increased suicide rate over the same period of time[3]" and
- "no deaths have been reported that are attributable to SSRI prescription[4]" and
- "overall, a stepped model approach is recommended for the treatment of depression in young people[5]".

These comments on the downloadable *Headspace Evidence Summary*[6] are not seen to be helpful by this author, and certainly do not paint a full, accurate or up to date picture. Some of these statements are misleading, and some directly disagree with previous statements in the same document. There is little or no mention of the lack of other interventions such as talk therapies and psychotherapy in discussions about increased suicide rates with declining rates of prescriptions and other statistical variables.

Headspace is funded by the Australian Government under the Promoting Better Mental Health -Youth Mental Health Initiative[7].

How can this happen?

How is this *allowed to* happen?

Blatantly, in clear view.

This is another example of one Australian government department's website and information disagreeing with the information on another Australian government website (Headspace vs. Therapeutic Goods Administration).

The downloadable *Headspace Evidence Summary* seems to say one thing and recommend another. At the least it is confusing.

The greatest shortcoming though, seems to be the fact that the *Headspace Evidence Summary* was last updated and current as at December 2012.

This Evidence Summary is out of date. And significantly out of date because it was written before the watershed *Restoring Study 329: efficacy and harms of paroxetine and imipramine in treatment of major depression in adolescence* was published in the British Medical Journal in September 16, 2015[8].

Since *Restoring Study 329* was published in the British Medical Journal a class action is being prepared in Australia[9] around the problems associated with prescribing antidepressants to children less than 18 years old.

Further information about this study, written by one of the study's authors can be found here: https://study329.org/wp-content/uploads/2015/09/Study-329-Final.pdf and https://study329.org/bmj-press-release-and-materials/ [10].

The TGA has approved two of the SSRIs (fluvoxamine and sertraline) for obsessive compulsive disorder (OCD)[11].

This is a very important chapter of this book, but need not be a long one.

Have you noticed any of the following alarming trends?

- Discussions about having doctors engaged at schools where they can see children without their parents'/guardian's consent?

- The advertising of early mental health interventions and mental health organisations in relation to school children (and/or children 18 years old or younger).
- The encouragement of children to seek mental health help from organisations that do not have up to date information on their websites and downloadable "factsheets"?
- The encouragement of children to seek mental health help where they may be given an SSRI script, while a class action is being prepared to question this behaviour in Australia, and the underlying evidence behind this behaviour.

Conspicuously, given the apparently alarming rate of mental health issues in younger people: where are the *non-drug* talk-therapy organisations? Psychotherapists? Supportive counsellors? Parent education bodies and the like, to help children have the *conversations* that need to be had, and receive the psychological/family/friendly *support* that they need when they find they have difficulties in their lives?

And where are the government initiatives to encourage independent organisations who want to help through *evidence-based* psychotherapy and counselling?

That's the disgrace.

Who do *your* children talk to when they have problems?

Do you listen to them, and treat their problems as valid, even if sometimes they stretch your patience? And our imaginations?

Or are we continuing to expect our children to be beautiful/handsome/hot (aargh...), high achievers in the areas *we* choose for them, get 99.99 in their HSC and the rest of it?

OMG, no wonder some of them are in strife.

But we are too busy to listen, too busy carting them to sport and social events, too busy taking them to piano lessons, beauty salons, sports events, parties.... just too busy all around.

And not too busy to do their homework for them, enabling them to cheat at school and university, covering up their mistakes, lying to their friends, putting on a brave face.

Will everyone just take it easy for a while, sit down, listen, go camping... get some real friends?

Bored? Well, who does that anymore? We need some of that introspection time. Reflection time, meditation time, time in nature or in your room just hanging out unwired.

Underachieving, even failing is quite OK.

This is all too obvious to discuss in detail.

If you don't get it... go figure!

Schools Teach Sleep Very Poorly

The George Institute on Global Health found that young adults who get less than 5 hours sleep on average are 3 times more likely to develop mental health problems than those who slept 8-9 hours regularly.

Sleep is mentioned in the NSW school's PDHPE syllabus for years 7-10, strand 4 under "Lifelong Physical Activity". (Yeah, curiously.)

It depends on the actual school how much importance is placed on the topic of sleep.

Knowing the inadequacy of the medical system, I believe that students should be taught extensively on sleep during school years as a priority. It is too late when their problem becomes so large that they have to see a doctor or psychiatrist ('cos we know what happens there). It should be a major part of their preventative health care strategies.

Young adults and students have to deal with puberty and sexuality, body image problems, electronic violent and sexualised video games, acne, the delayed sleep phase, hormone surges, peer group pressure and socialising, bullying, difficulty sleeping, pornography and pushy parents that want their children to achieve 99.99 in their higher school certificate.

I believe that school children have to contend with more than most adults, in their school years, so it is no surprise to me that they are developing anxieties and stresses at this time in their lives. In fact, it's nearly impossible to avoid them.

So sleep should not just be a topic in the curriculum: it should be sold to the students adequately.

Glamorised and made cool – whatever it takes.

The following connections are not being made in the school curriculums:

- How lack of sleep effects the brain, executive function, memory, cognitive processes, decision making etc.,
- How sleep is directly connected to performance – mental, physical and emotional intelligence,
- Lack of sleep's connection to mental health issues, depression, anxiety and stress,
- How sleep affects relationships, family relationships and resilience,
- How sleep affects eating, weight management, the ability and enthusiasm for exercising and movement,
- The stages of sleep: which ones integrate memories, are associated with super learning, release growth hormones, regulate the immune system, break down fats, grow internal organs, improve spatial memory, and improve happiness,
- How you can sleep your way to look better, stay slim, eat correct food etc.,
- How to read food labels, specifically in relation to what foods keep you from sleeping properly and are connected to mental health problems,
- Delayed sleep phase, melatonin production, circadian rhythm – all very important to teenagers and young adults,
- How energy drinks and high octane drinks effect your sleep and health,
- How to reduce accidents and risk taking behaviour,
- How to do better in exams using sleep and napping techniques,
- How good sleep clears out toxins in the brain,
- The direct link between lack of sleep, driving times and teenage driving fatalities,
- How the use of computers, tablets and mobiles with short wave light act to effectively put your body into a different time zone and exacerbate the effect of the delayed sleep phase,
- Different types of sleep disorders, sleep walking, sleep talking, breathing disorders, circadian rhythm disorders, nightmares, limb movement disorders, etc.
- The link between lack of sleep and psychological problems and substance abuse,
- How to manage the dark hours for success and safety,
- Who to talk to when you can't sleep properly, and
- What to say in a conversation when you can't sleep.

Motor vehicle crashes are the leading cause of teenage deaths in the US and globally, and drowsy driving accounts for 1 in 5 of those deaths.

In 2007 in Massachusetts they introduced stringent penalties for unsupervised night-time driving by 16 and 17 year old novice drivers, and mandated drowsy driving education. This study by the division of Sleep Medicine, Harvard Medical School, showed that restricting the hours that teenagers can drive in the night time hours resulted in a 40 percent reduction in fatal and incapacitating injury crashes observed for teen drivers.[12] That same study revealed that crashes decreased by 19 percent, and night-time crashes decreased by 29 percent.

Stop Calling Kids Mental

They are called feelings and emotions, they are not mental.

They are not mental health issues in most cases – they are just emotional times while growing up.

Just because some kids are up one day and a bit down the next does not mean they are bipolar.

They could have drunk an excessive amount of hyped up drinks yesterday, and feeling lower today.

The American National Institute of Mental Health says that seventy-five percent of all severe mental health illness begins before the age of 24 years[13].

There are often decades between onset of symptoms and when people seek treatment.

I'm wondering if people don't seek treatment because they don't have any confidence in the treatment systems, and/or if they would seek treatment if they went along and learned how to sleep better and feel better? Possibly in the form of simple online training.

Sleep is a Mental Health Issue

The underlying problems with sleep disorders are not necessarily physical. The mental health issues can include anxieties, depression, stress, unresolved emotional issues, PTSD, abuse, grief, etc.

The psychiatry profession's diagnosing and medicating practices have been questioned by many over an extended period of time. They include international research leaders such as Professor Peter Gøtzsche of the Nordic Cochrane Collaborative, Robert Whitaker (author of *Anatomy of an Epidemic*), and Professor David Healy.

Mental health professional practices raise obvious exposure questions into the future, including for Government departments responsible for the mental health of people in their care (e.g. the military, prisoners, etc).

And soon we will have corporate sponsorship of schools.

And doctors who can see your children without parental approval.

Ding-a-ling!

Career Choices for Students

One aspect of career choices that should be discussed more is the health, happiness and lifestyles of certain career choices. It's not all about being a doctor, lawyer, dentist or banker. Status careers in the 1950s and 1970s changed significantly at the end of the last century, and a new breed of ethical and technical entrepreneurs are disruptively occupying the large gaps created by ineffectual and unresponsive industries.

CHAPTER 16

What has Sleep got to do with Fatigue? And Other Scarily Common Organisational Questions.

C all me old-school, but if you think management has improved over the last few decades why do I *continually* get asked the following questions, and told the following lies by leaders in the human resources, fatigue and mental health fields?

- "What has sleep got to do with fatigue?"
- "Sleep has got nothing to do with mental health." (*Statement*, not question, from the office of the Mental Health Minister.) Yeah, scary.
- It's impossible to be fatigued at 9 am on Monday morning.

I was answerable to directors, financial controllers and treasury heads of listed companies in my 20s and 30s: now just mentioning the words "fatigue" or "sleep" will result in immediate screening by EAs.

"Disruptive thinkers" are apparently being celebrated, because we need them. I can't disagree with that. But is everyone with a brain now called *disruptive*?

Apparently organisations have "got it all under control".

Well, no. You haven't.

E.g. The Olympic Committee was apparently clueless that Stilnox was being prescribed to our elite swimmers. If you believe that.

Fatigue and Mental Health: Bedroom to Boardroom.

I need some help here, as I'm not an actuary. Loved maths, but that was going too far.

I've got a spreadsheet in Appendix 1 that I'd like someone to help me with.

Could that be you?

Yeah, you.

The aim is to quantify the cost of mental health, insomnia, and drugged employees to organisations.

With all the delightful side effects such as increased accidents, errors, violence, long term brain damage, etc.

This would be a significant contribution, because no one is doing this properly that I can find anywhere.

Will you help me please?

If so, please contact me and we'll have some fun together.

My contact details are at the end of the book.

"At Risk" Industries

I've included 'at risk' industries in *Fatigue and Mental Health: Bedroom to Boardroom* Appendix 1 because the exposures for these industries and careers are worse.

Some exposures are unexpected. For example, did you know that white collar workers are a lot worse at coping with overtime than blue collar workers?

When you look twice at it you might see it – but I wouldn't have guessed before I saw the evidence.

These sorts of discussions are not happening. I'm sure there are many more that will emerge when the general conversation is elevated from the present widespread ignorance.

Police Officers

As an example, let's have a look at the results of the *Sleep Disorders, Health and Safety in Police Officers* study published in the Journal of the American Medical Association (JAMA) December 20, 2011.

With a reminder that the NSW police force have recently voted to work consecutive 12 hour work days broken up with days off. A decision supported by the union.

They obviously must be looking at different data to me! And they're upping their fire power at the same time. Not a great combination.

Here are some of the results of the study which included 4,957 participants from the United States and Canada between July 2005 and December 2007[1,2]:

1. 40.4 percent screened positive for at least 1 sleep disorder.
2. 28.5 percent had screening scores that indicated they experienced excessive sleepiness.
3. Of the total 4,957 survey respondents 2276 or 45.9 percent reported having nodded off or fallen asleep while driving; 1,294 (56.9 percent of these, 26.1% of the total cohort) reported falling asleep while driving at least 1 to 2 times a month; and 307 (13.5 percent of them or 6.2 percent of the total group) reported falling asleep while driving 1 to 2 times a week! Now that is scary.
4. 33.6 percent screened positive for obstructive sleep apnea (OSA) – the most common disorder.
5. 6.5 percent had moderate to severe insomnia.
6. 5.4 percent had shift work disorder (14.5 percent who worked the night shift).

Positive screening of any sleep disorder was, not surprisingly, associated with increased risk of self-reported health and safety related outcomes such as:

- 10.7 percent with a sleep disorder reported having depression, compared with 4.4 percent who did not screen positive to a sleep disorder
- 34.1 percent (of the positive to sleep disorder group) experienced burnout/emotional exhaustion compared with 17.9 percent in the no-sleep-disorder group.

Positive OSA screening was associated with a diagnosis of diabetes, cardiovascular disease and high caffeine consumption.

Participants that screened as having a sleep disorder problem were more likely to report making important administrative errors; falling asleep while driving; making errors or committing safety violations due to fatigue; having uncontrolled anger toward a citizen or suspect; incurring citizen complaints; absenteeism; falling asleep during meetings.

According to data through the year 2003, more officers are killed by unintended adverse events than during the commission of felonies. It has been hypothesized that fatigue might be a significant factor in those 'unintended adverse events'.

That wouldn't surprise me at all.

The authors summarize by saying that "further research is needed to determine whether sleep disorder prevention, screening, and treatment programs in occupational settings will reduce these risks".

A pretty important step to move forward I'd say.

Shift Work

I often get asked by people about shift work and how to manage it in order to get a better night's sleep. It's a tricky one because no-one wants to hear that shift work is not something that I recommend at all!

That is usually the answer they don't want to hear, especially if they have spent years training and working in the field of nursing, for example.

Couple that with stressful, sometimes traumatic and violent situations at work. These careers are a very serious contribution to society, in more ways than one.

Other studies show other adverse results for night-shift officers including higher rates of metabolic syndrome, hypertension and glucose intolerance (an indication of diabetes), etc.

Sleep debt has been shown to have harmful impact on carbohydrate metabolism and endocrine function, which could contribute to metabolic disorders[3].

At risk industries also include, in my opinion, any that involve sleep deprivation, shift work, stress, observing traumatic events, long work hours, jobs where people's lives depend on your accuracy, etc.

Examples of at-risk industries, in my opinion, include:

- transport industry generally,
- trucking industry,

- air traffic controllers,
- nurses,
- doctors,
- hospital workers,
- emergency workers, helicopter pilots, etc
- emergency medical technicians,
- the military,
- police (pretty obvious now),
- security guards and services,
- website security workers,
- mining,
- journalists and morning television personnel,
- international banking and trading,
- government special branches (security, etc),
- ambulance drivers and administration,
- anyone carrying a gun or self-defence equipment,
- restaurateurs, chefs, cooks and wait staff,
- cleaners working night shifts, etc

And let's add to that the industries where employees are most likely to be drinking on the job, such as hospitality.

Then there are the alcohol-at-risk 'recent drinkers' which include transport services, education, construction (!), financial, defence (!).

... Knowing that people that can't sleep properly and/or have mental health challenges are more likely to be drinking and taking recreational and/or prescription drugs.

Carry on...

CHAPTER 17

Media Games and The Need for an Overhaul.

D rug companies in America spend over $ 5 billion a year on advertising direct to the public[1], with the greatest percentage on television and magazine advertising.

The US, New Zealand and Australia are some of the only countries in the world where direct to consumer advertising by drug companies is tolerated.

Although prescription-only medicines are not allowed to be advertised direct to consumers in Australia[2] (unlike the US and New Zealand), there has certainly been a push for it in the past.

The rules for advertising in Australia are found on the TGA's website, and they are rather broad.

They have been put together by the usual broadly based stakeholders that cover just about anyone who wants to play, so what do you expect?

Some of the problems cited are:

- Patients going to their doctors asking for a particular brand name of drug because they have seen it on TV, even though there may be cheaper and better drugs available.
- Drug ads are not reviewed by the TGA/FDA as to their relevance, effectiveness or appropriateness.
- Drug side effects are not being exposed in the advertisements, and when they are they are limited and even trivialised using comic characters for example.
- There is a promotion of drug based solutions rather than lifestyle, exercise and/or nutrition based solutions.

- No mention of clinical references or proof that the drugs actually work.
- The ads normalise drug taking.
- Little or no mention of drug interactions when several drugs are taken at the same time.
- Little or no mention of drug interactions with alcohol, supplements, etc.
- The large advertising budgets add to the cost of the drugs.

Advertising has many effects such as normalising taking medications. Especially when it now seems that some health ad is in every television ad break I see now, whether it's pain relief, vitamins, or a chemist chain making commentary, etc.

No longer do you need a medication just for a serious illness. Products are promoted for colds, flu, headache, pain of all descriptions, etc. It used to be families had some Dettol, bandages, a thermometer, and a simple pain killer in their medicine cabinets. Now they have everything from nasal douches and irrigators to heavy artillery pain killers that I thought you had to be half dead to take.

My full-fat eating and no-flu-injections-thanks parents lived till they were 97 and 99 so I need a bit more convincing of the raft of medicines out there. They weren't anti-doctor or anti-medications but there was a time and a place – not a career.

And extended media time is achieved, of course, with the continual conversations in the news on the latest "discovery" towards the cure of cancer, the "medical breakthroughs" of stem cell research and the like – when nothing will result for many years in most cases. If at all. There is certainly no proof that the discovery of "xyz" found in rats will translate to humans, and to a proven solution any time soon.

The pharmaceutical companies use "awareness campaigns" and the like to encourage you to go to see your doctor and talk to them.

Health advertising and editorial makes us all feel that we are unhealthy, rather than healthy. That we are lacking vitality, when most people should take health and wellness as a reasonable assumption when we look after ourselves, eat properly, exercise, socialise appropriately, get outside in the sun, etc.

Of course the greatest problem with advertising is none of the above.

The greatest problem with pharmaceutical and health companies' advertising is the influence they have over editorial.

I've seen blatant examples of exceptional medical investigations being bagged a few days after airing, where the program is forced to retract statements made, sometimes with adverse effects on the journalists involved.

No guessing why any of this is happening.

And unfortunately this has not been just the commercial stations.

With the government having significant conflicts of interest, the ABC and SBS are no longer totally independent.

Their mission is to uphold government policy.

I'm sure you've noticed.

Not every story of course, but enough to get my back up now and then.

I'm not going to mention specific examples as they are stories that have already caused large kerfuffle for ethical journalists.

We are not all as dim as we sim.

And then there's the raft of 'clinically proven' supplements that everyone needs if you want to grow up to be an elite sportsperson or even, if you're really healthy, a media personality.

Oh, please.

Lastly, there are the disturbing news stories that bring up emotional issues and problems for people. So disturbing that viewers have to be referred to Beyond Blue (for example).

OK if their services and websites reflected evidence based medicine.

Otherwise perhaps just marketing?

During the news and well respected journalistic spots: prime time in other words.

CHAPTER 18

Politicians are Not Capable of Doing Their Job

H ere's a very quick history of health governance in Australia:
1948: The Pharmaceutical Benefits Scheme started in Australia
with free medicines for pensioners and 139 medicines available
for other members in the community. It has gone through numerous policy changes and reforms since 1948, and now includes 793 medicines in 2,066 forms and dosages, sold as more than 5,300 differently branded items[1].

1953: If you want to read an account of parliamentary dithering, read and/or download *A History of Therapeutic Goods Regulation in Australia*, by John McEwan[2].

What started as a valid idea in November 1953 to test and monitor national health and therapeutic substances, Sir Earle Page introduced the *National Health Bill (Consolidate benefit provisions)* to the Australian Parliament, and the *Therapeutic Substances Bill (Quality of imported drugs)* in the somewhat prophetically, "Not Important" section[3].

Having been agreed in principal by both houses of parliament, a small change was made in the senate, and the bills went back to the House of Representatives to finally be approved in November 1953.

Sir Earle Page said "I regret to state that at present there is evidence that drugs are being supplied that do not conform to the requisite standards and, so, are incapable of carrying out the job which the medical profession believes that they will carry out. It would be criminal to allow such a state of affairs to exist and continue merely through lack of appropriate action."[4]

However, it didn't take too long before an amendment was gazetted (16 January 1958) and came into effect on 1 May, 1958, that meant that control on imports was largely limited to biological products and antibiotics and did not include most pharmaceuticals.[5]

1989: Therapeutic Goods Administration established finally! But still not good.

Do you assume that federal and state ministers and/or senators have a superior brain or even common sense?

If so, that's a false and sometimes dangerous assumption.

I've had a bit to do with pre-selection processes for politicians and it's a little depressing. Maybe a lot depressing. And I've also done a fair bit of communicating with politicians either personally, at branch meetings, or moving policy motions at annual conferences and the like. And hung out with some pretty cluey and savvy staffers.

The politicians first have to be elected by their local communities.

And sad to say, most people in the local community are not inspiring when it comes to their politically savvyness! That's the main reason we have so many dorks as politicians, sadly.

Many people in the community don't have a clue what is a state or federal issue, for example, and they might blame their state politician for something that is a federal matter. Or they have never, ever, spoken to their local politician – yet they expect the politicians to know what issues you are concerned with.

My favourite is when people blame the government for not getting a bill through when the people elected the 'patchy' senate that blocked the bill(s). I've voted for the patchy senate myself, but at least I knew what the ramifications would be. In those cases you can't 'blame the government' for not getting something through, you have to look in the mirror and take account of who you voted into the senate.

Of course the people with an agenda in mind will surely talk to the politicians and lobby their particular interests – but the general public is generally snoring.

So we get what we deserve really.

Not a thing I like to admit, but probably true.

So, in order to get a local person to be voted in at their local election the person that is picked/nominated/volunteered/pushed has to be a certain type. Friendly, somewhat professional, well presented, capable of giving 100 speeches at the drop of a hat, with a reasonably 'clean' background, that sort of thing. No nasty criminal records or misogynistic habits that might pop up during the campaign. (Well, there are exceptions.)

Notice I didn't say rocket scientist, nor even above average intelligence.

And they certainly don't need to know how to conduct a legitimate randomised control trial.

(Yeah, I can see you laughing.)

That local member that you just voted for in the federal election might end up being the Health Minister, or god forbid, the Prime Minister (or Deputy Prime Minister, perhaps, if you live in the bush and the Liberal/ National Party Coalition are governing).

If and when they are elected they generally have no background in the area of their portfolio at all: they enter without having a portfolio, of course.

For some it is a too-steep-learning-curve, and depending who is in the federal House of Representatives or Senate at any one time the brains trust can be pretty lean pickings.

It gets more complicated when you have a Federal Minister for Health, a State Minister for Health and Mental Health, and a Deputy State Minister for Health and Mental Health, and different responsibilities at state and federal level.

But even so, we as citizens have a right to expect that the health ministers have our best health interests at heart, and that they will figure out the computations and permutations of what is happening within their portfolio. And consult with bright sparks and truth tellers in order to do a great job.

And understand that in all portfolios, there are people pushing agendas to make bigger profits for their companies, lobbyists who may or may not be revealing the truth and vested interests that are happy to deceive people in power, and the people.

So why is it that in Australia, unlike other intelligent developed countries, do we appear to flagrantly ignore Cochrane and its recommendations? And allow pharmaceutical advertising in the media, for example (even when it's misleading and incorrect?)

How can we *require* ministers to get a clue?

It's a tough call, and the vested interests are having a field day.

What is democracy actually costing us? And is it an illusion after all?

I won't list here some soooo obvious examples of ministers who didn't have a clue ... let alone understand complicated drug and intervention trials that even Cochrane spends months, even years to decipher.

I won't get too philosophical, but I will give a few examples of my contact with federal and state ministers in Australia:

- One health/mental health minister's office told me that "sleep has got nothing to do with mental health" (in a very derogatory tone),
- Another health minister's office said I had the wrong number when I asked for contact details of the department that looked after sleep education. (Sleep had nothing to do with health either, it appeared.)
- When I asked the name of the person who I was speaking to in the minister's office she said "you don't need to know that".

So much for public service.

It turns out that there is NO section in the health administration that is dedicated to sleep education and sleep – none at all... not at the state level, not at federal, not in the local health districts, not in community health, not in preventative medicine (wherever that hangs out!): nowhere.

The experts tell me the 'doctors are looking after that' which I'm not buying.

And others are telling me that sleep clinics look after that – and I'm not buying that either. There are about 2 people educating adults on how to sleep better...

Yep, hard to believe.

If you don't ask the questions you won't find out.

The very small number of sleep institutions in Australia are not making the required behavioural changes within the industry, and not improving sleep and mental health outcomes.

So the government structures are set favouring incompetence and ... well, you can guess.

We're talking about the largest employer in Australia with 13 percent of Australian workers employed in Health Care and Social Assistance and we can't seem to come anywhere near getting it right for sleep and mental health problems.

The result is 1 in 6 Australians on antidepressants, over 35 million psycho scripts written annually and 95.2 percent of insomnia patients being prescribed a medication by their doctor.

And statements by the mental health industry that many more people in the community are undiagnosed mental health patients.

Really?

Are you buying this?

Because I'm not.

Accountability and Clinical Governance

Here is a list of organisations, ministers, government instrumentalities, companies, medical professionals, doctors, hospitals, health centres, training organisations, universities and individuals that should be held accountable for this mess.

Most of them have optimistic goals, glossy mission statements, administrative procedures, budgets to meet, projections, strategies ... with a list of KPIs that they're meant to meet.

Tell me how you think they are faring so far in relation to sleep and mental health?

- The federal minister(s) for health and mental health and his department.
- The state minister(s) for health and mental health and their departments.
- The Pharmaceutical Benefits Scheme (PBS), which subsidises, with our money, drugs that are being abused by the medical system.
- The Medical Benefits Scheme (MBS). The Four Corners *Wasted* program says less than 5% of the listed items are evidence-based.
- Clinical governance personnel at every local area health district in the state and country who have decided that sleep education is a waste of time.
- Your local GP, prescribing insomniacs in 95.2 percent of the cases drugs that the TGA attempted to move from schedule 4 to schedule 8 of the poisons schedule in 2012.

- Your local GP's administrative managers – listed on the stock market.
- Doctors being paid by activity. Good or bad activity. e.g. referring you to a sleep clinic or an x-ray when that may not be evidence based.
- Community Health. Where can I learn about how to sleep better? How to address my underlying issues that manifest as the symptom of insomnia? Who knew that there were a range of medications that cause insomnia? How do I find out about them? Where is sleep education and preventative medicine?
- The Diagnostic and Statistical Manual of Mental Disorders DSM-V. Who and how do they decide that it is not OK to grieve for over 2 weeks after someone dies? And the rest?
- The Fatigue Registered Training Organisations and government legislation that allow and enable trucks and other transport workers to drive for a 14 hour "shift" if they have the "xyz certificate". That piece of paper is sure going to stop you from having an accident on the roads....
- The police force with consecutive days of 12 hour shifts and more powerful firearms.
- Interns with dangerous shift hours in hospitals.
- Food labelling laws – obsessed with country of origin. Who cares if it's toxic?
- Drug companies.
- Off label prescribing.
- Clinical trials standards.
- Not all clinical trials are registered. If we get the result we want, we'll register the trial then!
- Universities accepting money from vested interests to conduct clinical trials.
- The media advertising drugs – which exposes them to editorial bias.
- The media plugging community groups and charities that have dangerously outdated information in their policies and websites.
- Medical websites that promote information that is not evidence based. Where do I start?
- Institutions with dubious procedures around mental health and drugs: prisons, the military, nursing homes, children's homes etc.

- Forced treatment of mental health patients, breaches of human rights.
- The loss of your right to choose your own medical treatment and approach.
- The lack of reporting systems for the public to complain about side effects of medications.
- The lack of reporting systems to complain about anything to do with health. No federal ombudsman.
- No whistle-blowing protection or facilities.
- Why aren't *government agencies* following correct procedures and duty of care towards staff who are traumatised, etc. Police, army, fire, emergency services, medical staff at hospitals, night-time staff at hospitals, ambulance drivers, all occupations that experience trauma situations, including volunteers and members of the public?
- The NPS that still does not recognise suicidal ideation is a side effect of antidepressants.
- The TGA that wanted to move all benzodiazepines to schedule 8 from schedule 4, but was overruled by the AMA and other interests.

Who can I talk to when I have a sleeping problem or a mental health problem? Where you can GUARANTEE I'm not going to be prescribed a medication?

A counsellor or an alternative healer.

No wonder people are going to them.

At least you get talk therapy and no drugs. (Talk therapy is evidence-based by the way.)

Other than that, you tell me, 'cos I sure as hell can't find them.

Conflict of Interest in Australia's Health Care System

Australia's performance in declaring conflicts of interest is derided even by our own *Medical Journal of Australia*.

Here is some of what is being said by research printed in the *Medical Journal of Australia* on conflicts of interest in Australian health:

"A recent study of 313 Australian clinical guidelines used between 2003 and 2007 found that almost 80% had no competing interest statement.

This lack of disclosure is inexplicably inconsistent with practices adopted by peer-reviewed journals and with guidelines for participation in meetings of some medical organisations.

... Rates of conflict disclosure on guidelines are so low that, at best, they may indicate that the profession is in a "precontemplative" phase, oblivious to the existence or extent of the issue."[6]

And continues...

"We were unable to quantify total sponsorship from pharmaceutical companies to guideline-developing bodies as institutions and to individuals on guideline-drafting panels. While organisations often disclose corporate supporters on their websites, information on how much is donated and where it is directed is neither easily accessible nor comprehensive. In some cases, the websites of pharmaceutical companies are more informative than developers' websites. For example, Pfizer Australia declares on its website a donation of $150,000 in 2010 towards the Heart Foundation's Career Development Fellowship. However, there is no corresponding statement on the Heart Foundation website or in its annual reports."[7]

Other findings in this study include:

- **"Only 15% of guidelines on the National Health and Medical Research Council (NHMRC) portal from the most prolific developers have published conflict of interest (COI) statements, and fewer detail the processes used to manage conflicts."[8]**
- "Pharmaceutical sponsorship of medical research and professional bodies is considerable, raising the spectre of influence, which should be unequivocally confronted by the profession."[9]
- "Comprehensive disclosure of conflicts is needed to safeguard the integrity of clinical guidelines and the medical profession."[10]
- "Peak bodies and clinicians should seek to promote an improvement in current poor practice."[11]
- The most common conflicts of interest are "authors having financial links with industry, including being paid consultancies or honoraria, or holding company shares".[12]
- "The NHMRC key principles for developing guidelines do not mention the management of COIs. The NHMRC standards and procedures for externally developed guidelines refers to the issue,

asking that drafting groups disclose their COIs, but is silent on the need to publicly disclose conflicts and how they are managed."[13]

- "It should be a condition of NHMRC guideline approval that competing interest declarations and processes are made public."[14]

All this just proves that the industry is incapable of clinical governance, and that it should be taken out of their hands.

Who knows how many wasted billions of dollars are being paid by the government and Australians to allow these inadequate practices, procedures and drugs to continue being included in supposedly "best clinical practice" guidelines.

How many lives are being shortened or lost, how much insurance is being paid and wasted, how much consultation time and effort is voided, etc etc.

You do the math!

Establishing **absolute independent evidence**, and ensuring that this is what is transferred into best practice guidelines should be priority number one.

This is where health reform should be done, not in moving the vested-interest-chairs on the Titanic.

Australian National Policy Changes: To Stop Australians being Sleepy, Suicidal and Cognitively Impaired.

1. **A full and scoping investigation should be conducted into how and why "energy drinks" are continuing to be sold and advertised in Australia.** Some "energy drinks" are registered as therapeutic goods, others as dietary supplements and therefore avoid food regulations. "Energy drinks" have been the subject of medical complaints in Australia and to the Food and Drug Administration (FDA) in America (including death); have been found to contain caffeine quantities outside approved guidelines; are known to impair sleep; and their advertisers have been successfully sued in the US for false advertising.

2. **A national definition of "addiction" should be established so that drugs of addiction include those where adverse reactions are experienced when patients withdraw from the drugs.** At the moment addictive drugs seem only to be defined as those where the patient wants and/or requires increasing amounts for a similar result. Many experts are advocating that drugs with adverse reactions in the tapering/withdrawal stages (such as suicide and suicidal ideation) be included in the definition of addiction. I believe that because of the inadequate definition of addiction many drugs are being treated as less harmful than they should be. This is possibly one of the reasons why benzodiazepines and SSRIs remain on schedule 4 instead of being listed as schedule 8 drugs in Australia, and why they are being prescribed so often.

3. **A full investigation should be made into why all benzodiazepines were not rescheduled from schedule 4 to schedule 8** when that recommendation was made recently by the Therapeutic Goods Administration (TGA) – but vetoed by the AMA, RACP and others.

4. **SSRIs literature and prescribing practices should be changed to reflect valid medical research and litigation.** If they continue to be available they should be listed as schedule 8 drugs because of their known dangerous side effects such as suicidal ideation, suicide, akathisia and aggressive behaviour, and their similar tapering side effects.

5. **A full enquiry is to be held into why, in 95.2 percent of cases, insomnia patients are prescribed medications against the recommendations of the TGA and the National Prescribing Service.** Procedures should be put in place to flag addicts, long term users, mental health patients, and other underlying physical health issues that are not being detected or addressed in sleep disorder consultations. Prescribing is masking the symptoms, delaying or preventing the solutions, and in some cases causing significant additional problems. The professionalism of doctors is questioned.

6. **Food labelling laws should be tightened considerably.** Present labelling does not clearly declare all adverse additives, nor contents that constitute less than 5% of the volume. Labelling laws should prohibit words like "natural", "wholesome" and "organic" without

well publicised rules. Many unsuccessful attempts have been made to achieve these changes previously.

7. **Fatigue policies in all organisations should educate on sleep, showing its *direct connection* to fatigue.** The word "fatigue" is so connected to legal exposure now, that many so called experts ask "what has sleep got to do with fatigue?" WHS laws do not recognise that a person could *arrive to work* fatigued. The proven quantifiable benefits of quality sleep should be part of the education to ensure that organisations understand the direct relationship to reduced accidents and deaths; improved performance; sharper mental acuity; elevated mood; reduced absenteeism and presenteeism; better executive functions of the brain; and the long term reduction of mental and physical illnesses etc. By avoiding sleep education and policies organisations are more liable.

8. **School curriculums should improve their education on sleep** – particularly in years 8-12, when lack of sleep, delayed sleep phase, and exam stress is causing and exaggerating psychological and physical problems (e.g. anxiety, substance abuse, weight problems, inappropriate eating, the misuse of caffeinated and "energy" drinks, etc). One study showed that students who sleep 5 hours or less a night are three times more likely to become mentally ill than those sleeping eight or nine hours.

9. **Cosmetics, beauty products and toiletries should be more regulated** because many products contain ingredients that are connected to adverse health effects including sleep disorders.

10. **Shift workers should be educated on the hazards of night work,** with career change assistance for long term shift workers. Shift workers in stressful and traumatic careers should be prohibited from excessive exposure to risk.

11. **Advertising of drugs and medical procedures directly to the public should be prohibited** in alignment with the great majority of developed countries. This should include social media, blogging and other internet platforms.

12. **A federal health ombudsman should be established** with broad ranging powers over all health issues. The ombudsman should oversee medical, health, nutrition, food labelling, exercise, drugs,

supplements, sleep issues, medical procedures, health products, hospital administration, drug scheduling, marketing practices, prescribing processes etc – at state, federal and local council level. The health industry is fragmented and complex and increasingly unaccountable and unsuccessful. Every measure is to be made to ensure that the ethics and independence of the ombudsman are beyond reproach, with associated tribunal and litigation arms.

13. **The Australian Government should establish an independent Federal Medical Research Centre where clinical trials and meta analyses would be funded to provide world class evidence based medicine.** Many times we hear that "there is no clinical evidence to support" an hypothesis, when it is clear that we need a definitive answer. This new centre would be separate from the National Health Ombudsman and would:

a) **Review the original raw data of all RCTs that relate to drugs and medical procedures that are already listed on our MBS and PBS to eliminate all drugs and procedures that are not evidence based** – saving billions to establish the ongoing funding for the centre and project.

b) **Perform RCTs and meta-analyses to ensure the correct spending on health where no relevant and correctly run RCT or meta analysis has established the validity of certain health methodologies.** This would not only include studies and reviews into listed drugs and procedures that have no real evidence base but would include preventative health measures, alternative health, supplementation, etc.

c) **Independently review food production standards and labelling laws.** Questions are being asked about manufactured and processed food, including toxic chemicals and colourings that affect behaviour and mood. Without proper clinical trials food manufacturers continue to insist that their methodologies are healthy and harmless. Many people and experts have opposing views.

d) **Independently review makeup, personal products and airborne chemicals (such as petroleum products and carcinogens) to establish higher standards of health for the**

Australian population. At the moment there are no rulings on what chemicals are allowed in makeup, hair treatments, etc., which is allowing toxic and carcinogenic ingredients to be absorbed into our bodies.

e) **Review the effectiveness and results of government grants and donations being made to charities and organisations** that may or may not be returning value for money on our investments: interpreted through real evidence of longer and better lives for our citizens.

f) **Establish effective, non-drug early intervention counselling/talk-therapy procedures and support centres for people who are suffering mental health challenges.** These systems already exist overseas but are unknown or non-existent in Australia. They are known to Robert Whitaker, Peter Gøtzsche, Peter Breggin, David Healy and other evidence based experts.

g) **Integrate and validate** the best value parts of preventative, allopathic, supplemental and alternative health modalities for the good of the nation's health through world class evidence and testing.

h) **Establish evidence based practices and centres for the rehabilitation of citizens** who are taking addictive drugs – prescribed, recreational and illegal.

i) **Establish new best practice guidelines for mental health and sleep,** so that Australians benefit from evidence-based science, and productive working lives.

j) **Establish truth in medicine, saving the country billions of dollars a year.**

k) **Finally establish clinical governance over our health system:** the drugs, products and procedures that are listed on the PBS and the MBS - now and into the future.

l) **Independently review the scientific evidence relating to all health related whistle blower cases in Australia.**

m) **Independently review all government funded bodies to ensure their medical information is based on evidence.**

n) **Collaborate with Cochrane for both RCTs and meta analyses.**

14. **The government should not fund any organisations, foundations or charities that allow or promote off-label prescribing of SSRIs to children under 18 years of age.** Or any off-label prescribing at all, or information which is wrong and/or outdated. We know who they are, why are we funding them? (There are many of them, not just the examples I have mentioned in this book.)

15. **Australia should establish a website where doctors, health professionals, hospitals and educational bodies declare income, incentives and funding they have received from drug companies and other organisations** similar to the US system and the website http://www.OpenPaymentsData.CMS.gov. This should include the sponsorship of clinical trials, payments made to doctors for advice or expert opinion, entertainment, conducting research for companies, shares in companies, speaker fees, free and sponsored conferences, advertising incentives etc.

16. **Doctors, medical professionals and psychiatrists should be retrained on what 'evidence-based' actually means.**
    This training would include:
    - the importance of Cochrane, its purpose and efficacy, and how to look up the Cochrane Library data;
    - the Cochrane training to learn how to decipher a good clinical trial from a biased and/or invalid one;
    - their professional duty to personally establish the value of every drug that they prescribe, beyond the present inadequate system, and beyond the information being presented by drug companies and vested interests;
    - A full understanding of bias in clinical trials and randomised control trials. From how the trials are randomised, braking the blinding, not publishing unsuccessful trials, ghost writing practices, misleading and fraudulent terms and procedures used, the lack of long term trials, epidemiology, meta-analysis etc.

17. **A royal commission should be established with wide ranging terms of reference** to investigate, report and bring to justice public servants, drug company leaders, doctors, medical authorities and others who are responsible for deaths, injuries and addictions to Australian citizens (including in prisons, institutions, the military,

hospitals, nursing homes, foundations, charities and other care); fraudulent clinical trials; prescribing without evidence; registering drugs inappropriately; and signing international and national trade deals that adversely affect the health of Australian citizens – including illness, deaths, suicides, homicides and addiction.

18. **Criminal proceedings should be brought against CEOs and directors of organisations whose activities lead to death, suicide, addictions or personal injury.** Personal liability should be enforced where business leaders kill, harm or injury members of the public including through misinformation and clinical culpability.

19. **A full investigation should be held into government-backed and maintained websites that are not up to date, and or include/ promote misleading health information.** This investigation should include inadequate information on the National Prescribing Service's website on the side effects of SSRIs, information on the TGA website, etc.

20. **A national drug database should be established to identify and monitor the prescribing and usage habits of doctors and patients - across medical practices: with state and federal cooperation.** This should help to minimise and prevent addiction, doctor shopping, inappropriate prescribing habits, crimes of addiction, suicide, homicide and homelessness. A number of coronial inquests have recommended this action, but nothing has been done about it.

21. **An education funding register is to be established and made public which lists all donations, incentives, scholarships (and the like) made to universities, schools and learning institutions.** This will help alleviate "incentivised" research results, biased education, and bias in education.

22. **An investigation should be held into why Australia spends approximately 4 percent of its health budget on preventative medicine, when it should be the other way around.** People clearly need encouragement to exercise, eat well, have meaningful relationships and be proud of their personal contribution in life. If we had a lot less sick people we would not need the huge medical treatment system that is crippling the nation.

23. **The Australian Government should joint venture with Cochrane to help fund, support and trial health and medical solutions that would be truly evidence-based.** It's not enough for the Australian Government to allow Australians access to the Cochrane Library, they should encourage more individuals to be trained in Cochrane methodologies and become Cochrane volunteers to help with their valuable research. Other countries collaborate with Cochrane to decide policy – we should too.

Most readers might be surprised to know that you do not have to be a doctor to be able to ascertain whether a particular RCT is valid or not. It's not rocket science when you know how to pick good and bad trials – Cochrane has online training to teach you how.

You have to be smart, but not necessarily medically qualified: an excellent way for many health enthusiasts to contribute to medical science. And for natural and alternative health readers, after you have been trained as a Cochrane volunteer, if you can find a properly conducted trial of a natural substance or supplement you can put it up for further investigation by the Cochrane teams. (You won't be on the final review team of course, but you can have input in the early review stages by putting forward legitimate studies of complementary medical options for further investigation – if they are valid.)

Yep, go do some more Googling (well 'Cochraning', can we make that a new word?), and contact them if you're interested. One of the least known and most valuable volunteer contributions available in my opinion, and great for people who are computer literate, intelligent and looking for something you can do from home.

This information wasn't lost on me when I found this out! Made me wonder again why so many medical professionals (who are "fully qualified") choose not to ask the *appropriate questions* of their drug representatives when they bring lunches to their practices, or when they attend conferences etc.

24. **The Australian government should review our ANZFA agreement to ensure that food items approved by New Zealand are**

not seamlessly brought into Australia to the detriment of our citizens' health.

25. **The contents of the Trans Pacific Partnership agreement (TPP) should be made public.** The fact that this agreement is secret is a problem. We need transparency so that we can see how this agreement will affect Australia's ability to design, develop and improve our health and medical system independently, if necessary, from international commercial forces. There are concerns that clauses included in the TPP will take away Australia's sovereignty in making its own decisions on what health care is allowed in Australia if it affects the commercial interests of listed companies and other international businesses. Other countries are already being sued for decisions being made by governments that 'restrict' the ability of companies and organisations to make a profit *in the way they see fit* in participating countries. If Australia is to keep its health care costs effective and manageable the TPP could be a conflict of interest. E.g. Banning smoking in Australia is a restriction of trade for tobacco sellers and opens up litigation opportunities that the government (i.e. Australian citizens) will have to pay for.

26. **Sleep education should be introduced across Australia so that people can learn how to sleep better without drugs and medical interventions.** The status of sleep should be improved and seen as a very valuable early warning signal of health issues. Education should cover inappropriate lifestyles, lack of exercise, obesity, bad eating habits, food labelling, sleep hygiene, recreational drugs, emotional problems and how to talk to people about them, Cognitive Behavioural Therapy, insomnia as a side effect of medications, the underlying reasons why people can't sleep, how to survive your school years, drugs of addiction, etc. This education should be run independently of the medical system so that the first line of solutions is common sense, not drugs.

Refer to appendix 2, *The Case for Sleep Education*. And I declare a vested interest.

27. **A national suicide investigation body should be established.** This organisation should register the circumstances of every suicide death in Australia, with details of the drugs that the person was taking

(prescription and otherwise), and the prescription patterns, specific drug names, drug interactions, source of prescription, nursing home/prison/institution name etc. They should also include drug tapering methodologies, drug dosage changes, detoxification and rehabilitation facilities, as we know that drug changes and drug tapering are serious problems, and causes of suicide and violence.

28. **Whistleblower protection should be significantly strengthened in Australia.** It is very difficult to know how to get whistle blower protection, with significant lack of information on where to go or what to do. There appear to be totally inadequate systems for members of the public working outside of government organisations, people in private enterprise, charity and foundation workers, unemployed or previously employed people, etc. There are also inadequate protections afforded whistleblowers, including compensation. Whistleblowers do not just reside in companies and governments, they can be anywhere, and this fact should be acknowledged. Many people who have left organisations because of ethical problems, for example, should be in a position to report criminal activity now they are outside of the organisation.

29. **Companies, organisations, charities and foundations that mislead the public about the efficacy and dangers of medications, or mention/promote off-label use of drugs should be brought to justice.**

30. **The National Prescribing Service should correctly show all side effects of medications on their websites, such as suicide, suicidal ideation and addiction.** Full descriptions of terms such as "akathisia" should be explained, so that the public knows that akathisia, for example, can be the forerunner of violent and/or suicidal behaviour.

The public is not capable of understanding technical terms, and it wouldn't be the first time that technical terms have been used to cover the truth and mislead. "Akathisia" is a very good example, as even on medical websites it is shown to mean very different things. (The NPS also quotes drug company research in their references, which is not a good look!)

31. **Off-label Prescribing and its Promotion Should be Illegal in Australia.** (See 14 above.) Since 'off-label' means that there is inadequate evidence that a drug or procedure works, and/or that it does

no harm - it should <u>not</u> be allowed to occur. It is *illegal* for drug companies to promote off-label prescribing, *legal* for doctors to prescribe off-label and *apparently legal* for registered charities, foundations and the like to promote off-label prescribing of medications in the media, on their websites and even *during the news*. These activities, individual professionals, CEOs, board members and organisations should be included in the royal commission.

Is it any wonder that the new trend is Overdiagnosis Conferences, Selling Sickness Conferences, and the upsurge in interest in alternative and complementary medicine and talk therapies?

CHAPTER 19

The Seventh Dwarf.

Warning: This chapter will hopefully offend. Not suitable for children (although it's quite OK to drug them and increase their risk of suicide). Read at your own risk.

This chapter is my psychotherapy and I'll vent, swear and cry if I want to.

So here's the rough storyline of the documentary I want to make.

Contact me if you want to play.

You'll notice I haven't referenced everything in this chapter. Bad luck.

You'll have to find all the references in the relevant chapters of this book, or Doctor Google it... you have my full permission to do that.

I'm too busy venting now.

Besides, all the brainpower in all the universities, clinical trials and professional associations with all their intellectual rules (and referencing systems) have amounted to a totally crap system that's killing people.

Asking Too Many Questions

Asking too many questions is a problem I have, if you want to see it as a negative. Some call it "disruptive".

My father brought me up to respect questions as a powerful way of finding out.

Probably the main lesson I got from Dad was his mantra "never be afraid to ask a question".

He sometimes followed up the mantra with the statement "when you stand up to ask a question there might be 100 people in that room that wanted to ask that question, but were too afraid". "You will be asking the question for them too."

And he celebrated "quality questions".

My father was effectively self-taught, and like me was a reading dyslexic for many years, before somehow fixing himself before I was born. (I knew him as an avid reader of high quality information.)

There was nothing dull about him. He was friends with supreme court judges, leading economic forecasters, university professors, as well as a lot of normal people and horsey types who loved his humble energy and smiling brightness. And sense of humour, mostly based on silliness, self deprecation and simplicity.

When he was 92 I remember visiting him in his aged care home and he said to me "I'm sorry I don't have anything interesting to talk to you about today". Wow, apology accepted.

I hope today that I have something interesting to talk to you about.

His favourite topic was banking, and their lending and other practices. Don't get me started.

Suffice to say he predicted the GFC decades ago, and the ramifications are far from over. They're still playing "pass the dodgy instrumentality parcel" to see who is sucker enough to take it. Governments generally. We have all watched as the bad banking practices have been passed on to the citizens by governments rather than make banks accountable for their dodgy practices. Fiat currencies, central banks and private banks, money laundering, creating money from nothing, were common conversations as I grew up. Dad was most disappointed that at Sydney University in my economics degree we learned just about nothing about banks, and certainly not the stuff he wished I had learned. Universities are increasingly becoming the play things of corporations and vested interests. And increasingly places where if you don't believe and accept what is being taught you fail.

(We won't go into wholesale cheating, that other new new thang!)

Students are not taught to think, or to question – they are taught to repeat the BS they are taught there.

And ironically, with world economies being compromised by various forces, it has become more and more attractive for governments to engage private enterprise to help them run educational institutions, finance them, etc.

My BS radar *particularly* goes off when I'm being told something is *incontrovertible*, and when the opposing opinion is being promoted as stupid. Both reactions get some serious question asking!

Because they reveal the "dumbness pressure" that manipulators want you to feel.

Sometimes it's *the reaction* to the question, not the answer, that is *actually* the answer.

So *listen up, watch up* and *sense up* when you ask your question.

Hold firm, stay strong - be confident in the way you think and the questions you ask. It's OK to question the status quo, even if they think you're an idiot, conspiracy theorist, alarmist, disruptive, mental and stupid.

"Mental" is a growing trend, you should totally get that by reading this book.

Watch the "mental" space over the next decade, it's already seriously in play.

The good news is that people are waking up to their innate intelligence, and critical mass is close approaching to upturn many institutions and beliefs.

Change has already been shown to occur in the wink of an eye over the last few decades. It works like magic when it finally happens – suddenly people really see.

What happened to the Berlin Wall exactly?

In the end it seemed like the blink of an eye.

Press on... but keep a sense of humour and perspective, otherwise it will adversely affect you.

By the way, let's recognise up front that the truth isn't ever easy to find, and can change over time as science and discoveries are made. But there is still, generally, quality information and misinformation to the best of our knowledge at a given time.

Let's go to the 'dark side' for a while, and the story of The Seventh Dwarf.

THE CHARACTERS

The names have sometimes been changed, or not: To expose the guilty.

Snow White

Works in the financial markets, sticks the snow white substance cocaine up her nose regularly to work long hours in the markets. Hence the name Snow White. Beautiful and superficially very successful, she's big on avoidance, and escapes to the bush when the bank starts chasing her for her mortgage payment arrears on her mega million dollar house in Sydney.

After meeting Bashful in the woods Snow White ends up keeping house for the dwarfs while they mine for jewels during the day. Old school. And at night they all sing, play music and dance.

I'm kidding, that only happens in Fantasyland.

What they're really doing is Snapchat and Tinder with lying size-enhanced-photos. Over stimulating behaviour, blue light coming off their computer screens and wrecking their circadian rhythms even more than their shift-work mining jobs.

Maybe that's why they never grew?

They have been stages III-and-IV-sleep-deprived for years, which is known to stunt your growth.

The lack of sunlight doesn't help.

In fact, long term, their sleep deprivation is going to lead to some serious problems which could include cancer. But let's not spoil a good story with some facts from Harvard and the Danish government payouts.

Eventually the wicked queen's huntsman found Snow White and gave her a Xanax (from the alprazolam group of drugs, which has since been moved to Schedule 8 - not before time) to calm her down.

It got stuck in her throat, which meant no more washing up and cleaning. Thank god.

A bit like having a Bex and a good lie down. Only a lot lot worse.

The Seven Dwarfs
Grumpy

Shift worker in the mine.

Never gets enough sleep and is a complete pain in the arse. Of course he doesn't have any friends.

He's not getting promoted at work, is very unproductive and vague, and prone to accidents.

He doesn't exercise and eats junk food to keep him awake at weird hours. Things just get worse and worse for him.

He went to the doctor and got a benzo, now he feels the drug hangover effect for hours a day and seems to live in a fog.

His mother died recently, and he's been mourning her death for over 2 weeks now. According to the Diagnostic and Statistical Manual of Mental Disorders he should be over it by now, so he must have depressive disorder.

Likely he'll be on antidepressants and stacking on the weight soon. That'll make him feel better... Sure.

Happy

He's the one that's getting enough sleep and is fun to be around.

He's got good friends, and they have real conversations about their problems.

Everyone has problems, and sometimes they crowd in on each other, which is really crap.

Which brings on some very real and revealing conversations.

They often joke about it and dig deep, which clears the air and strengthens the support he feels, and they feel.

They openly support each other.

He's an optimist and makes a difference in the world, because he sees things clearly and has the energy and vitality to make a valuable contribution. Often enough, not always.

He's also an endangered species because someone's going to put the fear of god in him soon and tell him that while he thinks he's OK, he's actually just one of the very large number of people who have a mental health problem that is *undiagnosed*.

35 million psycho scripts written in Australia a year is not enough.

Doc

The doctor only talks to people in 10 minute slots. Maybe sometimes a long consultation, but 10 minutes is usually enough time to deal with most problems a GP sees.

He maintains his healthy income by working the 'activity based' remuneration system by sending his patients for tests which lead to more procedures, and hopefully more tests.

Sure as hell someone will find stuff wrong with them with all those tests.

Doc worked at the "XYZ" medical centre (part of the large group of medical centres listed on the ASX). He was one of many doctors who bought shares in the publicly listed healthcare company. Of course companies on the stock market are profit driven, or at the very least capital accumulators (but that makes them takeover targets). So *profits* and dividends are king generally. Some of those listed companies operate as service companies to medical centres, others actually own them (in a share arrangement with the doctors in the medical centre). Some of the listed companies are international: for example their head office might be in the United States.

He was constantly under pressure to perform according to the guidelines and professional culture of his medical practice, in response to his and their shareholdings and connection to the listed XYZ medical centres.

And he worked within the time limits generally accepted as reasonable by the profession.

Time is the scarce resource, but there is time for prescribing and referring.

And he'd never heard conversations about conflicts of interest between this and the health of his patients.

Or he chose not to listen.

He didn't want to be prescribing and referring all day.

As a student he never dreamed this is what he would really be doing as a doctor. (And insurance forms…)

Clinical guidelines supported his behaviour: it was what other doctors did. He knew all the doctors were doing it too as they used to discuss it, and prescribing patterns were open to review.

Just no-one seemed to be doing the review. Just 'industry bodies'?

He hadn't seen the Four Corners *Wasted* Program on the MBS, and wasn't interested in any reviews of the PBS.

He's not diligent about asking about any side effects of the medications he has prescribed, and even less diligent about reporting drug side effects. And who the hell do you report them to, anyway… I don't have time.

Next.

Doctors have a very high rate of using drugs such as Ritalin at university to improve their performance under pressure. So many bought the bullshit even before they graduated.

(And they have significantly higher suicide rates than the normal population too. Women doctors are over double the normal rate.)

And then the system abuses them while they are interns, forcing them to work ridiculous hours in hospitals, for example.

Most of them must secretly wonder why the hell they studied so hard for so many years to become a pawn in a broken system.

By now they have invested so much time, effort and money into becoming a doctor that they continue even though it just about kills them.

And then they have uneducated patients questioning what they are doing.

You're kidding, right?

What possible rights do you have as patients to question my authority and my learning over the last 15 years?

I don't care who the hell you think you are, or what you have researched.

And don't bring me any of your Cochrane reports to our consultations.

You are a trouble maker.

I'm off to my pharmaceutical-company-paid-lunch.

Here's your script.

If this commentary brings up any issues for you call Beyond Blue.

Well, maybe not.

Bashful

Yep, he's the one with Social Anxiety Disorder.

"SAD" in DSM V - a cuter, more marketable brand than its previous "social phobia" name in DSM IV. The new name has moved the mental sickness line significantly, and a lot more people would line up for that one! SADly.

He used to be called shy.

And he was generally called shy by those totally noisy people who never thought about what they said before they said it, and who were quite happy to make fools of themselves in public, 'holding forth' on whatever random topic. Even if they knew bugger all about it.

He just wasn't born that way.

He thought that half the population were extroverted and half the population were introverted and that was OK. It kind of balanced things out.

And he never thought it was weird until recently when he found out from the Diagnostic and Statistical Manual of Mental Disorders that he had social anxiety disorder.

So now instead of forcing himself to go out to parties he stays at home and bonks his horse.

'Cos that's not listed as a mental problem in the Diagnostic and Statistical Manual of Mental Disorders DSM-V.

He's in a Stable Relationship.

But he's not going to cough that up to Doc in his next 10 minute consult.

Will shy Bashful ever ask his doctor if he's got a pill to make his horse less goddam hot?

The only reason they didn't try classifying the other half of the population with "Too Much to Say for Yourself Personality Disorder" DSM Blah Blah Blah - V was that we have enough lead in our pencils and outspokenness to tell them to go fuck themselves.

If you're going to be bully boys it's much more profitable to prey on the stressed, anxious, shy, depressed and vulnerable.

And the ones in institutions and ...

Kids and school children ... They've got more vulnerabilities than you can poke a stick at. Puberty, body image problems, social media, delayed sleep phase, peer group pressure, pimples and acne, pushy parents, youth sexualisation and porn, bullying, over-exposure to violent and disturbing media, hyper-consumerism, rubbish food, lack of exercise, desensitising and disturbing violent and sexualised video games, Kardashian complex... all that, possibly more. And we can't blame the drug companies for that. Get our mirrors out again wicked witches and warlocks.

Get 'em while they're down.

Sneezy

Sneezy isn't getting much sleep either.

He's got a stuffy nose, can't breathe properly, has clouded thinking and is generally not feeling that well.

He's got allergies and intolerances because of the junk food they bring into the mine each day.

He doesn't know how to read food labels and no one has explained to him that food labelling isn't good in Australia anyway.

The food manufacturers are streets ahead of legislation, in fact food labelling legislation is so far behind it might never catch up. (I remember coming into a room with formulae all over the board and asking what it was. The answer was 'a quiche'! Real men are right.)

We've got complicated international agreements too, to allow food coming in from New Zealand to be deemed OK under Australia New Zealand Food Authority (ANZFA) agreements and stuff.

And that's just Australia and New Zealand.

What could be in the Trans Pacific Partnership (TPP) agreement?

No idea because we aren't allowed to look at that. It's secret.

Ah choo.

Oh, maybe he should try a sleep apnea mask? Even though according to Cochrane there has been no long term study that proves their efficacy in improving mortality.

Who cares that his breathing problems actually relate to the food he's eating and the bad food labelling?

Let's put a mask on him and treat the symptom, not the underlying cause.

Ah choo.

Dopey

Dopey has been on antipsychotic drugs for so long now that he actually does have cognitive impairment and permanent brain damage.

Getting off the drugs is going to be really hard for him, and it will leave him with permanent problems that he does not know about yet.

Even when he finally gets off his drugs, some very adverse side effects will stay with him for the rest of his life.

He wasn't always dopey.

But he was dopey enough to listen to bad advice and not go outside "conventional wisdom" when he was medicated.

Sometimes you have to be a shit-stirrer if you want to survive.

Shit-stirring isn't dopey – they just want you to think that.

He's a victim of exceptional marketing that became best practice.

Sleepy

Sleepy is sleepy because he is on medications that have the side effect of insomnia.

Some of Sleepy's friends are sleepy because they have insomnia when they are coming off their benzos and/or antidepressants. His friends mistakenly think that when they get rebound insomnia from coming off benzos that the pills are actually working. They don't know that it is a withdrawal effect when you come off the pills and you have to stick with the process and the insomnia while you detoxify.

He's too tired to care.

THE CASTLES.

MORE POWER PLAYS THAN YOU CAN POKE A STICK AT. MAKES THE WICKED QUEEN LOOK LIKE A PUSSY CAT.

I'd like to slam some black box warnings on most of them.

TGA Castle (Therapeutic Goods Administration)

Supposedly protecting the public from the healthcare industry, but incapable and fundamentally flawed. They rely on dodgy clinical trials that are ghost written by drug companies, who have a vested interest in false positive results, and do not reveal the raw data or the clinical trial methodologies to anyone.

It's commercial-in-confidence, of course. Unless of course, they are found guilty of fraud in the courts (once every pancake day) and forced by the judge to reveal the raw data – a chance in a million and well worth the financial risk. This is how GlaxoSmithKline's Study 329 was restored.

Alternatively, if it's a supplement or herb or something – they can register with the TGA and it's seen to be fine until some shit hits the fan.

Well, very scientific indeed. But not clinical, I understand, when the shit does hit.

By the way, I'm not knocking all alternative and complimentary health systems – not much could be worse than the main stream system. And there's no wonder that it's the more intelligent and wealthier members of the public who are going there. In many cases there is no money for clinical trials to prove efficacy, the drug companies are the ones making billions.

However, the drug companies are now taking over the supplement companies, 'cos there's more than a buck in there now, so who knows what will be next.

Castle MBS (Australian Medical Benefits Scheme)

Federal government instrumentality that subsidises medical consultations and procedures for the good of the health of the nation. Well, that's the theory.

The problems with the Australian Medical Benefits Scheme were covered in *Wasted*, ABC Four Corners on Monday September 28, 2015, with Norman Swan and Jaya Balendra, presented by Kerry O'Brien.

In the program (full transcript available) it stated that the Medical Benefits Scheme has more than 5700 medical and surgical services that the Government will reimburse through Medicare, but there are 5500 items that are *not* evidence based.

That means that only approximately 200 of 5700 listed items, or *3.5 percent of our medical bills are actually supported by evidence-based science.* Some procedures are known to be harmful. All of them costly to individuals, insurance companies and the government.

It is beyond alarming!

Not only that, but efforts by certain medical professionals to stop the waste and procedures has cost them personally and professionally.

Please read the full transcript, or watch the program in order to understand why Australia is struggling to afford our medical system.

It's not about an aging population, and it's not about insurance costs, and it's not about whatever they're blaming.

It is about procedures that are not evidence based, activity based remuneration of doctors, procedures that do not work and create more problems, inappropriate solutions to medical problems that perpetuate the profitability of the system for some people and organisations.

My biggest question here is: With over 1.5 million people in Australia employed in the health sector, and numerous clinical governance employees in health, why are these problems being exposed by the *Four Corners* television program?

Federal and state health ministers are incapable of doing their jobs.

We need a Royal Commission in order to flush out the problems, and fast.

We need encompassing whistleblower protection for Australians who seek a better future for the health of our nation, and the courage to speak out.

Castle PBS (Pharmaceutical Benefits Scheme)

The PBS is the Australian federal government instrumentality that subsidises drugs for the good of the health of the nation.

Well, that's the theory.

The yearly expenditure by the Australian government on the PBS for the year ending June 30, 2014 was $ 9.1 billion which represents 82.5 percent of the total bill of the PBS. The remaining 17.5 percent is covered by patients – the cost for the same period being $ 1.5 billion. Total cost reported is $ 10.693 billion.

Following on from the *Four Corners* study of the MBS, we need a similar study of the PBS, with action being taken to take all ineffective and harmful drugs off the scheme, with penalties to doctors who prescribe medications that are not evidence based.

Many of the drugs listed on the PBS and subsidised are not good for the health of the nation at all, in fact they can bugger up your health big time.

Well, only if you think making you an addict or killing you is buggering you up.

And we pay for this.

We pay tax, we pay to subsidise dodgy drugs, we pay for the consultations where we are prescribed drugs, we pay for the rehab centres and we pay for the funerals.

Who's doing a cost benefit analysis on all this?

No one.

Castle Australian Government

The ASX 200 Healthcare Indexed stocks returned 247% over the past 10 years, compared to 54% for the all ordinaries.

Healthcare stocks are killing it.

Especially in Australia.

What could possibly be wrong with that?

The government keeps telling us we have the best healthcare in the world.

Or are they actually talking about "the most profitable healthcare system for private enterprise"?

Here's the problem with dumb politicians: If they're dumb you don't even have to bribe them, they'll probably do what you want them to anyway. It won't cost a cent, and there will be no paper trail. Easily confused, with no time to look at the finer print or think beyond the obvious, the world's your oyster if you have a barrow to push.

And sure as hell there are a lot of companies, organisations, charities, foundations and people with barrows to push through governments.

The chance of getting caught is minimal.

And then what?

Nothing much – as proven by the inaction after the release of Elizabeth Broderick's damning report into sexual abuse in the military.

Carry on.

Medical Journals' Castle

Where you publish the results of your dodgy clinical trials, and hope you get away with it.

Meant to be peer reviewed and the best that science can offer. In actual fact, not necessarily ... and the editors have been questioned on many occasions for printing material that did not stand the test of time, or the test of science. Obviously some good stuff gets published too, but who's to know what is good and what is polluted?

Who's going to argue the point with world leading scientific opinion? Less than 20 people on the planet probably. A risky road to take, duh. A major part of the problem.

AMA Castle: The Australian Medical Association

The professional association for Australian doctors and medical students. Presumably looking after the best interest of patients' health – but not if it gets in the way of their practice, profitability, reputation, etc. Why, for example, in 2012 when the TGA wanted to move all benzodiazepines from Schedule 4 on the poisons schedule to Schedule 8 did the AMA object? One of the reasons apparently, is that it would have increased their administrative workload (and been an impediment to business). Nice one. Most benzos are still on schedule 4 in Australia causing significant problems to many thousands of people. See Sleeping Pills, Chapter 9.

The drug companies would have no power at all if doctors didn't play their game. They know that, so they are keen to keep doctors happy, respected by the community, and doing what they are doing.

In America, health organisations can buy lists that link doctors' anonymous numbers with the actual names of the doctors. This helps the health organisations track individual doctor's s behaviours down to their individual prescribing patterns etc. Those lists are being purchased from the American AMA.

Nice?

DREAM Castle: Doctors Respecting Evidence, Against Manipulation

Dream on.

That's when they grow some balls and start advocating for their patients - instead of being told what to do by vested interests in all levels of the hierarchy.

Including being trained, and remunerated by drug and service companies through their various guises and activities.

Doctors aren't as smart as they like you to think they are.

Are they capable of saving their profession from going down the toilet?

Castle Diagnostic and Statistical Manual of Mental Disorders DSM-V

I'll keep away from this castle, thanks.

It's loaded and cocked.

Castle Drug Companies

Well if you haven't been under a rock for the last 50 years you will have noticed that drug companies are motivated by profits and are listed on the stock markets around the world.

You can't blame them for making a profit. That's what listed companies on stock markets aim to do. And you the shareholder compel them to make profits, to ensure you get your dividends and the stock price continues to rise, securing your shareholder asset base.

What gets tricky for the drug companies is the risk mitigation.

So we have a new drug, we know that eventually it might be established that it will kill someone (or a heap of people), and there is a risk we will be found out, and a risk we will be taken to court, and a risk we will be found guilty of negligence, or overlooking off-label prescribing or.... *insert options* ... and a risk that at the end of that long and drawn out trial (which they always seem to be) we might be fined.

Perhaps.

And a risk that that fine is low/medium/high in value.

Given all these factors, and being the only organisation to know the underlying facts of the clinical trials that we have performed, (commercial in-confidence information, you know...) what price will we charge for the drugs to cover these risks and future legal fees if it comes to that?

And what sort of insurance can we buy to mitigate the risk?

And then there is a risk that we may have to put labelling on the drug itself, perhaps a black box warning if we're unlucky enough for that to happen.

Or rarely that a drug be actually taken off the market – like Thalidomide.

Oh, actually that is now being used mainly as a treatment of certain cancers and of a complication of leprosy.

So maybe not that one.

What other ones can you think of?

By now I'm assuming that you've got with the program on this, so I don't have to give an exhaustive list.

I'll just state a few facts again here for you to think about:

- Prescribing antidepressants to children under the age of 18 is considered to be off-label prescribing in Australia.

- In 2004 New York Attorney General Elliot Spitzer filed a consumer fraud action against GSK based on mismatches between data and their marketing claims. In November 2012 GSK pleaded guilty and agreed to pay $3 billion, the biggest fine in corporate history.
- The next year, the number of prescriptions for paroxetine in the United States increased by 3%.

And yet, in March 2017 we still have doctors in Australia prescribing SSRIs to children under 18 years of age.

I wouldn't be taking them at any age.

GlaxoSmithKline has survived, is listed on the UK stock exchange, 97,000 employees worked there in 2015, and it looks like business as usual.

Carry on chaps.

I've only cited one example of many situations in this industry.

I'll leave it up to you to Google some more.

Stories like this are thick on the ground, but you have to be interested enough in life to search out the information and get informed.

Castle Randomised Control Trials (RCTs).

Covered in The Trojan Horse, chapter 6.

There's a large moat around this castle.

Castle Stock Exchange

The place which is motivated by profits and dividends.

And if you can do that without building up too much capital and leaving yourself open to a takeover even better.

Don't expect the drug companies, medical administration companies, medical servicing companies or medical training companies to overhaul the system.

That is not their job.

If you think it is, you're living in fairyland.

How many CEOs have you ever seen go to jail for gross negligence, misleading the public, misleading their employees, knowingly producing harmful products, etc?

How many CEOs have you ever seen take a profit hit because they fessed up to one of their products being faulty or dangerous and needed to be taken off the market?

About as many as I have.

This industry has taught me more than I wish to know. There are ethical ways of being prosperous and unethical ways of being prosperous.

Does your superannuation fund own shares in these companies? As I've said before, if you own shares in a company, you have to take responsibility for their behaviour, as you are the *owner* of the company. You are responsible as an owner.

Responsibility, it's such a cow!

Castle Media

Makes its money from advertising. Drug companies, pharmaceuticals, medical procedures, over the counter medicines and supplementation are all advertised in the media outlets and platforms.

Most clued up countries do not allow this advertising directly to the public. Of course Australia's media is biased because they are aligned with these interested parties, who make them profitable.

You are a media company and you're going to criticise a drug or a drug company that is bringing in income? No, duh.

Media companies are listed on the stock market: it's all about profitability.

And if you think the ABC and SBS are unbiased you are naive. They tow the party line for whatever government is in often enough. There are examples of journalists and programs that have been adversely affected when they expose the truth. It's risky. And there have been stories pulled before they aired too.

Castle Charities, Foundations and Community Groups

Watching the growth in their power base? And the amount of government funding they are receiving?

I'm most interested in the fact that they seem to be allowed to promote off-label prescribing.

On their websites, in the media – even during the news.

Through incorrect information, badly maintained medical factsheets, respected boards and brands, and selected spokespeople.

Castle Health Insurance

Yeah, some of them are listed companies too – how can that be good for your health?

And why don't more health insurance schemes give incentives for preventative medicine? Either they're thick, or they don't actually know how to keep their clients healthy. Either option isn't too pretty.

Castle Moats

Any technique or barrier used to protect the castles.

Endless candidates for moats include lies, fraud, incentives, dodgy RCTs, delaying tactics, not noticing, bribery, free conferences at exotic locations, special speaker engagements with high fees, promotions to boards of foundations ... you get the drift.

KPIs to follow, foundations and charities, tax deductible foundations and charities – even better.

The Wicked Queen

AKA the narcissist who looks at her Facebook image 6 times a day to check she's still "hot as"/the fairest of them all.

A very long while later the Wicked Queen heard of Snow White's trip to the forest.

Because it takes a long while for the established government to work out what is actually happening on the ground.

Years and years, even decades.

Then came years of thorough investigations, draft policy statements, calls for input from all highly qualified but not-so-bright-nor-practical professors and expert stakeholders (read vested interests), and add 4 years, impact studies, ground breaking policy reviews (but never a Royal Commission or anything that might have teeth), and then finally 'harmonization' between the states of Australia, She came up with the fully watered down and politically correct idea that Snow White had a problem - even though by now she didn't.

A newly formed and totally independent (ahem, ahem) National Snow White Foundation would draft Australian best practice guidelines and decide what to do, within the next 5 years, or so...

Aimed at preventing the mental health issue known as "tripping in the bush" for all international traders that take cocaine on night shift.

When the Australian National Harmonized Mental Health Act 2021 came into being it seemed to be a lot more broad brush that was originally intended. And a lot more people seem to now suffer from the mental health condition now known as Amorous Bushification DSM VIII.

And if you don't like that, you might have Female Sexual Dysfunction Psychiatric Disorder DSM V (yeah, that's a real one).

Hopefully other doctors will make that connection too.

But we would never notice off-label prescribing, of course. Well, not for another 40 years.

In the mean time, carry on.

The fine, if you are ever actually found guilty, will look nasty, maybe even billions – but promises to be proportionally small compared with how much you can make in the mean time.

The CEOs of the companies will never be jailed, and the shareholders (you?) won't complain because there was a 3% uplift in the share price last week. And who knows what companies my super fund or investment policy is investing in.

As far as turning up and asking questions at the AGM? You're kidding, right!

You'd rather get that horrible Amorous Bushification than do that.

(Are they working on Disruptive Dysfunction Psychiatric Disorder while we speak, or is that included in ADHD?)

Or the *Unqualified* Disruptive Dysfunction Psychiatric Disorder, which is far far worse, because they haven't had years of university training to eradicate all that, and come to their senses and fake KPIs.

Not *indoctrinated*? Funny word that.

Yep, I've got Unqualified Disruptive Dysfunction Psychiatric Disorder. Proudly.

Let's hope it's contagious.

The Glass Case

The dwarfs placed Snow White in a glass case and kept her there to stare at her and wonder at her beauty and now, totally agreeable nature.

She had gone from having some serious attitude to being a pussy cat (they didn't know about pink pussy hats back then).

And that was clearly a good thing.

So drug-fogged nothing would permeate through the glass case.

She was no longer making any trouble at all.

Very Snow White.

The Handsome Prince

He'll have to be more than handsome to crack through Snow White's glass case. Most nice guys would steer well clear of her. Maybe it was the money.

As fairy tales happen he smashed the glass, kissed her with enough tonsil work and suction to cause an air pocket that dislodged her schedule 8 Xanax tablet, and continued with a very slow withdrawal over more than 6 months.

A lot more, actually.

Otherwise she would have been really psycho Snow Bite with a very bad case of akathisia.

When she finally came up for air she changed her Facebook status immediately to "in a relationship" before he had time to get away.

The Poisoned Apple

Look closer on the apple's brand name sticker.

The poisoned apple might be any benzo or antidepressant that increases suicide rates or suicidal ideation, puts you into a deep sleep emotionally, causes addiction, results in permanent health problems, breaks up relationships and/or significantly impairs your life.

Or any of the 50 or so "chapter 9 or 10 side-effects".

CHAPTER 20

A Royal Commission with Broad-Ranging Terms of Reference.

Well by now you would see it.
But what will we do about it? And what is YOUR part in it?
We have a fundamentally broken sleep and mental health system that needs a complete overhaul, with no one with the intestinal fortitude to do anything about it.

Corruption and ignorance goes to the very top of government, all through the medical system, every so-called clinical governance body and member, to the listings on the MBS and PBS, the listed companies on the stock market, and finally best practice guidelines which are ... well, worst practice.

If death, suicide and permanent disabilities aren't your predilection.

The pack of cards is falling already, but unfortunately it is taking far too long, and too many lives are being lost or screwed over in the mean time.

Just last month, April 2017, GSK was successfully sued for $ 3 million in the case Dolin vs. GSK when Wendy Dolin successfully claimed that her husband Stewart's suicide death was attributable to taking the generic version of the antidepressant Paxil[1].

This case opens up opportunities for others, and at least informs the public who are watching that evidence exists of real harm and suicide. And proved in the US courts.

Anyone that would like to look further into the story might like to read the transcript of an interview with Wendy Dolin after the case was decided[2], and some background information on NBC Chicago before the case was decided in her favour[3].

During the case, the plaintiff's law firm Baum Headland presented *Plaintiff's Exhibit 347*: an exhibit where each picture depicts a real person who committed suicide while taking Paxil in a GSK clinical trial. The red "Vs" on the exhibit mean their specific suicides were violent in nature. There were multiple suicides using firearms, including a murder suicide by one patient. There were also two deaths from people jumping in front of trains. To see the document which contains a blackened portrait of 22 deaths, 16 of which were violent, see reference 4 for this chapter[4].

You might remember our previous discussions of the information shown on the Beyond Blue and Headspace websites that deny any suicide occurred during a clinical trial. There were 22 deaths in that one trial alone.

Institutional Corruption and Pharmaceutical Policy
Limitation to the Powers of a Royal Commission
There is an unfortunate limitation to the powers of a royal commission which was brought to my attention during Elizabeth Broderick's investigation into sex abuse in the military: its inability to hold individual perpetrators to account and to bring criminal charges to the offending people[5].

But let's have the Royal Commission just to see exactly what the dark forces are, and where they are housed.

By now I'm confident you will have a very good idea about exactly who some of those groups and people may be.

The royal commission into sex abuse in the military was not pursued by Defence Minister Marise Payne with one reason being that it could retraumatise victims[6].

I still believe this royal commission should proceed, because deaths and traumas continue to grow while the royal commission is not conducted.

Pharmaceutical Benefits Scheme (PBS)
A full and thorough investigation of the PBS should definitely be included in the royal commission.

Started in Australia in 1948 with free medicines for pensioners and 139 medicines available for other members in the community, it has gone through numerous policy changes and reforms since 1948, and now includes

793 medicines in 2,066 forms and dosages, sold as more than 5,300 differently branded items[7].

If it's anything like the MBS which was investigated in the Four Corners' *Wasted* program it will be a similar debacle.

Our Part in This

It leaves YOU and I no option but to buck the system in the mean time.

We (and YOU) have to refuse the solutions that the system is erroneously presenting you and your family so that at least you survive to figure out another way.

And after reading this book you know who to quote and where to get your information from.

Part Three: Sleep Mojo. You've Lost It, Now Get It Back.

Important Note for Part Three.

I have included some alternative solutions in part three that may or may not be evidence-based.

I'm confident that some methodologies, such as Emotional Freedom Technique (EFT), will change people's perceptions about how they think and why they might think in a particular way.

Exploring new non-drug methodologies enables people to step outside their predicament and form new ways of thinking around their problems and mental habits.

It also opens up learning pathways between mind-body connections that are now being seen and discussed in neuroscience.

The mind-body connection has been discussed for decades in alternative health and I believe it has validity, especially in the areas of sleep and mental health.

Most importantly these inclusions encourage people to take full responsibility for how they think and why they think in a particular way – which is a very important part of the healing process.

Meditation has been practiced for centuries, EFT has been around since the 1980s and music therapy is now reasonably well accepted by the mainstream. For people who have been watching the developments and efficacy of some of these techniques for decades they are soooo *yesterdays news*.

If you are going to go to an alternative healer, ensure that you pick only the best ones, and ones with years of experience. We need the combination of learning and wisdom through years of practice. You might start by reading very good books and doing quality research to see if the techniques suit you.

I'm having some challenges leaving out the more edgy and creative new stuff – but I don't want to bring on "Chapter 5 incidences" around the main messages in this book.

It's a double edged sword.

CHAPTER 21

The 10 Insomnia Types.

Why Bother Sleeping?

Lack of sleep:

- Has been associated with the following **physical health problems**: obesity, coronary heart disease, diabetes, impaired immune function, reduced grey matter in the brain and inflammation,
- Exacerbates **mental health problems** such as depression, all anxieties (including OCD etc), and stress, and
- Increases the likelihood of **accidents and errors** and involuntarily falling asleep – at work, in cars, working machinery, doing school exams, playing sport, competing in the Olympics and elite sports, etc.
- **Increases risk taking behaviours**, the probability of eating junk food, and **substance abuse** (nicotine, drugs and alcohol).

What Happens While We Sleep?

Our brains use more oxygen at certain stages of sleep than when we are awake. While we sleep we dream vividly and deeply, integrate spatial and long term memories, break down fats, make sense of the day, connect memory pathways, heal, recover, get restorative sleep, rest our bodies and parts of our brain, release hormones including growth hormones, grow, anabolically build tissue, clear toxins, regulate our immune system and regulate reproduction and sexual arousal.

The organ of the body most affected by lack of sleep is the brain, specifically what is called the "executive function". The brain is regarded as the most important organ of the body because that's where the instructions are controlled. Executive function includes working memory, task switching, planning, the ability to focus, attention span, decision making ability, verbal reasoning, mental flexibility, and making sense of things.

Frankly, if you don't sleep you become uncoordinated, anxious and stupid. Your mental health is challenged and you're prone to risk taking behaviour and substance abuse. Also you're more likely to become fat and die earlier of one of a number of serious diseases such as heart disease or cancer.

For more information about sleep and it's affect on your happiness and performance refer to Appendix 1 *Fatigue and Mental Health: Bedroom to Boardroom*, Appendix 2 *The Case for Sleep Education*, and Appendix 4 *Executive Function Report*.

Insomnia Types

There are at least 52 types of insomnia. They range from simple restlessness to the "fatal familial," an apparent genetic disorder that affects about two families in the world who can actually die from insomnia.

I have simplified the information as much as possible to make the types understandable and, more importantly, to provide practical and successful strategies and solutions by type.

I've devised 10 Insomnia Types, Type A to Type J, and suggest solutions matched to each insomnia type.

So, What's YOUR Insomnia Type?

TYPE A: Difficulty Getting to Sleep
TYPE B: Difficulty Staying Asleep
TYPE C: Waking Too Early in the Morning
TYPE D: Drugs, Food Additives, Food Colourings, etc.
TYPE E: Varying Sleep Times (circadian rhythm disruption, shift-work, jet-lag, etc.)
TYPE F: Muscles, Restless Leg Syndrome etc.

TYPE G: Illness and/or Pain (including sleep apnea, fibromyalgia, tinnitus and Meniere's Disease)

TYPE H: Mind Games (depression, anxiety, stress etc.)

TYPE I: Environment (snoring bed partners, overheating in bed, over-
stimulation, living next to the train track, etc.)

TYPE J: Decisions, Decisions (mortgages, relationships etc.)

Yes, you might suffer from more than one type of insomnia at a time. Once
you have identified which types apply to you, you will be equipped to decide
the best, most logical order in which to deal with them. Sometimes, by
dealing with one, the others will resolve at the same time.

CHAPTER 22

Why Natural?

We've talked about how insomnia is just the warning system our body is giving us, and how there are many underlying factors that contribute to insomnia.

The main problem with sleeping pills and psycho drugs, even as a short-term fix, is that they **never** treat the underlying cause of insomnia.

In this Part 3 we'll be talking about how you can start to solve your sleeping problems.

And thereby improve your attitude, productivity, mood and mental health.

Why Natural?

Because it works, and it is the best option you've got.

Natural IS evidence-based.

CHAPTER 23

Natural Solutions for Everyone.

There are some natural solutions that are applicable for most insomnia types. I say most, because occasionally I'll receive emails from people whose physical limitations keep them from being able to perform most exercise. I won't delve into all these possibilities, but if you have physical limitations, please do your best to find satisfactory alternatives to the suggestions.

The most important thing to remember in this chapter is that each healthy habit or emotionally balanced state you can cultivate will help you sleep better.

Exercise and Sun

I recommend walking for 45 minutes or more, at least 4 times a week, preferably in the morning. There is clinical evidence that supports exercise to reduce stress, anxiety and depression, which in turn aids sleep.

More exercise is fine, of course (within reason)!

I say "within reason" because I observe quite a few people using exercise beyond a healthy point. Exercise for some people has become an obsession, part of a new anxiety and a bit OCD. Hopefully you will know if you are one of these types. If the thought of NOT exercising for 4 days stresses you then you could be a candidate. The cases I'm talking about are usually accompanied with anxiety issues. Perhaps turning to Tai Chi or yoga from running might help you redirect that energy over time. I see excessive running as "running away from yourself" when I observe it in some people.

Sunlight, particularly at the start of the day, will actually help you wake up and will cultivate a good mood as you walk.

Enjoy the warmth and light that the sunlight brings to your day and attitude.

And enjoy the vitamin D from the sun, which helps as well.

Stress Relief

Stress relief is vital to good sleep. Please refer to the Stress Relief section in Chapter 31, Type H, Mind Games.

You and Your Pleasure

"Having a life" is a very important part of sleeping well. Neglecting time for yourself and your fun can affect your health and attitude substantially. Neglect over a long period can lead to larger issues, such as sickness or relationship problems.

This is particularly relevant to parents of many children or professionals who bury themselves in work!

I know some people who don't even *know* what they enjoy, and this can be a problem. Was your life designed by someone else?

Be cautious; it's not difficult to allow parents, a spouse, social or professional expectations, or the bank mortgage to start dictating whether you have the luxury of recreation.

Don't allow it to happen!

Eating Real Foods

Eating well is important, but the world is a little more complicated than you might think here. Many who assume they know about "real foods" are under misconceptions. To someone with intolerance to salicylates and/or amines, even some raw fruit and fresh vegetables can contain substances that are not good for deep sleep.

Read labels intelligently, and learn what the labels aren't required to show you. Learn all the different ways manufacturers and suppliers can hide nasty additives. For example, the 5% labelling loophole in Australia allows the inclusion of additives without declaring them on labels, provided they only amount to 5% or less of the content of the product.

We'll go deeper in Chapter 27, Drugs, Food Additives and Chemicals.

Hydration

Hydration is a part of overall good health, and certainly does affect sleep. Plain water is ideal for hydration. Bear in mind to hydrate earlier in the day; too many fluids right before bed can inhibit sleep for obvious reasons!

Avoid Fried Foods

Avoiding fried foods and trans-fats is especially important if you are waking up too early in the morning. I have read that fried foods get metabolized faster than omega-3 in our diet, diminishing the production of helpful long-string fatty acids in our body.

Dump the Duvet/Doona

Overheating in bed reduces your REM (rapid eye movement) sleep. Heavy bed coverings can keep you from getting your best night's sleep. For more on sleeping cool, watch a short video I put together some time ago.[1]

Using several lighter blankets is an ideal way to control your sleeping temperature. The trouble with a doona/duvet is it is either "all on" or "all off"—if you're too hot, you can't just peel back one layer of blanket. Using blankets instead, preferably natural fibers like pure merino wool, alpaca, or cotton waffle fabric, will help you stay just the right temperature throughout the night. The *first thing* I do when I can't sleep is remove a blanket and cool myself down. Try it!

For more information see Chapter 32 – Type I: Environment.

"Slow Time"

Especially if your recreation of choice is something active (or mentally active, such as internet browsing or playing video games), be sure to make time daily for "slow time." This could include reading for pleasure, listening to music, meditating, walking in nature or practicing Tai Chi or yoga. Any disruption to the cycle of stress and activity will help develop a more balanced lifestyle and a more relaxed, effective mental attitude.

This relaxation period could also include anything that aligns left and right brain, such as the 'Cooks Hookup' exercise.[2]

Your Strategic Life

Be vigilant about your life, your purpose, your contribution, your friends, your relationships, your health, and your attitude. By continually assessing all aspects of your life, you can recognise problems early and therefore avoid many root causes of pain, insomnia, breakup or breakdown.

Procrastination and avoidance will never solve problems. We have to face and embrace life, one way or another! Every day of our lives has challenges. We should recognize and make decisions today about the immediate issues. By keeping your mind in the present moment, you can not only be more effective at solving problems, but also avoid the stress associated with your mind drifting to situations in the past or future that are beyond your current control.

I've even read recently that couples that have arguments are more likely to survive. So get things off your chest without being vindictive. And not in front of the kids mostly: they need to learn reality but not if it gets nasty – it will add to their anxieties. Unfortunately some parents don't know when they cross the line.

Caffeine

I don't mean to be derogatory by including this oh-so-obvious solution. Don't just cut down on caffeine - perhaps take it out of your diet completely if you are overstimulated, nervy and can't relax or sleep.

In Chapter 27 you'll find more information about stimulants.

CHAPTER 24

Type A: Difficulty Falling Asleep.

"Difficulty falling asleep" includes the following types of situations:

- Being mentally over-active in general when you want to be falling asleep,
- Lying in bed, unable to "switch off",
- Being anxious or worried about something that stops you from falling asleep,
- Being nervous or jittery and unable to relax,
- Playing the day over and over mentally, pondering how you might have done certain things differently, worrying about what you have said, etc.,
- For those who work with detail all day, still thinking that way when trying to go to sleep (This includes what I call 'nerd-brain' for those of us who work late with computers and/or detailed technical material with a lot of variables and considerations). Just because you have closed down all those tabs doesn't mean your brain switched off like that too – it will still be processing,
- Not feeling tired when going to bed, inhibiting sleep.

If pain or sickness is keeping you awake, Chapter 30 covers more information to help your specific problem. Likewise, if you can't sleep because of Restless Leg Syndrome (RLS) or muscle tension, more information can be found in Chapter 29.

The good news about Type A is that in many cases, it's the easiest type to fix.

I'm going to discuss a lot of solutions here, in two groups:

Group A1 for easier, less stubborn cases, and
Group A2 for more stubborn cases.

GROUP A1: For Less-Stubborn Cases

- Have a definite end to your "questing" day. For example, decide that, from the time you arrive home from work, you are finished for the day. Do some reading, cook, go for a walk, or hang out with the kids. Avoid extending your day with more and more things to accomplish—kids aren't the only ones meant to have some play-time every day! And for their best development, playing with you is awesome.
- Set aside at least an hour of quality, relaxing YOU time every day.
- Investigate all food additives in your diet that might be associated with restlessness, insomnia, nervousness, anxiety, or ADHD. Refer to Chapter 27 – Type D for help with this.
- Avoid eating large meals late at night. Your body should be finished digesting by the time you "switch off" for the night.
- Don't play computer games, watch violent TV programs, or spend time on the computer for 2 hours before bed. No weirdoes, murderers, mind benders, sex offenders or psycho cases for several hours before bed. Do something low key or even boring instead, like polish your shoes (!), knitting, have a bath, light reading, review your goals book, sew that button on, read the kids a bedtime story, or listen to classical music.
- If you're an overachiever, try underachieving for a change. Many people get some of their most creative ideas when they're not working, but relaxing and having fun.
- Turn the lights down in the house as early as reasonable. Bright lights, particularly the blue light emitted from computers, inhibit the production of melatonin, which is necessary for sleep. At about 8:30 PM or so, start turning all the lights down or off, replacing them with lamps. Very eco-friendly, and will save money too.

- Sleep cool, not hot. Don't get into a warmed bed (we'll talk about this more in chapter 32, Type I). Sleep as cool as is still comfortable, without being cold.
- Parents, kids need some slow time before bed, too. Encourage some slower habits for evenings early in life, and they will serve your children in later years, as well!
- Don't forget all the suggestions from Chapter 23 – exercise, hydration, and so on.
- If you just feel you need some "soft options" look in Chapter 35. Many of the commonly known remedies that are useful in less-stubborn cases can be found there!

Group A2: For More Stubborn Cases

For more stubborn issues we have to re-train our brains into a new pattern.

Repeating a strategy over and over will help to re-pattern your mind to accept that you are serious about sleeping well every night. For example, playing relaxing music just for one night might not solve the problem that night, but repeated over some time will make a difference.

Similarly with a more healthy diet. There is not a lot of use cutting out a particular food item for a few days only, when you really need to make healthy eating your new lifestyle.

- Investigate each of the 50+ food additives, colourings and flavourings that are associated with insomnia, stress, anxiety, panic, depression, night waking, and other problems. It is very possible that intolerance to MSG, benzoates, synthetic and natural colours, or even naturally occurring salicylates and amines could be keeping you awake at night. Investigate them on the Food Intolerance Network's website http://www.FedUp.com.au.
- Listen to some sleep hypnosis cycles every night before bed, or actually when you are in bed (downloaded to your phone, mp3 player or device). My pick of audios that have been tested by customers are by Glenn Harrold.

- Utilize Cook's Hook-Up Exercise to balance your left and right brain activity.[1] (More in chapter 35.)
- Devise a special fall-asleep music playlist for yourself and keep it beside your bed permanently.
- Implement Cognitive Behavioural Therapy for Anxiety. (Explained in Chapter 31— Type H: Mind Games.)
- Use micro-movements to reduce stress and anxiety. If there is a part of your body that is stressed or hurting when you are falling off to sleep, move it just a few millimetres (no more), then make that exact movement with the other side of your body. Make the movement in the same direction if you have a difficulty with anxiety, but if not, you can do mirror movements. (Mirror movements, for example, would be moving your right hand a couple of millimetres towards your navel, and then move your left hand a couple of millimetres towards your navel. If you have anxiety issues, move your left hand a couple of millimetres away from your navel, in the same direction as you moved your right hand.) These micro-movements are a form of physical meditation, and help you relax at a deep level.
- Do a guided meditation, yoga exercise or complete relaxation.
- Use an alpha or theta metronome sound to force your brainwaves to a new pattern (brain entrainment).
- Use Thought Field Therapy to balance energy in your body.
- Take up journaling. Write down the things that are keeping you awake. Keep writing until the things you are writing about 'release their charge' on you. Keep a special sleep journal and pen beside your bed. The book has 2 covers, front and back. One way in the book is for journaling, front-to-back. The reverse way (back-to-front) is to write down good ideas and inspiring thoughts you get during the night, things to do tomorrow, what you've forgotten, etc. This way you don't have to get out of bed.
- Use Emotional Freedom Technique/Tapping (EFT) to reduce your anxiety or stress.
- Perform *Tap O' the Mornin'- EFT* with Brad Yates on YouTube[2] in the morning to feel better.

- Have a blood test to ensure you don't have a deficiency, irregularity, or health issue, such as anemia.
- Listen to your intuition. If something is absolutely aggravating, it needs to be acted upon. Mindmap the problem and then mindmap the solution. Google "Tony Buzan Mindmap" to find information on the subject if you don't know about mind-mapping.
- If you think your problem relates to a major decision or decisions that should be made in your life, refer to Chapter 33, Type J, Decisions, Decisions.

Still Not Happening for You? Here Are Some Further Suggestions:

- If you think your problem relates to depression and/or grief or anxiety, refer to Chapters 31, 9 and 10.
- Spend some one-on-one time with an expert counsellor to understand any unresolved issues in your life. Some of them can date back for years, even decades. I'm recommending talk therapies, not someone who will prescribe medications.
- An expert healer, therapist, kinesiologist or similar could help you go beyond old subconscious patterning. Talk therapies are preferred modalities for unresolved issues, because you are going to get the opportunity to open up in a supportive environment. Talk therapies alone can heal emotional issues. If they are performed by an experienced practitioner, the process is not traumatic, doesn't always require you to dredge through a whole lot of ugly stuff, and the solutions often come from left field. If you get release and relief it is worth it.
- Ensure that you are doing adequate exercise. Exercise alone can help many people move beyond sleep and mental health issues. It can include just regular walking for 40 minutes, 4 times a week.
- Psychologists, psychotherapists, counsellors and other practitioners are appropriate for moving beyond limiting beliefs and old patterns. A word of warning though, if you find you now have a new and long career visiting these people, it's time to look for a new

practitioner. And if you come out of sessions feeling worse about things than when you went in, it's time to move on, too. I've seen a lot of people who continue to have no resolution around certain issues in their lives, and/or the process takes them to hell and back. That may have been the system 40 years ago, but technology has moved on from that!

- Neuro Linguistic Program (NLP) is being used successfully to re-pattern old beliefs. If you are going to have an NLP practitioner help you, choose an expert. Check out their experience, not just their qualifications. Seems like I've met hundreds who have been to a couple of weekend seminars and now think they can solve anything for anyone. Sorry, but! And that advice goes for all practitioners that you trust your personal experiences and attitudes/beliefs to.

- One more thing. Hypnosis is effective for many people, but not everyone. And sometimes it may be "treating the symptom" but not addressing the underlying issue.

Making Decisions to Solve Problems

Some problems turn into mental masturbations because no decision is ever made and no change ever occurs. I've seen people dithering in the wrong job for years – it's always going to be next month, or after some milestone – and 5 years later they are still complaining about their crappy job.

Sometimes you deserve it if you can't activate and start having inter-views etc.

Procrastination is common and pretty deadly (and for the friends around you who have to listen to your story on repeat). Sorry, but. See Type J, chapter 33.

Most problems that are holding us back do NOT make sense. In fact most of them are in our subconscious mind – if we could pull them all out of there and see them face-to-face, we would realize that! Our subconscious minds (neurology, body, attitudes, motivators) cope as well as they can by making new pathways, new strategies, new beliefs and many become new habits. These new pathways, beliefs, etc. may or may not be helpful in the long run. Sometimes it is as simple as deciding that what happened in the past is just a memory, and that you aren't going to live your life based on that "ugly thing" anymore. Or you might write down a list of positive things you learned from it.

More often, however, it is good to seek gentle professional help to re-pattern unhelpful thoughts and habits. It is absolutely possible, and there are many qualified experts who can help you.

Learning to Relax

In this chapter, I have discussed using relaxation cycles, holosync/paraliminal audios, brain entrainment (using alpha and theta metronomes), and hypnotherapy to help you relax and fall asleep. If you have never used these techniques before, I suggest you start with a *guided* relaxation meditation where someone talks you through slow breathing, relaxing your body, etc., as it can take a little bit of practice.

When you start, you might find it a bit aggravating – that is quite common with a lot of people, because they haven't felt the benefits of relaxation and meditation like this. Please persist! Choose a particular time and place each day, and continue to push through. Make a daily habit of it. If you do, your mind will eventually get to the point of "not this again!" and, because it knows that resistance is not working, it will eventually yield! It is the same process as breaking any habit, really. When you eventually feel the clarity, refreshment and relaxation, you won't need convincing any more, and it will be like your own 'daily spa time'. Good luck!

Here are a few specific examples. For more information on music and sounds please see the Music and Sounds section in Chapter 35. Load them into your mp3 player and phone and you'll always have them with you – on public transport to work, at lunchtime, etc.

Of course, *don't use them while driving, doing things or operating machinery!*

Here are some suggested CDs/Audios:

Complete Relaxation, Hypnotherapy by Glenn Harrold
A Chakra Meditation, Hypnotherapy by Glenn Harrold
Deep Sleep Every Night, Hypnotherapy by Glenn Harrold

SLEEP DOJO - Type A

1. Ascertain if your problem is simply an overactive mind by implementing the steps in Group A1 above.
2. If falling asleep is still challenging to you, try the solutions listed in Group A2
3. If you are still having difficulties, investigate deeper reasons for your problem. My suggestion here is to visit an experienced psychotherapist, talk therapist, psychologist, counsellor or kinesiologist. There are other appropriate modalities. This decision is yours.

CHAPTER 25

Type B: Difficulty Staying Asleep.

This type of insomnia includes the following situations:

- Restless, light, and broken sleep
- Frequent waking
- Waking up during the night, unable to get back to sleep
- Waking up in the morning feeling exhausted, like you haven't slept properly
- Tossing and turning
- Anxiety and worry in the middle of the night.

Our brains cycle through different types and depths of sleep while we are asleep every night. The types of sleep include short wave sleep, REM (rapid eye movement) sleep, and slow wave sleep. There are also short periods of waking up that most people don't notice because they cycle down into deeper sleep shortly after the momentary wake up periods. However, if you disturb your subtle cycles (with alcohol and drugs for example), you can wake up totally during one of those short waking periods and find it difficult to go back to sleep. Sleep is a subtle thing and needs to be respected as such.

Difficulty staying asleep is associated with a number of problems, many of which are covered in-depth elsewhere in this book. Here are some general ideas about what might be causing Type B insomnia:

1. **Excessive alcohol consumption.** Consuming more than 2 standard drinks of alcohol at night can disturb your healthy sleep brain-wave

patterns. If you drink excessive amounts, you could wake up, wide awake, after a few hours. This is one of the body's direct responses to excessive alcohol consumption.

2. **Use of drugs, prescribed or otherwise.** More on this in chapters 27, 9 and 10.

3. **Food additives, colourings, etc.** There are over 50 food additives and colourings that are associated with sleep difficulties. Some additives and chemical problems are well-documented (such as MSG), but many are not. Some offending substances include natural colourings and naturally-occurring substances that are found in fresh fruit and vegetables and slow cooked food. See Chapter 27.

4. **Sleep apnea.** If you suspect you have sleep apnea for any reason, have a professional diagnosis. Read the sleep apnea section of Chapter 30 before asking your doctor for a referral to a sleep clinic for testing. Chapters 27 and 30 also mention the food additives and chemicals that have been associated with breathing problem symptoms that look like sleep apnea.

5. **Anxiety.** Refer to the anxiety section of Chapter 31.

6. **Depression.** Refer to the depression section of Chapter 31 and the additives information in Chapter 27 and Chapter 10.

7. **Compulsions.** Some methods to investigate for solutions include:
   - Cognitive Behavioural Therapy
   - Emotional Freedom Technique (EFT) and Thought Field Therapy (TFT).
   - Refer to chapters 9, 10 and 27.

8. **Emotional Imbalance.** Worried? Annoyed? Guilty? Ashamed? Stressed? Even excitement can wake you up at night. For emotional imbalances, investigate the following:
   - Visit an advanced kinesiologist for a one-on-one session
   - Emotional Freedom Technique (EFT) and Thought Field Therapy (TFT)

9. **Blood Sugar Level Drop.** Some people wake up because their blood sugar levels have dropped. If this happens to you, then have a boiled egg before you go to sleep, instead of sugary sweets. (Any lean, small piece of protein should do the trick.)

What Time Are You Waking Up?

Over 5,000 years ago, the ancient Chinese discovered a subtle energy in the body which can't be detected with our normal senses, one that is still not recognized by many modern medicines and sciences. The energy has been studied in yin/yang terms (feminine and masculine energies, and directional flow), as well as the 12-14 meridian systems that connect the energy flow to certain organs and functions of the body.

Most people call this energy Ch'i.

With the development of integrative and alternative medicines and mind-body connection, the information known about these energy systems (called meridians) has been extended in many ways into a range of natural health modalities, including Emotional Freedom Technique (EFT), Thought Field Therapy (TFT), general Energy Tapping, acupressure, acupuncture, etc.

If you have investigated most solutions provided in this book, and are still at odds with what might be the underlying emotion that is causing your body to "wake you up" it might be helpful to observe *what time you are waking up* during the night, and what emotion and/or condition relates to that waking up time in the Chinese meridian system.

The Chinese meridian system has a time dimension to it. There are 12 two-hour periods during a 24-hour day that relate to specific organs/meridians and their associated emotions.

Observe what time you are waking up, and what emotion is related to that time.

You may feel anxious, but what exactly are you anxious about? What sort of anxious are you?

Anxious because you want to do a really good job? Anxious every time you are around certain people, or if you have to make a speech? Anxious leaving the house, thinking you have left the gas on? Anxious with certain triggers? Anxious after a loved one died and you can't get rid of all the stuff in the house? Anxious about change?

This diagnostic method is a departure but could be helpful in finding underlying issues that are causing your symptom of insomnia and mental health issues. There are 12 times zones of 2 hours each and include liver, lungs, large intestine, stomach, spleen, heart, small intestine, bladder, kidneys, circulation/sex, triple warmer and gall bladder. Each time zone relates to a range of emotions. E.g. 11 pm to 1 am is gall bladder time on the Chinese clock and relates to negativity, gall, bitterness, constant sadness, anger, hasty decisions, etc.

No, you won't find this in Cochrane – sometimes we have to look at *emotions and feelings* and try to recognise what they are first, and then try to see where they come from, in order to move through them and beyond them.

A competent counsellor or healthcare professional will be able to help you look further into these challenging thought patterns.

But do some homework first, by yourself, to hone in on how you are actually thinking, and what can trigger you, etc. Write down your thoughts and emotions, and any further thoughts that come later.

More in chapter 31.

SLEEP DOJO - Type B

1. Write down a list of the emotions, triggers and possible history of your worrying thoughts.
2. Write down the factors that could be leading to your difficulty staying asleep.
3. Investigate each possibility one by one.
4. Keep a notebook and pen by your bed to write down your thoughts when you wake up in the night. Write down any problems you are having, any worries that have woken you up, anything that you need to put in your diary, anxious feelings, etc. Then address them the next day. Problems always seem far worse in the middle of the night. You might also write down something(s) that you intend to do tomorrow to help solve the problem. That gets it out of your head and on to the paper so you can forget it for now and relax again to go to sleep.
5. If anxiety and panic issues, depression, or obsessive-compulsive disorder are factors, please refer to Chapter 31 and the solutions listed separately for those problems.

CHAPTER 26

Type C: Waking Too Early in the Morning

A t least 80 percent of depressed people experience insomnia. They have difficulty falling asleep, and more often staying asleep and/or waking too early in the morning.

In fact, early-morning awakening is a virtual give-away of depression. Fifteen percent of depressed people sleep excessively. Some think that early waking is more than just a symptom of depression, it may in fact unleash the mood disorder and/or be an early indicator of it[1].

You already know that if you are feeling low you should be looking for counselling help, psychotherapy, Cognitive Behavioural Therapy, exercise, support groups and the like.

Trying to tough it out by yourself is not the best option; but don't let your friends talk you into inappropriate drug therapies either.

Work with a supportive professional to establish the underlying reasons for your depression and unmet expectations.

And you should also be reviewing the side effects of any medications and foods, food additives and lifestyle choices that you are currently making.

It's all about the underlying reasons for depression.

Remember that depression is a symptom, not the root cause.

SLEEP DOJO - Type C

1. Consider depression and grief as possible causes for your insomnia. Refer to Chapter 31.
2. Research any recreational drugs you are taking, including alcohol.

3. Look at the side effects of your existing prescription medications for indicators of depression. Look up your medications on the www. rxisk.org website.

4. Exercise for an hour a day, 4 days a week. Walking is fine, it doesn't have to be punishing – in fact it's time to look after yourself.

5. Get professional counselling help urgently if your depression or grief is getting on top of you. Early action is preferred. You'll feel better having someone on your team to help you.

6. Tell your partner/friends/family that you are not going well and ask them for appropriate help and support.

7. Go to chapter 31 (then 9 and 10 if you missed them).

CHAPTER 27

Type D: Drugs, Food Additives and Chemicals

Type D includes a number of reasons why you might not be getting your best night's sleep:

- There are over 50 food additives, colourings, chemicals and substances which adversely affect sleep. The inability to fall asleep, restlessness, sleep disturbance, anxiety, panic, depression, sleep apnea, snoring, ADHD (Attention Deficit Hyperactivity Disorder), restless legs ('the jumps'), weird dreams, nightmares, night terrors, headaches and migraines, premenstrual symptoms, sleep walking, sleep talking, irritability, oppositional defiance, mood swings, breathing difficulties, itching, chronic stuffy and runny nose, heart palpitations, hot flushes/flashes, even bedwetting, head banging and seizures[1].
- Insomnia, depression, anxiety, restless sleep and other sleep symptoms are the side effect of a number of prescription drugs. You will have to check the drugs you are taking to see if and how they affect your sleep, anxiety, depression, etc.
- Insomnia and other sleep symptoms are the side effect of many non-prescription and recreational drugs, including alcohol.
- Salicylates are natural food substances that effect sleep. They are contained in fresh fruit and vegetables, dried fruits (e.g. sultanas), honey, and some multivitamins (citrus bioflavonoids and concentrated fruit flavour). Salicylates can be inhaled as well, especially through flowery smells and pine smells (including air fresheners), even hairsprays.

- There is one natural colour, annatto (160b) that causes as many problems as the artificial colours!
- The food and product labelling laws in each country will prevent consumers in many cases from identifying exactly what the solution to their diet problem might be.
- Cosmetics, VOCs (volatile organic compounds) such as tooth moose and lip moisturizers can cause sleep problems in some people.

So if you're saying to yourself now, "I've got a healthy diet, this chapter's not for me", think again! What is commonly perceived as a "healthy diet" might actually be keeping you awake, and eroding your health. You might also be interested to know that a UK study in 2003 (in Cheshire) indicated that two in three children responded favourably after an additive-free fortnight both at home and at school.

For information on the effects of food chemicals and food items on snoring, sleep apnea etc, please refer to the information in Chapter 30, Type G, Illness and Pain.

So, this is type D, everything that's a drug or an additive that is synthetic, and sometimes natural, that you are putting into your system.

Whether prescribed or not, we're going to have a look at it.

I want to recognize and thank Sue Dengate and her husband, Dr. Howard Dengate, again for their amazing work with food additives, chemicals and natural substances that affect our lives. Most of the information presented here is taken directly from the *Food Intolerance Network's* website[2], or from her presentation *Fed Up with Sleep Disturbance* on *Sleep with the Experts*.

List of Additives and Chemicals to Avoid for a Good Night's Sleep

Here is the list of additives to avoid as presented by Sue Dengate[3].

Colours	102, tartrazine, E102, yellow #5,104, 110 Sunset Yellow, 122, 123, 124, 127, 129, 132, 133, 142, 143,151, 155
Natural Colours	160b (annatto)

Preservatives	Sorbates200–203 Benzoates 210-213 e.g. Sodium Benzoate, E211 Sulphites 220-228 e.g. Sodium metabisulfite, sodium hydrogen sulfite E222, sodium pyrosulfite Nitrates 249-252 Propionates 280, 281, 282 Bread preservative calcium propionate, 283
Synthetic Antioxidants	310-312, 319-321e.g. BHA 320
Flavour Enhancers	Monosodium Glutamate, MSG, 621, 627 & 631. These two can boost the effectiveness of MSG up to fifteen times!
Flavours	Trade secrets! Many flavours cause problems, including mint flavouring.
Volatile Organic Compounds	Chemicals that smell at room temperature and include perfumes, furniture chemicals, air fresheners, pesticides, and building materials.
Wheat and Gluten	Sometimes refined (white) wheat flour is better than wholemeal. Yes, you read that right – it is the opposite of the conventional wisdom!
Natural Food Chemicals	Salicylates in plant foods, including fruit and vegetables. High salicylate foods to investigate further are sultanas, mint-flavoured sweets, tomato sauce, oranges, strawberries, vinegar, megavitamins with citrus bioflavonoids, and very concentrated fruit flavours. Salicylates also occur in flowery smells, pine smells, air fresheners and hairsprays. And yes, salicylates can make your reactions appear to be 'seasonal'.
Natural Amines	In protein foods, increase with age, and length of cooking. In chocolate, cheese, processed fish, bananas, vacuum-packed meats, slow-cooked foods, especially slow cooked tomato based foods.

Natural Glutamates	Cheese, tomatoes, mushrooms, stocks, sauces, meat extracts, yeast extracts Highest in tomato sauce, juices, grapes, broccoli, Vegemite, Nutella, cola drinks.

List of Sleep-Related Disorders linked with Additives, Colours, Flavours, etc.

(In alphabetical order of sleep difficulty)

Please note – individuals have different systems, intolerances, allergies, etc. Use this list as a *guide only*. Groupings give you some clues to follow. You will need to do your own research for your own particular situation. The list is not conclusive, but instead presents a starting point.

These are shared from Sue Dengate's Fed Up website and book and the *Sleep with the Experts* webinar where she was my featured expert in 2009.

ADHD and possible incorrect diagnosis	Salicylates, All listed items
Anxiety	Investigate all those listed
Babies Not Sleeping?	Calcium Propionate 282, Tartrazine colour 102, E102, yellow #5, Salicylates
Bedwetting	Calcium Propionate bread preservative 282
Depression	Calcium Propionate bread preservative 282
Difficulty Falling Asleep	MSG Monosodium Glutamate, Benzoates 210 – 213
Frequent Night Waking	Calcium Propionate 282, MSG Monosodium Glutamate, Benzoates 210 – 213, Salicylates
Headaches and Migraines	Amines in vacuum-packed meat, processed fish, cheese, etc.
Insomnia	Benzoates 210 – 213, MSG Monosodium Glutamate, 621, Calcium Propionate 282, Salicylates

Irritability	Artificial colours
Nightmares	Salicylates
Oppositional Defiance and Aggression	Salicylates
Night Terrors	Salicylates
Restless Legs, Twitching, The Jumps	Benzoates 210 – 213
Restlessness, Sleep Disturbance	Artificial colour 102, (tartrazine, E102, yellow #5)
Sleep Apnea and possible incorrect diagnosis	a1 milk (proteins), Sunset yellow (110), Calcium Propionate bread preservative 282, MSG Monosodium Glutamate 621, mattress fumes Investigate everything on the nasties list
Sleepwalking	Antioxidant BHA 320
Sleep Talking	Antioxidant BHA 320
Snoring, Snorting, Blocked Ears, Sleep Apnea, Difficulty Breathing	a1 milk (proteins), Sunset yellow (110), Calcium Propionate bread preservative 282, MSG Monosodium Glutamate 621, mattress fumes and furniture fumes.
Weird Dreams	Salicylates, green food colouring.

Did you know that the following sleep related issues have been connected to food additives, colourings and chemicals?

- Sleep walking and sleep talking
- Difficulty falling asleep and staying asleep
- Weird dreams, night terrors, bad dreams
- Bed wetting
- Sleep apnea-like symptoms and snoring,
- Insomnia and restless sleep.

Follow these references to find specific factsheets on the following symptoms[4] from the Food Intolerance website www.fedup.com.au:

General Sleep Disturbance and Insomnia factsheet[5], and the symptom-specific factsheets on ADHD and Diet[6], Bedwetting[7], Chronic Fatigue[8], Depression[9], Joint Pain and Arthritis[10], Oppositional Defiance Disorder[11], Sleep Apnea[12] and Teeth Grinding[13].

Then, if you like, you can continue on to the additive-focused-factsheets, such as the factsheets on MSG, 621, and glutamates[14], and the others including propionic acid (the bread preservative)[15].

You'll need to read the whole factsheet, as there is amazingly detailed information on the labelling laws. MSG can be named a number of ways apart from "MSG"—look for the words hydrolyzed or formulated, hydrolyzed wheat, Chinese seasoning, vegetable, plant, soy or wheat protein, HVP or HPP, yeast extract or just yeast, or broth. If MSG is one of your offending items, you have to research very thoroughly.

That's a start, and there is plenty more on that website, it's awesome. Get involved!

The above information relates to babies, children and adults.

Mothers, remember that if you're **breastfeeding**, the additives can go through your system into your milk, then to your baby, e.g. Artificial colour 102, (tartrazine or yellow #5). And when I say that, please don't think that I'm advocating giving up breastfeeding, because I'm *definitely* not. It just means that you have to be vigilant about your diet while you are breastfeeding.

Sue Dengate reports that the average consumer eats 20 additives a day, and if you cook at home, which most people regard as healthy, you will, on average, consume 19 additives a day[16]. Interesting? Some takeaway meals are actually better than some things you make at home if you have intolerances.

How do you know if you have an "intolerance"?
It's important to understand the difference between allergy and intolerance. Allergies can be confirmed with laboratory tests, and are usually quick reactions to the proteins in foods, such as peanuts.

Intolerance reactions, on the other hand, can happen hours or even days later. And because of the delayed response, many people blame the reaction on the *last* thing they ate. This is not generally the case.

Food reactions are a dose-related response, so if you have enough of the offending item, the effects can last for more than 24 hours. The effect is cumulative, so that if you continue eating a particular substance, the reaction can build over hours and days. The good news here is that for some people, just reducing the intake of the offending items might make a noticeable difference without having to totally eliminate the item.

Intolerance reactions include asthma, eczema, hives, rashes, itching, swelling, bloating, heart palpitations, seizures, arthritis, irritable bowel IBS, sleep disturbance, airways symptoms (stuffy and runny nose, colds and ear infections, asthma), head banging, bed wetting, etc. See the list above for sleep-related reactions.

Intolerance is now a lot more common than allergies.

There are no scientifically proven laboratory tests to tell what you are reacting to, and that is the reasoning behind the Low-Chemical Elimination Diet. The scientifically-sound Low-Chemical Elimination Diet was introduced by Dr Ben Feingold in the 1970s in the USA, and has been refined over many years by Sydney's Royal Prince Alfred Hospital Allergy Unit. By using this diet, a lot of people start improving almost straight away, some after 2 days, etc.

There are withdrawal symptoms when you eliminate certain food items, because *food chemicals are addictive*. The good news on withdrawal symptoms is they normally indicate that the diet will work.

The FAILSAFE diet is recommended on the FedUp website. It is a

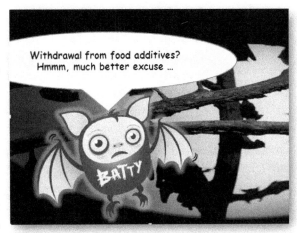

Withdrawal from food additives? Hmmm, much better excuse ...

Food Additives are Addictive

diet Free of Additives, Low in Salicylates, Amines and Flavour Enhancers. There are many FAILSAFE stories on the Food Intolerance Network's website.

It is very encouraging to know that simply reducing the intake of offending items can improve your situation. For many people though, it's just better to bite the bullet and do the FAILSAFE diet. Why put off your best sleep and elevated mood any longer?

People who use the FAILSAFE diet usually get very good results within 3 weeks.

To start the FAILSAFE diet, you can visit the Food Intolerant Network's website[17], become a member of their helpful forum, and/or order their newsletter[18].

International Food and Labelling Standards

My apologies for being a little parochial, being an Australian. To study the labelling laws in each country would be an impossible task, and the best general references I can find is from the Food Intolerance Network.

Don't believe what you read on the label!
If the label says 'No artificial preservatives, artificial colours or artificial flavourings'
it could be misleading or simply not true.
e.g. MSG is a natural flavour, so it won't show as artificial.
There is also the 5% labelling loophole that
allows any items that is less than 5% of the content to not be shown or declared at all.

Good Brands and Preferred Products?

Now that you know about the 5% labelling loophole, I'll share a few of Sue Dengate's good brands (from *Sleep with the Experts* 2009, go to her website for the most current information):

Bread brands in Australia that don't contain calcium propionate 282 are Bakers Delight, Brumby's and Banjo's. You could make your own bread if 282 is one of your problems.

These breads are preferred because vinegar (high in salicylates and amines) is used as a bread preservative in many breads, but not these brands[19].

Frozen Chips (French Fries) without BHA 320: Woolworth's brand[19]

Oils Select brands and Logan Farm[19]

Alcohol recommendations for people intolerant to salicylates and/or amines: vodka, gin and whiskey[19].

If you react to **dairy products,** the best milks to try are a2 milk (comes from Jersey cows), soymilk or rice milk[19].

"Healthy foods" such as yoghurt, crackers, cooking oils, canned soup, ice cream, pasta, rice dishes, lemonade etc can all contain nasty chemicals. Don't assume anything about processed foods and what they contain.

As for medications: just because a drug is approved by the Food and Drug Administration (FDA), or an item is passed by the Therapeutic Goods Administration (or your country's equivalent), it is not necessarily OK.

Other issues arise when people *mix* medications, legitimately or otherwise.

Food Intolerance Network Nasty Food Awards

This page will probably raise your blood pressure too! Go to the Food Intolerance Network's website to see further information on foods that are being watched and commented upon by the Food Intolerance Network and given 'Nasty Food Awards'[20].

If you have (or suspect) a food intolerance, then you need to get to know Sue Dengate's website and information inside and out. Every time I go there, I learn something new. Today, for example, I learned that *slow cooking* (which appears to be healthy cooking) can increase the potency of amines and glutamates. And if your problem is amines and/or glutamates that is not a good thing.

Sue's book *Fed Up* is recommended to you, refer to *Recommended Reading* at the end of the book.

Prescription and Non-Prescription Drugs and Other Substances That Affect Sleep.

There are a range of prescription and non-prescription drugs and herbs that affect sleep. They include:

- Psychotropics and antidepressants e.g. selective serotonin reuptake inhibitors, SSRIs.
- Stimulants.
- Cardiovascular drugs.
- Bronchodilators used in the treatment of asthma and chronic bronchitis. Insomnia and sleeping problems are listed as side effects.
- Decongestants, flu and cold medications. Some that you are giving your children. Reactions can include insomnia, drowsiness, sedation, nervousness, sleep disturbances, sleeplessness, and central nervous system stimulation, e.g. pseudoephedrine.
- CNS (central nervous system) stimulants, e.g. pemoline, used to treat narcolepsy and ADHD, dextroamphetamine.
- Cold remedies contain pseudoephedrine, and are available over the counter.
- Respiratory medications (e.g. theophylline, albuterol).
- Diuretics.
- Steroids.
- Antihypertensives (which have been associated with both sedation and sleep difficulties) Beta-blockers, Alpha-blockers (e.g. those used to reduce blood pressure).
- Some slimming tablets, diet pills containing pseudoephedrine.
- Hormones (e.g. corticosteroids, thyroid).
- Herbal agents (e.g. ginseng).
- Painkillers.
- Cough Syrups (look for tartrazine, colour 102, E102, yellow #5).

The effect of a drug or substance can be either direct or indirect. Some drugs have negative side effects that lead to stress, which then affect sleep.

Other drugs and substances that may affect sleep because of *associated stress* include drugs that:

- decrease libido,
- cause sexual dysfunction (including anti-depressants),
- cause diarrhea,
- cause headaches,
- bring about overheating and/or sweating,
- bring on nausea,
- are linked with depression,
- are addictive, including sleeping pills: knowing they are addictive adds to your anxiety and stress levels while you wonder how long you can be taking a medication, how you will withdraw from them, where you can find help in the process, etc.,
- Cause weight gain or loss, and/or
- Are associated with stomach ache, or any other pain etc.

More specifically, here are some groupings of substances and their sleep relationship:

Drugs with a Side-Effect of Depression and/or Anxiety, and therefore affect Sleep:

- The Contraceptive Pill. "Use of hormonal contraception, especially among adolescents, was associated with subsequent use of antidepressants and a first diagnosis of depression, suggesting depression as a potential adverse effect of hormonal contraceptive use."[24'27] Adolescent girls who use the mini pill are 2.2 times more likely to be on antidepressants, and adult women are 1.3 times more likely.[25] With about 30 percent of Australian women taking the pill[26], this is a serious consideration – and should be included in mental health and suicide discussions.

- Some cholesterol reducing medications have the side effect of depression. (e.g. if you are newly on a cholesterol reducing medication, and you start waking up earlier in the morning, investigate that. This can be an indicator of depression as a side-effect of this medication.)[21]
- Some anxiety medications have side effects of either depression or anxiety. The side effect of anxiety when you are taking anxiety tablets is concerning.[22] It becomes more difficult to help yourself if you don't actually know whether the anxiety is coming from you or the medication.
- Immunomodifiers used to treat hepatitis B and C.
- Amphetamines, cocaine, ecstasy, crystal meth, ketamine (special K).
- MS (multiple sclerosis) drugs, carcinoma drugs, some interferon drugs, HIV drugs.

Freely available and commonly used substances that affect sleep:

- Alcohol
- Nicotine
- Energy drinks
- Caffeine. See the special section on drinks marketed to teenagers in the Teenagers Section in Chapter 34.

Going Organic?

Truly organic foods do not have nasty chemical additives, pesticides, growth hormones and the like.

Organic diets are obviously advantageous, but be aware that labelling that claims to be organic may or may not be. Similarly, packaging that claims to be "gluten-free", "natural", "healthy" and "additive-free" may just be "good marketing" and may not be true at all.

Foods imported from overseas where production standards are not as high as Australian standards can also be suspect.

You cannot tell the origin of a food item by the bar code on the product. The barcode indicates where a product is *produced*. This means that the raw vegetable, for example, could be shipped from China to Canada and Canada can add the barcode that is relevant to their production company. The product "looks Canadian", but actually is not in the full sense of the word. Countries that have low growing standards use these techniques and laws to hide what is really going on with your food.

If you Google "organic cheater brands" and similar terms you will also find more anomalies that hinder our ability to eat the quality of food we choose to eat.

The other thing to keep in mind in relation to organic foods, is that if you are intolerant to salicylates and amines, they occur naturally in healthy foods, such as strawberries and saltanas (salicylates), and slow cooked tomato based foods (amines).

Please don't get put off by the overload of information. Once you know the information you can sort your lifestyle around the products, quality items, meals and exercise habits that suit you and that help you get a great night's sleep, and therefore help you feel and think better.

SLEEP DOJO - Type D

Food Additives, Colourings, Flavourings and VOCs (Volatile Organic Chemicals)

1. Make a copy of all the additives to eliminate from your diet (including their numbers and alternative names), and keep them in your wallet.
2. Educate yourself on the full ramifications of food additives, flavourings, colourings, natural flavourings, perfumes etc., and their connection to sleep and mental health.

3. Choose a dietary strategy such as the FAILSAFE diet or the Elimination Diet to ascertain exactly which substances are your problem triggers.

4. Pre-plan strategies around withdrawal symptoms when eliminating offending additives and colourings. They are addictive, and side effects need to be managed.

5. Drink water as your drink of choice.

6. Reduce citrus and tomato products.

7. Avoid artificial colourings and flavourings.

8. Eat preservative-free breads (Brumby's and Baker's Delight and Banjo's Brands in Australia)[23].

9. Avoid salicylates in vitamin supplements (e.g. citrus bioflavonoids, concentrated fruit flavour).

10. For supportive dieticians email confoodnet@ozemail.com.au and ask for help.

11. For more information and to access Sue Dengate's Food Intolerance Network and her newsletter visit www.Fedup.com.au

Medications and Drugs

12. Go easy on the alcohol. It disturbs your normal sleeping brainwave patterns. It might knock you out so that you fall asleep, but it can also wake you up in a few hours after the first effects have worn off. Alcohol is also a depressant. Your problems will not be solved with alcohol; it's an unsuccessful strategy.

13. Investigate the side effects of every single prescription medication you are taking on www.rxisk.org.

14. Investigate any medications/drugs/substances you believe might be affecting your sleep.

15. Ask your healthcare professional about the MIX of medications you are taking. Take care that they are aware of the full spectrum of what you are taking. How drugs interact with one other is another story altogether. Unfortunately a lot of this information is simply unknown.

16. Are there any better ways to approach the medications that you are on? You need to be proactive in your dealings with your doctor and medical professionals. If you don't tell them that it's affecting your sleep or ask about it, they may not know, and could wrongly assume that you are not having any difficulties.

17. Polypharmacy (taking 4 drugs or more) should be avoided totally.

CHAPTER 28

Type E: Varying Sleep Times, Circadian Rhythm

This chapter is dedicated to anyone who finds it difficult to sleep because of jet lag, shift work, varying sleep times ("on call" situations), etc.

Circadian Rhythm and Melatonin

There are a number of time rhythms that cycle through our day. The most obvious one is the 24-hour rhythm called the circadian rhythm.

Simply put, the pineal gland in the centre of the brain secretes a hormone known as melatonin. This hormone controls the sleeping/waking cycle and is itself controlled by the daily light-dark cycle. Melatonin rises and falls in a distinct pattern known as the circadian rhythm, which generally follows a 24-hour cycle. Interestingly, in studies done on people deprived of environmental day/night cues, the cycle is actually closer to 25 hours rather than 24. It has been shown that when we wake up each morning and 'see the light' we reset or 'entrain' the cycle back to the 24 hour period.

As your circadian rhythm declines (as you get more tired at the end of the day), your ability to metabolize stimulants declines. This magnifies the disruption caused by that late night coffee, cigarette, or violent movie.

And you can see why, when you might go to sleep when the sun is coming up, or wake up at 3 pm in the afternoon (for example) your inner circadian rhythm clock becomes "all over the place" and disrupts your sleep (and a lot of other things too, like eating times, etc.)

Ultradian Rhythm (UR)

Whilst there is general familiarity with the 24 hour circadian rhythm, many people have never heard of the Ultradian Rhythm (UR). The UR is a mini-cycle of melatonin secretion that operates within a 90 minute period (there are 1.5 hours between peaks on this cycle). Knowledge of this cycle can help us to manage our sleep more effectively at certain times.

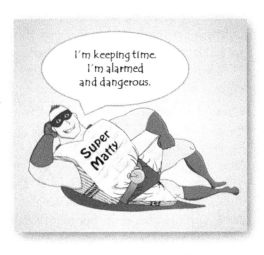

Our Bodies have Timing Mechanisms

A good way to demonstrate the effect of UR is to consider a familiar situation such as watching the Sunday night movie. If the movie runs from 8.30 – 10.30 PM, you may notice that around 10 PM that you are having trouble keeping your eyes open. In this situation both your Circadian and Ultradian rhythms are probably well on the way down to their respective low points. You might be enjoying the movie and decide to watch till the end before going to bed. After brushing your teeth etc, you may find you have trouble falling asleep, when half an hour ago you had trouble staying awake! What has happened is that you pushed through the low point of your UR and are now on the "upswing." Your next opportunity to get into some reasonably sound sleep may not be until 11.30 PM (90 minutes from your last UR trough).

Putting sleep off for 15-20 minutes may actually cost you 90 minutes of quality sleep, at the same time as reinforcing your unfortunate mind-pattern of "I can't fall asleep straight away when I go to bed."

I recommend experimenting with different sleep times. E.g. 10.00 pm, 10.30 pm or 10.45 pm? Which time helps you fall asleep the fastest?

Melatonin

Melatonin is a natural hormone-like compound produced in the pineal gland. This hormone is involved in numerous aspects of general circadian and physiological regulations. It sets and maintains the internal clock governing the natural rhythm of body functions. The amount of melatonin produced by our bodies seems to lessen as we get older.

Clinically, melatonin supplements have been used in rhythm disturbances and sleep disorders, as the chemical has been reported as useful in resetting the body clocks of shift workers and people suffering from jet lag.

Melatonin supplements are not suitable for pregnant women. Reports from users include vivid dreams and sometimes slightly 'freaky' dreams. Follow the instructions on the label. If the time to take melatonin is not stipulated on the label, then start at about 7 pm (for a normal day). Getting the timing right may be a matter of experimentation.

Shift Work

The Danish Government has commenced paying compensation to women who have developed breast cancer after years of working night shifts.

There appears to be mounting evidence that shift work could suppress the production of melatonin in the body. Melatonin is believed to have some beneficial effects in preventing the onset of cancer.

A report by the BBC shows a link between nurses who worked shifts and breast cancer, with a comment that the level of evidence is really no different than it might be for an industrial chemical.[1]

One of the reports published in the journal of the National Cancer Institute showed a 36% greater risk of breast cancer for women who had worked night shifts for more than 30 years, compared with women who had never worked nights.[2]

There's also mention of cardiovascular disease and gastro-intestinal disadvantages... which is old news... and also low birth weight in babies and longer pregnancies for women.

Jet Lag

Jet lag occurs following air travel across many time zones. It is experienced as lethargy, sleepiness, difficulty concentrating and moodiness during the day, as well as difficulty sleeping at night at your overseas destination. If you do nothing to reset your body clock at your destination you will feel like falling asleep in the middle of the day. You will then awake in the middle of the night and be unable to fall back to sleep for the rest of the night. If it is necessary to stay awake during the day for meetings or work you will struggle to maintain concentration and to stay awake.

Jetlag is caused by your body clock still on home time and not "in-sync" with your new destination time.

It is generally easier to adjust to a lengthened day than a shortened day. Specifically East-West travel is easier than West-East—unless, of course, you travel to a time zone 12 hours displaced from your normal one; then it doesn't matter which direction you go.

94% of passengers suffer from jetlag. It can last for up to 2 weeks. It has been stated that 1 recovery day is required for each time zone crossed.[3]

I have seen recommendations to organize your flights to arrive in the afternoon or evening.

When you get on the plane turn your watch to the time of your destination and start eating and behaving as close as possible to the time zone you will be arriving into.

If you are a frequent traveler who frequently stresses your rhythms, buy any relaxation audio that suits you and the 10-Minute Supercharger to download into your iPod or computer.

Time Reset Process

There is a tapping process that uses the Chinese meridian time-related pressure points to tap yourself into your new time zone when travelling.

This is outside the scope of this book, and won't be found in Cochrane, but you might like to investigate it.

Like changing your clock, always wind yourself forward, not backwards when you do this process.

Bright Light Therapy

In the early 1980s, Dr. George Brainerd's team at Thomas Jefferson Medical University identified a photo receptor in the human eye responsible for reacting to light and controlling the production of melatonin. Light in the range of 447-484 nm (nanometers) is responsible for suppressing melatonin production.

It is for this reason that we are promoting the use of light and darkness (and red lights vs. blue) to help with sleep, and even mood.

Lights and sunlight can be used to reset circadian rhythms and to shut down melatonin and increase serotonin and alertness.

Professor Leon Lack from Flinders University (Australia) has spent years researching the circadian rhythm, sleep and bright light therapy.

To read about the work being done at the sleep labs at Flinders University visit http://www.flinders.edu.au/sabs/psychology/research/labs/sleep/ (accessed June 5, 2017).

To read *The Diagnosis and Treatment of Circadian Rhythm Disorders* by Professor Leon Lack go to http://www.sleep.org.au/documents/item/417 (accessed June 5, 2017). You'll see that they are prescribing the use of bright light and their re-time glasses to adjust for jet lag and shift work circadian disturbances.

Bright light therapy can be used for Seasonal Affective Disorder (SAD), Winter Blues, Delayed Sleep Phase (like that experienced by teenagers and adolescents), Advanced Sleep Phase (mature age sleep) and Night Shift Work.

Experimenting with different LED light options and lighting is very valuable. You might buy the Re-Timer glasses (see http://re-timer.com/) or experiment with your own home lighting arrangements.

Be careful using strong blue lights, because some can be harmful.

Certainly the information on light makes walking in the sun in the morning and turning the lights down low at night valid suggestions. And remember red-based-LED lights are more conducive to sleep, and the blue-based-LED lights are the ones that suppress melatonin and keep you awake.

SLEEP DOJO - Type E

1. It is advantageous for shift workers to vary their shifts less often if at all possible, so that they can manage a rhythm as best they can.

2. Use the Time Reset Process to align your internal body clock to *present time* when you suffer from time-lag problems (the start of a new shift, when you get on a plane to travel to another time zone, etc.)

3. Use light as much as possible to readjust your circadian rhythm, and 'manipulate' melatonin production. Use both bright light/blue spectrum and low lighting/red spectrum, depending on your intention.

4. Avoid long-term shift work if you can. E.g. Look for day time administrative positions in your current line of work if at all possible, possibly becoming a consultant to the profession you work in, or something similar.

5. When travelling, try to stay up until the normal sleeping time in your new country/time zone, if your travel time is not really long.

6. Eat and drink healthy foods while travelling and re-adjusting, and time your meals as much as possible to your *destination time* as soon as you get on the plane. This will give your body a better chance to readjust.

7. When you travel, or work shift work, be more conscientious about sleeping at the right hours, walking in the sun in the morning (to reset your clock), sleeping in a very dark room etc. The more you can do to normalize your hours the better.

8. Go to "Your Pitch Black Bedroom" section in Chapter 32 – Type I: Environment if you want to blacken out your bedroom for great results.

9. Melatonin supplementation is used quite often for circadian rhythm problems. Look up the Cochrane Library to review its efficacy.

10. Download the free f.lux program, developed by Michael and Lorna Herf in 2009, to reduce the blue light being emitted from your screens at night time. www.justgetflux.com

CHAPTER 29

Type F: Muscles and Restless Legs Syndrome

R estless leg syndrome (RLS, also known as Willis-Ekborn Disease) and muscle problems may be related, and the underlying problem is different for different people.

It is interesting to note that there is no specific diagnostic test for RLS. However, there are so many people putting out different 'solutions,' it is bordering on a joke.

Here are some options to try:

A. Look at the side effects of every single medication you are on. You already know that RLS is a side effect of some. Look up any medications you are taking, and review reports being made on the www. rxisk.org website while doing this. Muscle problems are a side effect of a number of prescription drugs including drugs to treat high blood pressure, heart conditions, nausea, colds, allergies and depression.[1] Similarly, research the side effects of any herbal or 'natural' supplements you are ingesting.

B. Use the correct elimination diet described earlier in chapter 27 to establish if you are intolerant to any food additive, colouring, chemical or VOC that is causing your muscles to behave irregularly. Eliminate the offending food additives and chemicals from your food and environment.

To access the factsheet on Diet, Sleep Disturbance and Insomnia (including restless legs) go to this link on the Food Intolerance Network's website: http://fedup.com.au/factsheets/

symptom-factsheets/sleep-disturbance-and-insomnia   (Accessed June 4, 2017.)

Additionally in *Sleep with the Experts* Sue Dengate mentioned benzoate preservative, which is contained in tooth mousse and some children's medications, as a possible offender to investigate. If you have ANY sleep problems that are listed by Sue, then you need to eliminate and test ALL the nasty additives listed in Chapter 27. It may be a discipline to do this, but from many of the case study reports on Sue's website, it could change you and your family's lives significantly and permanently.

C. Magnesium amino acid chelate combined with vitamin E (Source: Phil Alexander, Naturopath, Radio 2UE Australia). I have personally observed success and anecdotal support, but cannot site any evidence-based clinical trial.

D. Check to see if there is an underlying iron or vitamin deficiency, and then perhaps supplement your diet with iron, vitamin B12 and/ or folate.[2]

E. An excess of phosphorus, and a shortage of calcium circulating in your blood system (Source: American National Sleep Foundation www.sleepfoundation.org, accessed 2010). Avoid carbonated sodas and drinks.

F. Limit your caffeine and alcohol intake.[3]

G. Warm baths.

H. Relaxation and/or meditation.

I. Acupressure and massage.

J. Iron deficiency (anaemia) might suggest a change in diet. This can be relevant for pregnant women. I personally prefer diet changes rather than supplementation for iron, and I wouldn't recommend pregnant women to take pills and supplements without rigorous research.

Cravings are a great way to see what your body might be lacking when you are pregnant: and of course a great dietary solution. Leg cramps seem to be more prevalent in the third trimester of pregnancy.

K. Folic acid deficiency.

L. Vitamin B deficiency.

SLEEP DOJO - Type F

1. Review the side effects of all medications you are taking on www. rxisk.org.
2. There is no direct solution that is recommended across the board for RLS. It is a trial-and-error situation in my opinion.
3. Look at the side effects of any natural supplements you are ingesting.
4. The combination magnesium and vitamin E is a rather easy trial you could do; certainly easier than the food additives elimination diet. But that would be my next suggestion. See the FAILSAFE elimination diet spoken about in Chapter 27.
5. Follow with the other suggestions listed before the Sleep Dojo.

CHAPTER 30

Type G: Illness and Pain

This chapter covers:

- Sleep Apnea
- Arthritis and joint pain
- General pain
- Tinnitus and Meniere's Disease

I've included Type G in this book, because there are a lot of different sicknesses and illnesses (and other things) that are going on in our bodies that are *really* the problem, not necessarily sleeping. Some are brief references only, as they go beyond the scope of this book. I've included some information to help you with your research.

Other medical conditions that impact sleep—particularly in senior years—are dyspnea (shortness of breath or uncomfortable breathing) of cardiac or pulmonary origin, gastro esophageal reflux, obesity, nocturia (frequent urination), incontinence, and neurodegenerative diseases (e.g. Alzheimer's disease and Parkinson's disease). These are beyond the scope of this book.

Sleep Apnea

If you feel that you are being woken up by your own snoring, you wake up a number of times during the night, or you have disturbed breathing patterns, you should seek expert advice for sleep apnea. It is a very serious condition, and needs to be addressed promptly.

The British United Provident Association has stated that not all individuals who snore have sleep apnea, and that not all individuals with sleep apnea snore.

According to the American National Sleep Foundation sleep apnea may be present in up to 40 percent of those adults who experience snoring.

Children can have sleep apnea. Because children grow while they sleep, growth spurts have been known to happen after children with sleep apnea have been treated.

This area of sleep is one that is being serviced quite well. I'm not saying that sleep apnea sufferers are happy, only observing that there are a lot of people in the industry trying to give the service!

Being diagnosed with the problem is the first step, but the solution is not easy. CPAP (continuous positive airway pressure) masks are not enjoyed by anyone that I have ever met. They are worn reluctantly (if at all), the pressure settings seem to be a problem with many people, it's expensive, the style choices seem pretty daunting (shape, full face etc), and the relationship and self-esteem issues are a significant challenge.

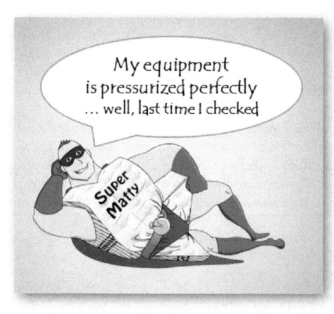

The whole thing seems to take away people's mojo. Even though you can travel "anywhere where there is electricity that you can plug into", it's never as easy as that with embarrassment issues and relationship considerations. It's a tough call. And I'm pretty sure there are some of you not taking the tests because you don't want the answer. I understand that (although I don't agree).

Sleep apnea has associations with depression and being overweight, as though you needed more problems!

There is a list of food additives and chemicals (even dairy products) that have been associated with sleep apnea and snoring symptoms, so it is definitely worth having a look at the information on the Food Intolerance Network's website. Go to www.fedup.com.au if your child (or you) has problems with snoring and sleep apnea.

The Food Intolerance Network's factsheet on sleep apnea is here: http://fedup.com.au/factsheets/symptom-factsheets/sleep-apnea

Also read the section on snoring in Chapter 27.

Sue Dengate cites a few case studies where people have gone on the "FAILSAFE Diet" and actually fixed those problems, because it wasn't actually related to their breathing, in the "publicized sleep apnea" sense.

Cochrane

The Cochrane Collaborative, as discussed in Chapter 4, has very high quality information on sleep apnea and CPAP machines.

To access the general search page in Cochrane go to: http://www.cochrane.org/evidence (Accessed August 17, 2016).

By investigating through that search page you will find the following sorts of articles and research:

- Continuous positive airways pressure (CPAP) for relieving signs and symptoms of obstructive sleep apnea, which discusses the different sorts of machines and how motivated sleep apnea patients are to use them – thereby pointing to their actual use and effectiveness. There are many such quality studies.
  http://www.cochrane.org/CD001106/AIRWAYS_continuous-positive-airways-pressure-for-relieving-signs-and-symptoms-of-obstructive-sleep-apnea
  Accessed August 17, 2016.
- The effects of different pressure delivery interventions for improving use of continuous positive airway pressure (CPAP) in the treatment of obstructive sleep apnea.

http://www.cochrane.org/CD003531/AIRWAYS_the-effects-of-different-pressure-delivery-interventions-for-improving-use-of-continuous-positive-airway-pressure-in-the-treatment-of-obstructive-sleep-apnea
Accessed August 17, 2016.

You may also wish to search Cochrane for any evidence that CPAP machines improve mortality rates.

American National Sleep Foundation

`General information on sleep apnea, from the American National Sleep Foundation can be found at https://sleepfoundation.org/sleep-disorders-problems/sleep-apnea (Accessed August 17, 2016). They also have a Pillow Talk forum that you might find useful http://answers.sleepfoundation.org/forum/topics/alternatives-to-cpap

Accessed August 17, 2016.

Remember that the US National Sleep Foundation is sponsored, and the website doesn't provide much detail about it. https://sleepfoundation.org/funding-sources-and-editorial-independence

Accessed March 20, 2017.

Arthritis and Joint Pain

We suggest you have a look at both salicylates and monosodium glutamate (MSG, in all its forms) in your diet, including airborne salicylates, etc. There is a relevant factsheet prepared by the Food Intolerance Network[1].

Please notice, on that website, that slow cooking can increase the potency of amines and glutamates, so be aware of this challenge.

Get the full story on MSG, the labelling loopholes in Australia, the different names they give MSG on labels, etc.

In naturopath Phillip Alexander's book *It Could be Allergy and it Can be Cured* he states that 70 percent of arthritis sufferers responded to a nightshade exclusion test[2]. Others have nominated various intolerances and allergies as a possible lead to a solution.

Go to the Music and Sound section of chapter 35 for information on using music to distract from pain.

Tinnitus and Meniere's Disease

Sometimes described as "ringing in the ears", tinnitus is the medical term for hearing sounds within the ear when there are no external sounds present. Hearing buzzing, hissing, roaring, whistling, or humming are all indications that something has gone awry in the auditory system. Ranging from constant to intermittent, the level of symptoms can vary from annoying to very severe and debilitating.

Our 6 top strategies for Tinnitus are:

1. Look at the side effects of your medications, and at the https://www.rxisk.org website.
2. Download the salicylates factsheet from the Food Intolerance Network's website. See if you could have an intolerance that affects tinnitus, reversible hearing loss, vertigo, or symptoms of Meniere's disease. See Chapter 27.
3. Introduce a low salt diet.
4. During your investigations, use white noise in the background to help. It's not a solution, but it keeps the annoyance levels down slightly for some.
5. The Dr. Oz show, aired on Australian Television on February 2, 2011 claimed that tinnitus was a vitamin B12 deficiency. He recommended cutting caffeine, quinine (found in tonic water), aspirin and alcohol from your diet. I have not investigated the evidence base of this claim, but I can leave that to you now, can't I? You have all the capabilities.

Tinnitus Retraining Therapy

My interest in neuroplasticity lead my curiousity into this possible solution.

In my previous book I mentioned tinnitus retraining therapy, specifically Neuromonics Tinnitus Treatment (Curtin University of Technology, WA), as a possible solution to tinnitus. The treatment involves providing a pattern of sounds to re-train neural pathways involved in tinnitus.

However, only one study of tinnitus retraining therapy has passed the inclusion tests of Cochrane, and more study is required before this solution can be recommended[3].

Cognitive Behavioural Therapy, while not showing as a solution to the loudness of tinnitus, has shown benefits in managing the emotional aspects of tinnitus, namely depression scores and quality of life[4].

Meniere's Disease

If you have tinnitus coupled with hearing loss and vertigo please investigate Meniere's disease with your medical practitioner. Symptoms of Meniere's disease can include the feeling of ear fullness.

Be aware that vertigo can be an adverse reaction to some drugs, such as anti-viral agents; it may not indicate that you have Meniere's disease. Please refer to your doctor for full testing, and look up www.rxisk.org for listed side effects of medications you are presently taking.

Low-Salt Diets

Low-salt diets can be effective for sufferers of vertigo (a component of Meniere's disease). Tinnitus may respond to some degree (for some).

Salt has also been associated with elevated blood pressure, heart disease and fluid retention. It is estimated that about 10% of the salt in the average diet comes from that naturally found in food, 15% is added in cooking or at the table and 75% is added to processed foods. Generally, taste is no guide.

Salt Matters By Dr Trevor Beard is an excellent book for those who are wishing to reduce their sodium intake. Low-salt cookbooks also contain valuable information.

Cochrane does not have any published studies, that I can find, that support a low-salt diet to alleviate Meniere's disease. Because Meniere's disease fluctuates, it appears that trialing solutions can be challenged.

Potassium-Rich Foods

I have also read that foods high in potassium oppose the effect of sodium (salt). Potassium-rich foods include bananas, oranges, sunflower seeds, beans, squash, mint leaves, potatoes, mung beans and nuts.

Again, I see nothing in Cochrane that supports this solution.

Pain and Other Illnesses

Pain is obviously a reason some people can't sleep, and it generally comes with other medical problems that are beyond the scope of this book. Please refer to the Music and Sounds section of Chapter 35 for suggestions on pain distraction. We aren't talking pain relief, but there is evidence to suggest that distraction can help.

SLEEP DOJO - Type G

1. Look into the possible chemicals, food additives, or dairy products that might be associated with your breathing problems, tinnitus, snoring, joint pain, etc.
2. Review all your medications and the combinations of medications to see which are adversely affecting your sleep and mood. You can ask your chemist/pharmacist for a list of the side effects of each drug you take, they will be happy to oblige. When drugs are taken in combination it is very difficult, even for the experts, to tell you

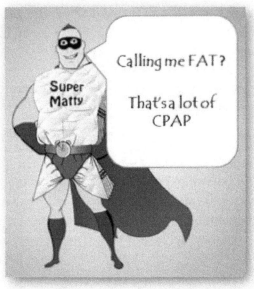

how they are interacting and the possible side effects of the combinations themselves.

3. If you are overweight your snoring and chances of sleep apnea are reduced significantly by losing weight. Try this solution because it will help many other aspects of your life as well.

4. If you suspect you have sleep apnea, look up the Cochrane research website for any evidence that long term use of CPAP machines improves mortality. If you like what you see, visit your doctor and get referred to a professional sleep clinic to be assessed. Some sleep clinics are better than others, so do your own research before asking your GP for a referral.

5. A healthy diet, exercise and lifestyle will positively affect your general and mental health and sleep.

CHAPTER 31

Type H: Mind Games

> "I should have been madder.
> But, as doubtless happens with most people,
> she had found this out too late."
> *Veronica Decides to Die*, Paulo Coelho

Lack of Sleep Relates to Mental Health.

I'm sure you already know that there is a significant connection between lack of sleep and mental health issues. Even common sense tells us that after a bad night's sleep we are emotionally less robust, less resilient, more inclined to be grumpy and moody, etc. (Even though our mental health ministers' offices have told me that sleep has got nothing to do with mental health! Refer to Chapter 18 – Politicians are Not Capable of Doing Their Job.)

Not only do anxious and stressed people find it harder to fall asleep and stay asleep, but insomnia is a side effect of many of the medications being given to mental health patients.

When antidepressants cause people to put on weight (which they do) their probability of suffering other sleeping problems, such as sleep apnea and snoring increases.

And of course, overweight people are less likely to exercise, and have poorer body images and lower self esteem which exacerbates their mental health problems.

They may spend less time in the sun each day, which can further adversely affect their attitude and feelings of wellbeing.

There have been a number of studies linking grief and depression specifically to waking too early in the morning, therefore limiting sleep hours.

Lack of sleep in adolescents has been linked to mental health problems.

It's common sense really, I won't go on... but who has ever felt better after they had a bad night's sleep?

And who has felt more anxious, less confident, more jittery after a bad night's sleep, making it difficult to concentrate and impairing your performance generally?

And making you more grumpy and less resilient?

Mental Pain

We all recognize that physical pain is an indication that something isn't right.

Somehow though, when it comes to mental pain, we aren't so motivated to find out what's causing the problem, talk to our friends about it, or "have it looked at".

Let's just say it straight: at some point in our lives EVERYONE is going to have to deal with some pretty big stressors, and we ALL need to have some great tools to deal with it all when our time comes around. Personally, I'm VERY OVER people pretending that life is just one jolly, tidy, abundant, healthy, glamorous occasion!

There will be times in everyone's lives that are sad, challenging, stressed, broke, lonely and even shocking. Hopefully they will be balanced by joy, creativity, achievement, fun, love and abundance at other times - or even at the same time. You can experience the sadness of someone dying in the same week as the joy of a newborn baby. Or be given the sack the same month that you celebrate a major birthday.

It's called "having a life"!

We are supported and challenged by different people throughout our lives. The support might make us complacent, and the challenge might call us to our highest order. Everything is not exactly as it seems – especially in hindsight. Some of the worst times lead to major positive changes in our lives. Though we might need a few years to see it that way.

Once people understand that, the conversation changes – and I'm noticing a change for the better, at least in Australia.

Some people react to bad situations more strongly, and it affects them more. These people seem to have less resilience to deal with stresses when they come along. We ALL have to have some good strategies around depression, anxiety, stress, and other mental conditions.

Be aware here that I believe there is a mind/body/neurology connection with all the problems discussed in this chapter, It is not just "in your head," and, luckily, there are new technologies coming forward to help.

Oh, one more thing: there are a million organisations and people who are hypnotizing us to become dull. We are born into an advertising world, told at school that we have to get good grades (knowing that most careers are reinvented 3 or more times in a lifetime), are taught to be good employees (in jobs many don't like), believing that the whole world is dog-eat-dog and competitive. Most of what we learn at school and university is a complete waste of time. Most people are 2 months from being evicted from their homes if they were to lose their jobs. And then there is the media with its dose of bad news every night followed by hours of violent and weird television shows!

No wonder so many people are stressing out, feeling anxious, devoid of spiritual happiness, not exercising, not eating well, not even contributing.

Every family group consists of "life's rich tapestry" of good one, bad one, alcoholic, depressed one, the one that pretends to be deranged just to get attention, the high achiever, the loser, the intellectual, the crook, the rich one, the addict, the gambler ... Why are we pretending that this isn't the case?

And mightn't some of us move to another "persona" if we hadn't invested so much time and effort creating this one?

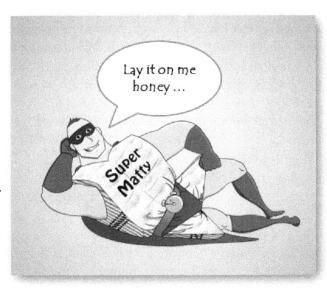

We need to wake up and get real.

There is more at play than we are lead to believe.

And we need to be openly talking about it more.

Wake up to sleep better. It's is all related.

Psychiatric conditions that impact sleep include depression and other mood disorders, anxiety disorders, adjustment disorders, alcohol abuse or dependency and drug use or dependency.

In this chapter we are going to address depression, anxiety, ADHD and stress.

Depression

Depression can be caused by a number of factors. Research has shown a connection to trauma, grief, concussion, genetics, childbirth, creating a life for yourself that you no longer enjoy, unrealistic expectations, emotional and spiritual pain (spending your life doing things you don't find uplifting or rewarding), and exhausted adrenals.

It is proven to have correlations with insomnia, sleep apnea, waking too early in the morning, and certain prescription and non-prescription drug-taking.

I am a strong believer that not taking responsibility for your own life and actions can lead to depression in the long term. If you are a parent, allow your children to feel the pain from the decisions that they have made that didn't end with a good result. People need to understand the sequence of action and consequence, and take full responsibility for it.

Feeling pain is a normal and important part of life. So are the other emotions we feel. We should recognize and feel the full spectrum of emotions throughout our lives: joy, love, peace, shame, guilt, despair, enlightenment, acceptance, neutrality, grief, fear, ecstasy, frustration, pride, desire, anger and the rest.

We should be continually vigilant of the circumstances we find ourselves in – because every day there are challenges to face, and every decision has implications. That thought might put pressure on some people, but for others it is a statement of ultimate freedom.

Unfortunately, because of the problems with antidepressants and SSRIs (Selective Serotonin Reuptake Inhibitors), and the medical and psychiatric professions' willingness to prescribe them, it is vital that you become informed *before* you develop an emotional disorder, if possible.

Here are some references for you to read and/or watch today, hopefully before you develop a mental health problem.

Professor Peter Gøtzsche, the co-founder of the Cochrane Collaborative, in his presentation *Mental Health, Overdiagnosed and Overmedicated* in Australia in 2015 (about 50 minutes in)[1] says:

> "People I know, psychiatrists,
> have weaned off very many people from ben-
> zodiazepines and antidepressant drugs:
> all of them tell me it is far less to stop heroin in a street junkie
> than to get people off benzodiazepines and SSRIs.
> These are terrible drugs that we should use very, very little.
> So, we should focus on psychotherapy…"

The information in these references could save your life, or the life of your child, or someone else's child, or a loved one.

- Gøtzsche, Peter, C, Professor, Co-founder of the Cochrane Collaborative. *Mental Health, Overdiagnosed and Overmedicated*[2]. https://youtu.be/ZMhsPnoIdy4
- Whitaker, Robert. *Mad in America*[3].
- Whitaker, Robert. *Anatomy of an Epidemic: Magic Bulletts, Psychiatric Drugs and the Astonishing Rise of Mental Illness In America*[4].
- Gøtzsche, Peter, C, Professor, MD, DrMedSci, Msc. *Forced Admission and forced treatment in psychiatry causes more harm than good (short version)*[5], available through this link http://www.deadlymedicines.dk/wp-content/uploads/2016/03/Abolishing-forced-treatment-in-psychiatry-short-version.pdf.

We need to learn to speak about our problems more, to engage in talk-therapies, to seek non-drug solutions, and to develop effective family and community strategies to deal with, manage and help our friends and family members who have mental health issues and/or emotional problems from time to time.

I have previously mentioned *Doctor Mercola's Interview with Robert Whitaker on Mental Health,* which is available on YouTube[6]. I would recommend you listening to this interview as well.

Interestingly, apart from talking about the value of exercise, he also says that whether you get treatment or not, you're going to get better in approximately 90 percent of cases. And if you had listened to Professor Peter Gøtzsche's presentation in Australia[2] (above), he says that even *a week* will improve most people's mental health, even after a psychotic episode.

Here are some other concepts and research sources that you might find helpful:

Concussion

A number of studies, such as that performed by the Indiana Sports Concussion Network[7] and by the University of North Carolina's Centre for the Study of Retired Athletes[8] show a link between sustaining concussions and developing depression during your lifetime. According to the research, published in the journal *Medicine and Science in Sports and Exercise,* National Football League (NFL) players surveyed who had sustained three or more concussions were three times more likely to develop clinical depression than players who had not suffered concussions[7,8,9].

Loss, Grief and Shock

Please visit my *Loss, Grief and Shock*[10] reference page on the Sleepless No More website, it may have relevant information for you.

Post-natal Depression and Baby Blues

Most mothers, even fathers, can become overwhelmed after the birth of their baby. Though important, "baby blues" is not as serious as post-natal depression, and it is important to be able to tell the difference. Another trend I notice in Australia is mum's having their babies at an older age. I have also heard that mothers who are super competent and may have had good careers before having babies can feel the challenges more, as their self-worth has become dependent on many other factors – which have never included KPIs such as "being a good mum"! This is possibly another factor in being able to cope well in those first few months. I remember being exhausted after the birth of my baby, and it went on for quite some time. I also felt that I wanted to achieve more in a day than "caring for my baby" – which, looking back, was an internal pressure built from years of wanting to achieve in my career. Some mothers don't feel like they are bonding with their babies, and they should seek professional support and help before it gets more tiring and serious.

If you are struggling it is most important to tell people, your partner, your family, your friends – someone who understands how you are feeling and coping. Don't let your problems be ignored or misunderstood: persist until you find proper help and support. It will be worth it.

I also recommendation you contact the professionals at Karitane in Australia[11], who have a wonderful reputation around mothers and babies. They would be able to help you. And do it early rather than wait, as they will make you feel better just because they will "have your back" in the early stages. They are there to help parents just like you.

Waking Too Early in the Morning

Please refer to Chapter 26 – Waking Too Early in the Morning, and the Sleepless No More website[12].

Psychological Health

Every day everyone has some sort of stress in their lives[13]. This can lead to anxiety, overwhelm, emotional outbursts, substance abuse and other coping mechanisms. If you are generally healthy, fit and have a good social network and family support you will probably cope better. However this is not always the case. For some, where there is family violence and/or abuse, their families are part of the problem.

Over the long term, and in extreme situations, such as watching or being part of violence, wars and so on – these problems become more severe and our coping mechanisms are often strained beyond what they should be.

Talking to people and getting it off your chest is a vital and effective solution to your problems. Talk therapies are actually old-school, but also the new new thing. Of course, who you talk to, and how they support you is vital in finding solutions.

As previously discussed in this book, medication is generally not going to solve the *underlying problems* that have caused you to be sleepless, stressed, anxious or depressed.

So chose your counsellors very wisely.

If you have to try a few different people, do exactly that – until you find someone who is respecting your thoughts, listening to what you say, and working with you in a gentle way to relieve your mental and emotional stress.

I have read reports from the most distinguished mental health professionals that indicate that even *during* psychotic episodes people actually say things that are *revealing the underlying problems* being experienced.

So don't dismiss conversations as 'mad'. Listen up and ask some kind and open questions to see what is underneath the conversation.

SLEEP DOJO –Depression

1. Eliminate all food additives, colourings and chemicals from your diet that are associated with depression. Refer to chapter 27 for the exact links to Sue Dengate's website. Seek out assistance with eliminating these problem substances, as most are addictive and will have withdrawal symptoms associated with them. There are specific ways to find out exactly which chemicals are the offending ones, so take advice from the experts on exactly how to isolate them.

2. Exercise is a great solution for depression. It does not have to be punishing and exhausting, it just needs to be regular and for a reasonable amount of time. If you were to walk for an hour at least 4 mornings a week, great benefits would be gained. I've seen figures that exercise ALONE can help as many as 50 percent of people.

    Walk in the sun, exposing your skin to absorb vitamin D. Exposure to UVB radiation is necessary to produce vitamin D. Now here's where it gets a bit kinky! According to studies if you wash with soap within 48 hours of the correct sun exposure, you will wash away the vitamin D before it has had time to assimilate into the blood stream. So minimize the use of soap and don't be a clean freak. For the readers who are detailed and would like to know more, refer to a fuller explanation from Dr Mercola's website[14]. You'll note that Dr. Mercola says that sunlight coming through windows is not the same as the sunlight directly from the sun, outdoors. Things can get pretty complicated, but it's a good reason to just get out more, eh!

In addition to cheering you up, the light will also help in re-setting your circadian rhythm for the day, especially if you didn't sleep so well the night before. Specifically, if your circadian rhythm is not 'clear', I'm speculating that your walk in the sunlight early in the morning will tell your body to wake up, and set your internal clock for morning, therefore perhaps making night time and "sleeping time" a clearer transition.

3. Cognitive Behaviour Therapy (CBT) has been proven to help with depression. Some distinguished Australians have developed an online clinic to help you, called Virtual Clinic[15]. This organisation works to help sufferers using CBT, which is basically training you how to think better in your life, and deal with your mental health issues in ways other than medications. Read the CBT section later in this chapter (in the anxiety section). Perhaps not surprisingly, anxiety, depression and social phobias often happen together, so any work you do on one aspect can improve a number of areas of your life.

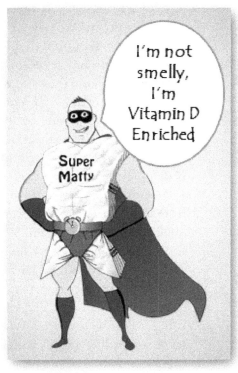

4. Avoid fried foods and watch your diet[16]. Eat plenty of wholesome, fresh (including raw), chemical-free food. I'm sounding like your mother, but you should be doing this anyway!

5. Refer to Chapter 33 – Type J: Decisions, Decisions. If you are in a job you hate, a toxic relationship, or are

crushed under a huge mortgage, no amount of walking or healthy eating is going to get you out of your problem. Procrastination is a killer. Do something about it. If you feel overwhelmed, you might engage a coach or mentor to help you – they are generally independent and can encourage you to see the problem from different angles to get resolution. Having problems with your relationship? Your parents? Your school? You need to talk to someone now.

6. Do something for your community. The Australian television documentary *Making Australia Happy*[17] drew attention to research that indicates helping people in your community will help you feel better and have a more positive outlook on life. It isn't to do with realizing that other people might be having it rougher than yourself. The results were measured through a variety of scientific monitoring processes including saliva samples, pain intolerance tests, etc.

7. Review the side effects of your drugs. I recommend www.rxisk. org[18] where individuals report their drug side effects and the results are not affected by Google rankings, the TGA and FDA, the insistence of 'clinical trials' to support certain disclosures, and other problems and vested interests. An alternative is to Google *your drug name* and the word *depression*. Also *your drug name* and the phrase *side effects*. And *your drug name* and the word *insomnia*. And *your drug name* and the phrase *waking too early*. These sorts of enquiries will help you establish if your medications are associated with your lack of sleep and mental attitude challenges. There is definite evidence of a connection between some prescriptions and depression, anxiety, insomnia, and restlessness – including from anti-depressants, sleeping tablets and SSRIs. Some of these medications are very commonly used and prescribed. Refer to Chapters 9, 10 and 27 for more specific information on drugs.

8. Talk to someone and ask for help. Get it off your chest instead of bottling it up. There are a stack of people with similar problems to you. You might find some new supportive friends, and/or you could help someone else. There is nothing to be ashamed about, it's a fact of life, and incredibly common. In fact everyone goes

through rough times in their life, at one point or another. It is normal. We all feel, and we all have emotions.

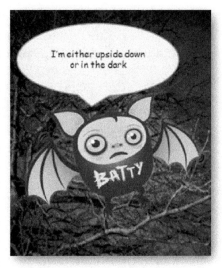

9. Supplements suitable for depression? Check any that people suggest in Cochrane. And be mindful of interactions between medications, supplements and food items that can be unknown and adverse. If you are looking at supplements as a quick fix, like popping a pill, think again. Are you avoiding making the effort to address the underlying problem?

10. In BBC One's *The Doctor That Gave Up Drugs* television program it was suggested that swimming in cold water (13 degrees) can help with depression and anxiety. Is it just because it feels so good when you get out? He was also teaming up the patients with fun and challenging exercise (their choice of martial arts) which would have been a significant factor in feeling a lot better too.

And remember, if you have serious depression and mental health problems you need to talk NOW to qualified counsellors and professionally trained experts. If you are at risk, call a service immediately in your town or city, and if there is no such service available, ring a friend and tell them that you have a serious problem and that you would like immediate and urgent help, today.

Anxiety And Panic

> *When we are faced by something*
> *that really threatens us,*
> *it's impossible to look around,*

even though that is
the safest and most sensible thing to do.
Chronicle: At the End of the Dark Tunnel, Paulo Coelho

In *Sleep with the Experts* Dr. Nic Lucas revealed that, in Australia and similar studies overseas, it was found that the majority of people who have anxiety do not seek formal help for two reasons. First, they don't really believe that anything can help them, and second, they don't really want to admit that they have anxiety. [20]

The good news is that there are a number of natural solutions to anxiety, and people who are anxious can go beyond the problem with the correct strategies.

Dr. Lucas, a medical researcher and previous anxiety sufferer, said that while Cognitive Behavioural Therapy (CBT) was effective in treating all types of anxiety disorders, it appeared to be more effective for generalized anxiety disorder and post traumatic stress disorder than social anxiety. Interestingly, CBT was **not** better than "relaxation treatment" which he added is actually one version of CBT. By that, he actually explained that relaxation treatment is a training on *how to relax*, and is less extensive than having formal cognitive behavioural therapy[21].

Insight produced a television program on Anxiety that was shown in Australia. Of note in this program was Professor Gavin Andrew's opinion that CBT is better for anxiety sufferers than the use of medications[22].

After having watched the progress of "positive thinking" (a supposedly fringe and hippy idea when I was first introduced to it in the 1970s), I am amused to see the term "Cognitive Behavioural Therapy" being totally accepted today.

By the way, I'm not impressed with this *not-sexy brand* – the nerdy name probably turns more people off using it.

Who else *doesn't* want to know about Cognitive Behavioural Therapy? ... Let's just get pissed or do drugs.

Get my drift?

I also watch with interest as "neuroscience" becomes the new new thing – recognizing the connection between the body and mind, and now "mindfulness meditation" another new branding of what "alternative heal-ers" and "hippies" were promoting way back when.

For goodness sake!

Very old school, actually.

So let's just do it.

Cognitive Behavioural Therapy (CBT)

Cognitive Behavioural Therapy (CBT) is a way to discipline ourselves to think about how we think. To step back from our thoughts (of panic, for example), so that we can understand and cope better with our feelings and thoughts, eventually changing our response to negative situations. Most cognitive behavioural therapy includes, eventually, exposing the sufferer to more and more of the "problem situation" in order to desensitize the person, and make them gain confidence in the situation that used to cause the nega-tive physical and/or mental response.

Easier said than done, I get that.

CBT has been clinically proven to be beneficial for anxiety, panic disor-der, depression, social phobia, worry disorder, post-traumatic stress disorder, obsessive-compulsive disorder and social disorder - to name a few psycho-logical challenges.

Read my blog post on CBT[26], and note that Crufad has developed and is now *This Way Up* (www.ThisWayUp.org.au).

As mentioned above, the *Insight* television program in Australia[22] on anxiety, incorporated some very valuable information related to depression, social disorder, and panic disorder with some leading Australian experts in this field, including Professor Gavin Andrews and Dr. Sarah Edelman.

I absolutely recommend that anyone with any of these problems watch this full program – there is MUCH to learn and be encouraged by!

Some interesting facts from this television program included:

- Anxiety is the most treatable of all mental disorders.
- Anxiety is the most common psychological disorder – 15% of the population is the figure quoted by Dr. Edelman.

- The physical and psychological feelings of the panic experience include the feeling of being out of breath, even "going to die" for some people.
- "Inside your head is the enemy."
- Is there a trigger or tipping point for an anxiety attack?
- It's not the event that causes anxiety, it's what you think about it.
- As you grow older you get calmer. Anxiety is 3-4 times higher in 20-year-olds than in 70-year-olds.
- Anxiety is not increasing (I was surprised by that fact)! We live in a safer society now than during the depression in 1929.
- The difference between anxiety disorder and being anxious.
- The pros and cons of medication, and the new medications being researched.
- How being the devil's advocate for your own thoughts is recommended.
- And interestingly, anxiety disorder people are reactive, arouse quickly, and are not stoic. They may have had some problems in their childhood which make them think they are vulnerable.
- Very encouraging success figures from the 1000+ people who have participated in the online program. 75% are better, and in Prof. Andrews' quirky words, after another 6 months they are "more better", so it appears that it is not a "temporary fix."

Let me introduce you to the very successful online Cognitive Behavioural Clinic that is run by Professor Gavin Andrews (psychiatrist and head of St. Vincent's hospital Anxiety Clinic, Sydney, Australia), Dr. Nickolai Titoy, and Dr. Blake Dear. This organisation, previously crufad.org is now, at September 2016, www.ThisWayUp.org.au.

In Chapter 34, *Mature-Age Sleep*, I refer to the downloadable report *Sleep Disorders in Older Adults*, Table IV "Components of Cognitive Behavioural Therapy for Insomnia: Stimulus Control Therapy, Sleep-Restriction Therapy, and Sleep Hygiene Education[27]. Locate the link from the references, download the PDF report, and look at the table on page 28 of this report.

In the *Sleep with the Experts* program, we covered aspects of anxiety in 3 different episodes, and combined them in an *Anxiety Training Pack*.

Dr Sarah Edelman, featured in the *Insight* Anxiety program, has compiled an audio CD recommended for people suffering from Anxiety. It is available from Amazon and is called *Letting Go of Anxiety Meditation*.

Emotional Freedom Technique (EFT) and Thought Field Therapy (TFT)

Emotional Freedom Technique and Thought Field Therapy are alternative therapies based on the Chinese Meridian energy flow systems.

If you are feeling anxious *right now*, you might like to try this exercise from YouTube by Dr. Franzi Ng, to see if it improves your state[23].

The discipline of Thought Field Therapy was started by Dr. Roger Callahan over 30 years ago, and since then the basic principals have been spread to many practitioners and evolved through a number of developing alternative disciplines[24] including Emotional Freedom Technique (EFT) and Kinesiology. Dr Callahan died in November 2013.

I have no intention of arguing the point about the lack of an evidence base for his techniques in this book, but I include the information for those of my readers who enjoy pursuing alternative solutions, and who have derived benefit from them.

Recognition of the body-mind-brain connection is only just being recognized, after having been spoken about in alternative circles for over 4 decades (possibly more).

The Chinese meridian system and acupuncture have been recognized in oriental medicine for centuries, but apparently still not proven by clinical trials[25].

SLEEP DOJO – Anxiety and Panic

1. Ascertain the underlying cause of your anxieties, whether through counselling or talk therapies or some other alternative.

2. Daily exercise (as discussed earlier) is very beneficial for anxiety and panic sufferers.

3. Learn to relax, and set aside special time every day when you do your relaxation exercises.

4. Eliminate and/or reduce all chemicals from your diet and inhalants if you suspect that you might be intolerant to them. Refer to the factsheets listed in chapter 27 for the food additives and chemicals that might be linked to anxiety and panic. Do a complete, supervised elimination diet if you think you have intolerances to some food additives and chemicals that are mentioned there, and isolate the exact offenders.

5. Cognitive Behavioural Therapy. Investigate *This Way Up*, the Australian online clinic that is useful for anxiety, depression, OCD etc.

6. Read the excellent book *The Anxiety and Phobia Workbook*, by Dr Edmund Bourne. This award-winning workbook is detailed, giving solutions and strategies for a lot of different anxieties and phobias, and a section on sleep. Written by a PHD, but doable and incredibly practical. Highly recommended.

7. Emotional Freedom Technique (EFT) is very effective in reducing anxiety and panic. Related disciplines include Thought Field Therapy, etc. Refer to the EFT section in Chapter 35. Like all alternative therapies, ensure that you see a well respected and experienced practitioner to get the best results. Do your homework.

8. Breathing exercises, meditation, Yoga, Tai Chi and other slow movement, brain-relaxing methodologies are all helpful.

9. Insomnia is one the most common conditions that can aggravate anxiety disorders. Yeah, OK, so that's why you're here...

Stress

If the strings of an instrument are always taut
they go out of tune.
Manual of the Warriors of Light, Paulo Coelho

Stress is experienced in a number of dimensions in our lives, some of them more obvious than others. And each day we all experience stress, whether minor or major, or both.

Stressors can be very complex in our consciousness, subconscious, physical makeup, genetic predispositions, etc.

All this is complicated by our subconscious minds, our belief systems, and often our inability to understand exactly how all this integrates to make us who we are, and who we think we are. What part of our lack of confidence is inherited or wrongly adapted because of circumstances? Can we change any of it? And if so, how?

And the opposite thoughts: how do we develop our abilities, strengths and creativity? What processes brought us there, and was it all an accident?

With all the personal development courses, psychological analyses, advanced research on how the mind works: does any of this really make a difference to improve the quality and meaning in most people's lives? Does it bring people the peace, contentment and success that we apparently all want and need?

Without getting too philosophical here, I think we all agree that we need to have some pretty good techniques to be able to survive and enjoy our lives as best we can.

It is while we are sleeping that some of the day's stress is resolved, our bodies rest and repair, new connections are made in our minds, emotions are worked through, our day is sorted, and our imagination is let loose.

Good sleep is vital.

Emotions

A significant factor in stress is unresolved emotions.

Guilt, sadness, fear, frustration, resignation, shame, regret, grief, happiness, excitability, tenderness, fear, apathy, scorn, jealousy, blame, humiliation, embarrassment, trust … we know that they affect our daily lives. We are constantly dealing with them.

They are in our conscious, and our subconscious.

We should observe the kinds of emotions that are most common in our lives. Before you go to sleep at night, are you re-playing parts of the day that you regret? That you were embarrassed about? That you felt shame for?

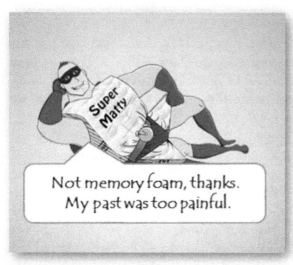

These are common thoughts, but they need to be addressed as part of your self-diagnosis around getting a better night's sleep.

Most of us will admit that unresolved emotions affect our energy levels and our health.

For many years people have been associating different parts of the body to different emotions. Some of these connections are obvious and used often (e.g. the heart with love) and some are less obvious (anger with liver, sadness and grief with lungs, fear with kidneys, etc).

The Chinese associate different emotions to different energy meridians and pressure points in the body.

Healing modalities such as yoga, Tai Chi, Qi Gong, meditation, Emotional Freedom Technique (EFT), Thought Field Therapy (TFT), acupressure and acupuncture have developed systems to help with emotions and general health. In fact, there seems to be an endless array of healing modalities, and it is possible to combine a number of modalities/platforms in order to achieve positive results.

SLEEP DOJO – Stress

1. Like all of the emotional reasons why you are not sleeping well, you must address the underlying reasons why you are feeling

stressed. Firstly identify the reasons, then get some professional help (if necessary) to work out a strategy to address the underlying problem – either to reduce the stress, or to eliminate the stress. This could involve counselling, a life change, lifestyle change, a large decision, finding new friends, or working out a strategy to deal with the stress better – if your stressor is a permanent problem that you can see resolving.

2. Daily exercise.
3. Clean up your diet and lifestyle - refer to Chapter 27.
4. Even half an hour a day of a new habit could be helpful over time, in retraining your routine to more self care and relaxation. If you are really stressed, the first few times that you might listen to soothing music, for example, may feel like it isn't making any difference. However over time, you might find that that same music will put you to sleep, because you have entrained yourself to relax to the sound of that music. Similarly this can happen with meditation, guided meditations, Tai Chi, etc. A visit to the beach to listen to the crashing waves for half an hour a day might be meaningful to another person, or a walk in nature in the evening.
5. Investigating new alternatives is recommended. You might take up art, or music or help in a community group, investigate different healing modalities. Anything that gets you away from your normal stress patterns.
6. An example of a new modality is Neuro-Training. Reference 28 will lead you to an eye modes and breathing exercise that might help you with your problem[28]. Think of what you are stressed about while doing the exercise.
7. Use EFT to tap-out your stress (see Chapter 35 - Emotional Freedom Technique section.) I recommend that you get the help of a leading practitioner if you want to use EFT to help.
8. Make some tough (or easy?) decisions in order to get the stress out of your life. Refer to Chapter 33.

Attention Deficit Hyperactivity Disorder – ADHD

My most recent research into this problem came from Professor Peter Gøtzsche's presentation *Mental Health, Overdiagnosed and Overmedicated* in Sydney in early 2015. You might be interested to learn that he basically stated that ADHD was not a well defined psychological problem and that most of the high achievers he knows would possibly/probably qualify as having the problem[29].

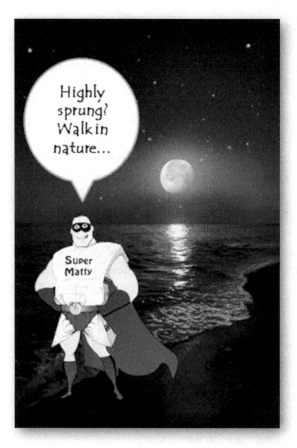

Sue Dengate, founder of Australia's Food Intolerance Network has isolated many food additives, colourings, and chemicals that are associated with ADHD[30], and some are very similar or the same offenders that are causing other problems mentioned in this book.

I've also seen ADHD described as "hyper vigilance", which might be a pointer in your family to something going on that is causing your child to be wired too often, then becoming exhausted, which leads to further nervousness. A vicious cycle of stress that is not being relieved.

How long has your child been hyper vigilant? Have you correctly eliminated all food intolerance options? Is your child being neglected, bullied, isolated or abused? Is your child spending hours a day on computer games, video games and/or with violent and disturbing images and ideas?

Did you know that our subconscious mind can't tell the difference between reality and what we watch on television or violent games? Our brains have to "integrate" that rubbish somehow – which of course puts stress on our bodies and minds.

Frankly, I'd prefer not to integrate it – so I don't watch violence at all.

Even watching television is disturbing for adults – let alone innocent children. It is so full of rubbish.

The other overlapping research is with omega-3 supplementation. Dr. Natalie Parletta (previously Dr. Natalie Sinn) from the University of Adelaide has seen significant positive results for about half of the ADHD sufferers taking omega-3 supplementation[31][32] over a significant period of time. Even though Cochrane does not support omega-3 (yet?) I'm open that future research might support it.

In a previously cited interview with Newshub Auckland, New Zealand[33] Natalie Sinn mentioned a study that showed evidence that long-term use of stimulant medication (often prescribed for ADHD sufferers) has been associated with stunted growth and increased risk of juvenile delinquency and connections with offences and jail time. Convincing reasons to have a look at food additives (Chapter 27), and do your own experiments with appropriate omega-3 supplementation.

You might be interested to see how the laws were developing in the FDA in 2011 around synthetic food colourings and their perceived (or actual) effect on behavioural problems in children:

"In 2011 an FDA Food Advisory Committee heard expert comment and then voted by a four-fifths majority that the evidence did not support a causal relationship between consumption of synthetic colour additives and adverse behavioural effects in children in the general population. By a much smaller majority (8 to 6), they decided against interim warning labels for products containing synthetic colour additives. But the FDA has not closed the issue and is reportedly collecting data on current dye levels in foods with an eye toward revisiting estimated daily intake levels."[34]

The full article is very interesting if you are keen to know more.

SLEEP DOJO – ADHD

1. Establish the underlying cause of the problem that is manifesting as the symptom of ADHD, or ADHD-like-behaviours.

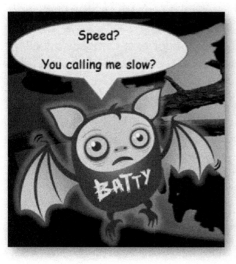

2. What is the reason for 'hyper vigilance' in this specific case?

3. Do one of the respected full-elimination diets under supervision to isolate exactly the offending food additives or chemicals, if applicable. Refer to the Food Intolerance Network for recommended dieticians.

4. Get one-on-one help from a well-qualified practitioner, talk therapist and/or counsellor.

CHAPTER 32

Type I: Environment

Your sleep environment is very important. You should sleep in a dark, clean, chemical-free, quiet, and cool room, with fresh air and where you feel totally safe.

Snoring and Snoring Partners

The most common sleep disorder is snoring. There are a few different ways people breathe while they sleep. We breathe differently when we have a cold, when we are in different positions in bed, if we are overweight, if we breathe through our nose or mouth, if we have some obstruction in our airways, etc. Different sounds and noises are made with different issues. E.g. the noise made by the vibration of the pharynx in your throat made during breathing, generally with the intake of air.

Nearly 85% of snorers exceed 38 decibels of sound, with loud snorers getting up to about 90 decibels, which is similar to a loud yell[1]. At that level it affects hearing, including the hearing of your bed partner.

Infants

Snoring affects 18-20% of infants, which is a higher percentage than other childhood snoring – they seem to grow out of it gradually, and then only return to snoring as adults.

Breastfeeding for longer than a month has been shown to reduce snoring at aged 8. The study, reported in the Cochrane Library, was performed on a cohort of children with a family history of asthma[2].

Children and Adolescents

According to the American National Sleep Foundation most children snore on occasions, with about 10 percent snoring most nights[3].

The data indicates that children with poor sleep and snoring will have a lower IQ, not just during the sleep deprivation period, but subsequent to it.

A study in America found that children who were identified by their parents as snorers at ages 4 and 5 had lower-than-average IQs[4].

Another study, published in *Pediatrics* showed that persistent snorers showed higher incidence of behavioural problems, particularly hyperactivity, depression and inattention[5]. That same study showed the highest predictors of the presence of and persistence of snoring were socioeconomic and the absence or shorter duration of breast milk feeding as infants[6].

Adults

Snoring afflicts about 44% of men and 30% of women. (About 45% snore occasionally, and around 25% snore habitually[7]).

Snoring is linked with sleep deprivation, depression, aggression, daytime exhaustion, hypertension, cognitive impairment, obesity, cardiovascular disease, hearing loss, digestive dysfunction and even impotence.

People tend to snore when they are on their backs, according to Edward Stepanski, director of the Sleep Disorder Center at Rush-Presbyterian-St. Luke's Medical Center in Chicago. He suggests placing a tennis ball in a sock and pinning it to your pyjamas right between your shoulder blades. It sounds punishing, but he says it will prompt you to roll back on to your side, without waking you up.

Numerous studies indicate that snoring is more likely in overweight people, and generally gets worse with age.

According to the British Medical Journal 1997, about one-third of adults over the age of 30 are snorers, that number increasing to about 40% by middle age.

The American National Sleep Foundation states that sleep apnea may be present in up to 40% of those adults who experience snoring.

You probably won't appreciate it when I tell you to lose weight, but I'll say it anyway. This is a pretty obvious solution for many snorers, and there are many other health benefits from having a healthy body mass index and diet, with improved energy.

I've seen studies that link being overweight to depression (although I'm not sure which comes first).

As little as 10 to 15% weight loss can reduce or eliminate sleep-disordered breathing, and may curtail the cardiovascular risk associated with sleep-disordered breathing.

Respondents whose body mass index exceeds 35 (described as 'obese') experience the highest rates of insomnia.

Having a lean and fit body improves your emotional well being, and motivates you to keep active.

The last solution for snorers who may not have noticed special information in *Chapter 27 – Type D: Drugs, Food Additives and Chemicals*, is that there are foods and dairy foods that are associated with snoring in babies, children and adults!

The Bad News about Overheating in Bed

This discussion rarely comes up, but it's a very important one, as you'll see.

Our normal body temperature is 37⁰C, but when we sleep we should be significantly cooler than that.

Sleeping cool is better for your sleep, and your health generally:

- Overheating in bed reduces your REM (rapid eye movement) sleep, and causes disturbed sleep patterns. Temperatures above 32⁰C (which is pretty cool, actually) begin to adversely affect REM sleep[8].
- Overheating in bed has been associated with the following adverse skin conditions – doona eyes, facial dermatitis, peri-oral dermatitis, Grover's disease, facial excrescences, atopic eczema, acne, and hair and scalp problems[9].

- Overheating is associated with problems in the first trimester of pregnancy. Hot spa baths and saunas have been associated with foetal abnormalities. Sleeping cool during this period is recommended.
- The ultimate temperature for sperm production is 35.5 degrees C, temperatures above that can affect fertility[10].
- In order to fall asleep our core temperature needs to reduce by 0.3 of a degree. This temperature drop is actually a trigger to switch our bodies to sleeping mode. It's one of the reasons people recommend having a warm bath before getting into bed, to effect that temperature drop. And it's also a reason why we don't recommend warming your bed with an electric blanket (or other methods). If you do pre-warm your bed, turn the electric blanket OFF before getting into bed.

So we need to sleep cool, right? But what happens if one partner in bed is hot, and the other isn't?

We have noticed that in about 80% of couples, one partner is hotter than the other. Men are usually hotter than the women, for example. We have also noticed that women after menopause can become hotter than the men, reversing the situation.

This situation was the catalyst years ago for inventing the *Compatibility Blanket™*. How do partners "sleep cool" when one has a different idea of "cool" than the other?

The *Compatibility Blanket™* has pure cotton sheeting on one half (for the person who feels hot) and pure merino wool blanketing on the other half (for the person who feels cold).

Put the *Compatibility Blanket®* on top of your top sheet, with the cotton half over the hot person, the woollen half over the cooler person. When it gets colder just add more bed coverings. One side will always be warmer than the other. No more arguments!

The Compatibility Blanket is unique in the world, only available through the Sleepless No More website. We ship internationally, and are looking for distributors in Europe and the US, because freight is costly.

For more information about the Compatibility Blanket visit https://www.sleeplessnomore.com/compatibility-blanket/ (Accessed March 22, 2017)

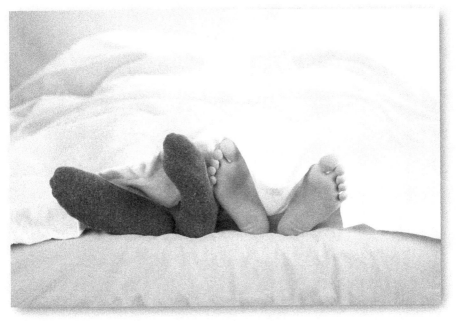

One's Hot, One's Not?

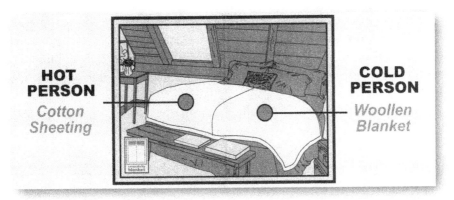

End the Nightly Battle of the Bedclothes

Fresh Oxygenated Air and a Chemical-Free Environment

I've read a number of articles over the years about people having difficulty sleeping, or sleeping when they shouldn't, because of chemical fumes in new furniture, mattresses, television chairs, lounges and carpets, even office equipment.

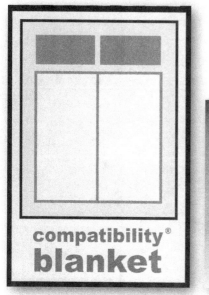
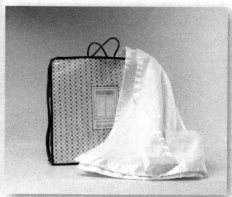

The Compatibility Blanket®

"Sick Building Syndrome", a term used by Steve Brown of Australia's CSIROs Department of Building Construction and Engineering, is one person who has highlighted a variety of chemicals that are emitted in and from newly built houses, paints, carpets, air conditioners, VOCs (Volatile Organic Chemicals – not the good "organic"), toxic chemicals in building materials and furniture materials, pillows that have been treated with fire retardant, etc[11].

Studies in Australia and Britain, and others published in *New Scientist* have found high levels of toxic chemicals leaking from newly built houses.

In Melbourne, a CSIRO study found that houses less than a year old had up to 20 times the safety limit of volatile organic compounds (VOCs) recommended by the National Health and Medical Research Council (NHMRC)[12].

In Britain, concentrations of VOCs in homes less than a year old were twice as high as in homes built 10 years ago.

Quite apart from disturbing your sleep patterns, chemicals used in construction materials that leach into the air in your environment include the possible carcinogens formaldehyde (from manufactured wooden flooring, plywood, pressed wood products, particle board and furniture), and styrene (new carpets). More and more carcinogens are being added to lists now, including chemicals used to perfume bathrooms and houses, and makeup components that are not regulated at all in Australia (that's another topic, refer to the Environmental Working Group's website http://www.ewg.org/skindeep/, accessed March 20, 2017, which is USA-centric, but some brands sold in Australia are listed on this site).

VOCs give intolerant people headaches, or make them feel instantly sick[13]. Not thinking I was one of 'those people', the other day I was sniffing expensive soaps at a plant shop and felt a headache coming on while I was doing it! Interesting.

Consequently I do not promote buying a new pillow and/or mattress every other season/year for whatever "profit-for-the-pillow-and-mattress-industry-reason".

It's not all about the mattress.

If people can sleep well, they can sleep on a concrete floor, or camping out. It is rarely about what you are sleeping on, and often about industry promoting what is profitable. (Super Matty disagrees – for him it's all about me, me, me, the mattress.)

Yep, same old story here too. Let's keep it real.

Dust mites don't make much noise, nor emit toxic carcinogenic chemicals.

Clean Air Solutions

Maximizing the oxygen in your bedroom and home is going to improve your sleep and health significantly.

The first list of air-purifying plants was published by NASA in 1989.

The NASA Clean Air Study found that some plants have the ability not only to help oxygenate an environment/room but can clean certain chemicals from the air including benzene, formaldehyde, trichloroethylene, xylene, toluene and ammonia[14].

What's not to love about that?

Refer to that study (and others since) for a list of indoor plants that might improve the value of your sleep through improved air quality. The plants include peace lily, English ivy, mother-in-law's tongue and florist's chrysanthemum. Many of the best air purifying plants can be toxic to animals (if they eat them, for example), so watch how you implement this strategy.

Further research will even help you calculate how many plants you should have inside, depending on the size of the house and pot size.

Those peace lilies and spiky mother in law's tongues we see around aren't just decorative.

Your Pitch Black Bedroom

If you aren't doing it already you'll be surprised at how awesome having a completely dark black bedroom will make you feel. I've experimented with this idea personally, even using black cotton sheets on the bed – and I'm a convert.

I personally don't think eye shades over your eyes compare to having a completely dark black room.

I suspect that being in the dark is a whole-of-body-experience, not just limited to our eyes/retinas etc.

Ever since I read about the circadian experiments done by the University of Virginia in Charlottesville, using light shone behind knees[15], and another report about how our skin changes in bright light, I am convinced that there will be significant future developments in the science of light and circadian rhythm.

The retina of the eye is only one place where light is sensed by our bodies. So, OK, use those eye shades on plane flights and other places where the options aren't great – but at home create a completely dark and peaceful world to sleep in.

Black out curtains, no light from anywhere.

Just thinking about it and visualising it is relaxing.

If you're a shift worker (and hopefully after reading this book you won't be a *long term* shift worker – like ever, duh) it's even more important.

Completely black rooms should be universal for shift-workers, travellers, pilots, airline industry workers, emergency crews, mine managers and workers, ambulance personnel, medical emergency professionals, hospital workers, nurses and security personnel.

And this black room can double up as an awesome napping room or meditation room too.

SLEEP DOJO - Type I

1. Your bedroom should be quiet, dark, clean, uncluttered and used for sleep and sex only.
2. Sleep cool, rather than hot. Sleep under layers so that you can regulate the temperature. Throw out any heavy doonas. If you wake in the night, take a layer off as your first option. If you sleep in air-conditioning, ensure the temperature is set low.
3. If you sleep with a snorer or sleep apnea sufferer and you can't sleep successfully in the same bed, go to another bed, or another room if necessary. It is not an ideal situation, but if you're not sleeping properly, that is worse. In 2007 a survey of the National Association of Homebuilders predicted that by 2015, 60% of custom built homes in America will have two master bedroom suites[16]. That didn't happen to my knowledge, but for snorers, bed hoggers, wrigglers, and sleep apnea couples I think it's a great idea. And for your pets too, by the way.
4. Save electricity – start turning the lights down or off early. Download the f.lux free software to your computer to reduce the blue light coming off your screen at the end of the day. Set up a peaceful environment for the later hours of the day, and use that environment to prepare for sleep.
5. Fresh air! Reduce all chemicals and volatile organic chemicals, perfumes, and sprays – particularly if you are intolerant to them. Use oxygenating and cleansing plants to improve the air quality in your home and bedroom. Dump all those toxic perfumes, room deodorisers, plug in room scenters and harsh cleaning chemicals and opt for a more natural and healthy environment.
6. Select peaceful, clean, and cool colours for your bedroom e.g. blues, off-whites, pale greens, greys, browns and neutrals. Black is great for your sleep if you're creative enough to make it work in your home. I've seen some awesome black bedrooms, one with a Venetian glass chandelier: get creative.
7. Get rid of all the clutter in your bedroom (preferably in your whole house too), and in your mind. Some people who are "collectors" need to simplify, as their behaviour could indicate obsessive compulsive

disorder (OCD), anxiety, unresolved emotional issues or other psychological problems. Certainly hoarding is associated with anxiety and stress (if you don't believe me try suggesting that you come around and help your friend declutter). Get some help simplifying your house if you need to, before it becomes overwhelming. Don't put off the decision. My observations are that procrastination also comes with hoarding. If you do get a bit anxious about decluttering, schedule it just for one hour at a time, regularly each week, and make a promise that if you bring a new non-consumable into your house, you have to dump something in return. You will be surprised that you can make great progress by chunking the job down – you might even start enjoying it when you see and feel the difference it makes to you.

8. Remember to use black out curtains and other props to ensure that the bedroom is really dark or black where possible. If you're a shift worker, a black room should be compulsory.

CHAPTER 33

Type J: Decisions, Decisions

When we postpone the harvest, the fruit rots,
but when we postpone our problems, they keep on growing.
The Fifth Mountain, Paulo Coelho

ot being able to sleep is often a result of not being happy in our lives.
One out-of-balance area can adversely affect all the other areas.
Do this simple exercise now:

Consider the following statements, and rate them 1 – 9 (from 1 strongly disagree, to 9 strongly agree, 5 being the neutral position):

A. I love my job. It is rewarding, challenging, and fun, and I enjoy my workmates a lot.
   1   2   3   4   5   6   7   8   9
B. My partner is my "soul mate", we are friends and lovers, have great fun, and get along really well.
   1   2   3   4   5   6   7   8   9
C. My children and extended family feel supported, loved and encouraged by me.
   1   2   3   4   5   6   7   8   9
D. I contribute significantly to my community, and offer a worthwhile service that I am proud of.
   1   2   3   4   5   6   7   8   9

E. My friends are honest and fun, and we get together often in a very positive environment.

1 2 3 4 5 6 7 8 9

F. I treat people with respect, show love, and vice-versa.

1 2 3 4 5 6 7 8 9

G. I have great health because I look after myself, exercise, eat properly and think expansively.

1 2 3 4 5 6 7 8 9

H. When I have problems in my life, I take full responsibility for them and spend time and effort to work through them to create a better life.

1 2 3 4 5 6 7 8 9

I. When I have difficulties, I ask for help from positive, friendly, qualified talk therapists.

1 2 3 4 5 6 7 8 9

J. I am open with my emotions when I'm happy, sad, lonely, or challenged. I allow people to know the real, vulnerable me.

1 2 3 4 5 6 7 8 9

K. I spend my time doing activities that uplift and contribute to society, my family and friends.

1 2 3 4 5 6 7 8 9

L. I recognize that discipline, endeavour, hard work, persistence and a willingness to learn are important for my success.

1 2 3 4 5 6 7 8 9

M. I work continually to encourage and leverage my natural talents.

1 2 3 4 5 6 7 8 9

N. I enlist others to help me in areas where I don't excel, so that I can still have a rounded and successful life.

1 2 3 4 5 6 7 8 9

O. I set goals and take action to achieve what I want in all areas of my life.

1 2 3 4 5 6 7 8 9

P. I value money and wealth, and work towards contributing more through those accomplishments.

1 2 3 4 5 6 7 8 9

Q. We keep our lifestyle balanced with our income so that my family and I aren't stressed about bills.

1   2   3   4   5   6   7   8   9

R. I have good self esteem, accept myself as I am, and think I am physically and otherwise attractive.

1   2   3   4   5   6   7   8   9

S. I pick myself up when I fail, and try again, knowing that failure is part of success.

1   2   3   4   5   6   7   8   9

T. My life is challenging, rewarding and a lot of fun.

1   2   3   4   5   6   7   8   9

U. When I think that I'm stuck in my life, I have the courage to make the hard decisions to change, even when it affects other people.

1   2   3   4   5   6   7   8   9

Of the 21 questions, how many 1-4 answers did you rate? How many 6-9? How many 1s? How many 9s?

What insights, aggravations and reactions did just seeing those questions bring up? Did you bother to answer the questions? Did you avoid any of the questions? Did you think some of the questions were stupid? Did you think some of the questions are naïve or only for people who believe in fairy tales?

Now, write down your emotional and other reactions to doing that exercise.

Keep that list, and write down in more detail exactly what was going on for you while you answered the questions. Knowing that there will be some reactions, note whether you were making excuses why you could only rate a 2 here, or a 1 there. Or blaming other people or your circumstances for why you couldn't possibly answer an 8 or 9 for some relevant questions.

Do you procrastinate and make excuses instead of making decisions? Do you always have to be right, refusing to recognize the problems around you? Is your mortgage keeping you awake? Is your primary relationship toxic? Is your work a total drag? Negative friends? No work-life balance? Unethical behaviours? Domestic violence? Manipulation? Victim mentality?

These are all very good reasons why you don't sleep well at night, and good enough reasons to make a change!

This exercise, if you choose to go into it in detail, will reveal some areas that you could work on in order to achieve a happier and more fulfilled life. And remember: if you are happy and fulfilled, those around you will be much happier and fulfilled, too.

What's the other side of the coin? Somehow, life seems to come up with the balancing act whether we like it or not. It might take a bit of time before it does, but sometimes the balancing act is a Mack Truck that we cannot avoid, and it is VERY painful. If we hate our work for 5 years, can't stand our boss, but don't take the risks to move somewhere else or do something else (or both), one day, whammo!—we have been given the sack. Somehow, our attitude was affecting our work, output, and co-workers. It's not too hard to see the "whammo effect"— especially in *other people's lives*, is it?

By the way, did you know that couples that argue stay together longer? But there are good ways to argue. A perfect relationship doesn't necessarily mean you never argue.

And what about YOU, mums? Are you spending your whole life looking after the kids, keeping the house clean, shining the shoes, mending the school uniforms, and doing the laundry at midnight? If so, you'll wake up one day and ask, 'where did my life go?' Hmmm, it isn't necessarily a midlife crisis. Maybe it just took that long to see what we were doing to ourselves!

My theory is that we have quite a few challenges continually. Don't leave the challenges so long that they pile up and become unbearable and insurmountable.

And generally addressing one problem positively affects the others. Well, often enough.

Denial doesn't work. For example I've known dishonest people who "get away with" their dishonesty for a while, and then later find their life not working. They wonder, twenty or so years later, why they're depressed, and have very few genuine friends to talk to.

Authenticity is required to sleep well, and so are all the other aspects of having a good life.

Having great friends, who you openly converse with, showing your vulnerabilities and challenges is a very precious thing. Generally friends who genuinely support each other emotionally and are open with each other find and give support when each other needs help.

By the way, if you get lonely, keep in mind that you don't have to be 'better' to have friends, you just have to be open and loving. Showing your vulnerabilities is an endearing quality to other people who start relaxing with you, and allowing you in to their friendships and life.

Kind of the opposite to the bragging and BS we do on Facebook and social media. Sure you can talk about your trip to Fiji (if you're lucky enough to go), but balance it with real world stuff, fun and interesting valuable information .... or don't bother at all.

SLEEP DOJO - Type J

> *The warrior of light knows that he is free to choose his desires,*
> *and he makes these decisions with courage, detachment*
> *and – sometimes – with just a touch of madness.*
> The Manual of the Warrior of Light, Paulo Coelho

1. Write down 3 things you'd like to improve in your life.
2. Write down next to that what ACTION you are going to take to bring it about.
3. Tell someone close to you about your new plans, and ask them to help you be accountable for your new changes.
4. Set a date.

P.S. If you can't find things in your life you would like to improve then I don't think you're being real.

CHAPTER 34

Age Related Sleep.

The required hours of sleep vary with age. Not only that, but at certain ages the natural sleeping patterns seem to change, such as the delayed sleep phase pattern of adolescents and teenagers versus the advanced sleep phase syndrome that can occur in mature age. Discussion of these changes is often accompanied by the question of "the ultimate number of hours sleep" for different people. This chapter addresses these questions.

Some people seem to survive well on only a few hours' sleep, like Margaret Thatcher and Winston Churchill, who could run a country at the same time.

Recent studies by Ying-Hui Fu at the University of California, San Francisco indicate that the Dec2 gene is one gene that is mutated in people who survive well on very little sleep.[1] This genetic mutation follows through families.

A word of warning here, because I often hear people bragging that they do fine on very little sleep. And they often quote people like Winston Churchill and Margaret Thatcher (like I have above) as reasons why we don't need much sleep.

Winston Churchill was both depressed and an alcoholic, and napped during the day. Margaret Thatcher suffered from dementia and a series of minor strokes from her early 70s[2], which I believe precludes her from being a "lack of sleep hero", in spite of the fact that she previously had an incredible mental capacity. That could make her case even less convincing.

I'm not buying the general conversation that "lots of people do well with very little sleep", and I never encourage people to go without a decent amount of sleep.

I especially don't encourage children and adolescents to reduce their sleep, as I believe that mental health issues are exacerbated by lack of sleep – adding to anxieties, stress and muddled thinking.

I see *no evidence* at all to promote a less-sleep strategy (except in the case of investigating narcolepsy and people who want to sleep all day).

What I do see is a *supposed* rise in mental health issues - many of which would be fixed by good sleep, proper food, some healthy exercise outside and reasonable social engagement with family and friends.

Pregnancy and Unborn Babies

It's very common for pregnant mothers to get out of bed a number of times a night to go to the bathroom. In fact, by the end of pregnancy 97.3 % of soon-to-be mums wake up an *average* of 3.11 times[3].

It is most important during pregnancy to be aware that the baby is responding to the foods you eat, the sounds that you hear, the medications you take (preferably none), the alcohol you drink, etc. It is a great time to improve your diet and lifestyle in preparation for when the baby arrives! Do not take any unnecessary substances or medications before checking the impact they might have on your baby from a very reliable source.

SLEEP DOJO – Pregnancy and Unborn Babies

Here are some of the tips that I've read to make it easier to sleep:

- Sleep on your left side, avoiding lying on your back for extended periods.
- Restless Leg Syndrome and leg cramps – see the solutions in chapter 29, including avoiding carbonated sodas and drinks.
- Be a bit *more* sensitive to your health and wellbeing. There is a lot of change happening, and it is affecting your whole family.
- This is the time to establish good habits *before* the baby is born. Optimize your health now, because when the baby is born you will

have less time for "you" and you could be tired and a little emotional for a time after the baby is born.

■ If you feel like having an afternoon nap, just do it. Look after yourself; you are doing it for the two of you now!

Babies and Toddlers

Babies and toddlers definitely need the most sleep of anyone. Newborn babies may sleep on and off for as many as 16 hours a day. Not only is the amount of sleep different for babies, but they also have a shorter sleep cycle (40 minutes, instead of adults' 90-minute cycles). You will appreciate this sleep time as parents, so that you can recover from what is often a very demanding and exhausting day, especially when the baby is first born.

There are many reasons why babies cry. Most of them, thankfully, are "normal" feeding cries, over-tired cries, or "feeling uncomfortable" cries. One of the hardest things for stressed-out new mums and dads to achieve is to distinguish between normal crying and crying that might indicate a more serious condition. Unfortunately, there are no hard-and-fast rules here, so you do have to be vigilant. Generally, it will eventually become clearer, but the first week or so can be challenging. And sometimes for a lot longer.

It's also a time when everyone else will give you their opinion on how the baby should be looked after, which adds to the parents' stress. Mothers-in-law, sisters-in-law, grandparents with their old-fashioned ideas, even friends who mightn't have a clue! New evidence shows that fathers (not just mothers) can be depressed during the early years of parenthood; in fact, a study reported in the online journal "Pediatrics," indicated that as many as 7% were clinically depressed. The clinically-depressed dads were 4 times more likely to report spanking their child in the last month, and were less likely to read to their children 3 or more times a week. Fathers interactively playing with their children is associated with attachment security in later childhood, and the exposure to speech and language by reading is associated with language development.

It's most important that you try to fit in some time for yourselves when the baby is tiny. I personally found it one of the most challenging times of my life because I like to be productive. I felt like I wasn't doing anything except feeding the baby, getting meals, washing and home duties.

Make sure you verbalise your challenges to your partner, family or friends – someone might volunteer to look after the baby one afternoon so you can have a very big sleep, for example.

You don't have to become a whinger, but you can get mentally low when you are exhausted – and fathers are in this group too. Suddenly they have gone from the most important person in their partner's life to somewhere a long way down the list after doing the washing! It isn't pretty and it is a very challenging time all round.

It's great to join parent's groups, or meet your friends for coffee – no one really gets what you are going through, except your friends who are in the same place. If you don't have any friends who have young babies ask your community health nurse, or the local council and other places to see if there are any groups you can join. They will be very pleased to have a new friend in you.

And don't confuse exhaustion with depression, they are different things.

Post natal depression is a serious condition, so watch to see if you are showing symptoms of feeling emotionally separated from your baby, crying and generally feeling low.

Bringing a new child into the family is a big event, so be easy on your-selves, your partner and all the family around this time.

If you are a family member wanting to get involved, offer some help rather than your opinion on "how it should be done". Hang the washing out, clean the house (without making the new parents feel inadequate), take the baby for a walk to let the parents have a sleep, or offer to take the baby or the other children for a set period each week so that the parents can begin to look forward and plan for that time next week or next month. Even the time to watch a movie together is something to look forward to when you have a baby in the house.

Other issues include colic, reflux, teething, jaundice (where babies often sleep more often), reactions to injections/immunizations, and food additives and colourings that pass through the milk of breast feeding mothers.

Please refer to the sections on snoring and sleep apnea for children.

Each baby is different, even within the same family, and they change their sleeping habits reasonably often. Fortunately, there has been much written about the baby-sleep arena. I'm not going to repeat it all here, but I'll make reference to some areas that you might want to investigate further.

Karitane

The Karitane Mothercraft Society is famous in Australia for helping mothers and babies. Karitane started in New Zealand in 1907 with Sir Truby King helping mothers who could not breastfeed when there were no available successful formulas. In 1923, the Australian Mothercraft Society was established in Coogee, Australia. It has also been known as the Plunket Society.

This organisation's help has expanded greatly over the years beyond baby-feeding problems, and includes sleep and settling routines, immunization information, weaning, toilet training, management of gastro-oesophageal reflux, development, toddler behaviour management, childhood illnesses and problems, perinatal and postnatal moods, anxiety, stress, and depression.

People who have gone to Karitane with their unsettled babies have joked to me that they "must put something in the air conditioning" because their babies seem to improve as soon as they enter the building! So if you have access to their help and information, do it.

The Karitane website is a wonderful place for information that you can access, including downloadable factsheets on a wide range of topics that will interest you. Here are the links that I think you will find most valuable:

Website: http://www.karitane.com.au (Accessed March 22, 2017)

My baby and me information page: http://karitane.com.au/mybabyandme/ (Accessed March 22, 2017)

Parenting advice and downloadable factsheets, in different languages: http://karitane.com.au/karitane/parents-overview/ (Accessed March 22, 2017)

Look around in there, as there is a wealth of information –the organisation has grown since I looked there last.

It's very important that you feel OK when the baby is born and that your baby feels safe and warm and gets the attention that he/she needs to feel comfortable and loved and relaxed.

There's no replacement for the love and care of a mother and parent when they are tiny and growing.

Not a PC statement for some, old-school for others, but if you get the opportunity you will not regret it. And I'm sure your child will benefit throughout their life.

There's information on sleep needs, tantrums, feeding advice and a whole lot more. What a great resource.

Good luck – it is challenging, but well worth it.

And yes, if you want to know, I'm a breast feeding enthusiast. For a long time. Just sayin'.

After having a baby it takes a while to get your time back, and your independence (and your brain, that was my challenge!).

Apparently it is harder for women who have had good jobs and are very independent.

I found that out much later! I wish I had heard it earlier.

Karitane is there if you want to call them, email them a question, whatever. They understand and are awesome.

Their 7 days a week CareLine is 1300 227 464.

The Food Intolerance Network

Talking about breastfeeding leads me to the work done by the Food Intolerance Network.

Did you know that if your baby is intolerant to certain food additives, colourings and chemicals it might come through your breast milk and cause them sleep disturbances and other problems?

Likewise any medication you are taking while breast feeding, alcohol, etc.

I recommend that you visit the website www.FedUp.com.au for more information. Also refer to Drugs, Food Additives and Chemicals, Chapter 27.

There is also a forum on the Fed Up/Food Intolerance Network website that you can join if you need some help.

Sounds and Music

Many babies and young children find the heartbeat sound very comforting. There are cuddly toys and other baby-friendly comforters that I think have benefits, as well as playing soft calming music in the house generally.

I'm not a fan of a lot of digital equipment, wifi beams and electronics near babies as I don't see the point, and I'm seeing some troubling speculation and developments.

Simplify rather than complicate their environments, and you will find it less complicated too, I expect.

Massage and a few Random Ideas

Warm baths, massage, gentle homeopathics, calming music, and aromatherapy are often used successfully with babies and toddlers.

And organic foods (where possible, and within your budget) are always preferred.

But the overriding idea is to keep it simple and do the best you can while trying to get some sleep yourself. It's not all about them, though it often feels that way.

SLEEP DOJO - Babies and Toddlers

1. If you are breastfeeding your baby, be mindful that certain food additives and colourings pass through your milk to the baby.
2. If you suspect that your child is intolerance to something he or she is eating (See Chapter 27), eliminate that item from their diet—and yours, if you are breastfeeding.
3. Seek professional advice if you have a baby who suffers from colic, is continually restless, or if you can't really understand why they are restless. When mums and dads are tired and stressed, it is easy to make some inappropriate decisions.
4. Organic food is ideal, and highly recommended for babies.
5. Look out for your partner and other members of the family as well. It is not all about the new baby—the new arrival changes the dynamics of the whole family, so make sure that every member is happy and well-adjusted during this period. Follow up any signs of depression in either parent immediately!

Teenagers and Adolescents

"Insomnia is both common and chronic among adolescents. **The data indicate that the burden of insomnia is comparable to that of other psychiatric disorders such as mood, anxiety, disruptive, and substance use disorders.** Chronic insomnia severely impacts future health and functioning of youths. Those with chronic insomnia are more likely to seek medical care. These data suggest primary care settings might provide a venue for screening and early intervention for adolescent insomnia."[4]

Researchers measured 14 aspects of personal well-being and found that adolescents with chronic insomnia were much more likely to have problems with drug use, depression, schoolwork, jobs and overall perceived health.[5]

Adolescents are a very maligned group of young people. They have a lot to deal with: physical change in their bodies, peer pressure, entering the confusing realm of relationships, end-of-school exams, their competitive parents pushing them to achieve good grades, all accompanied by the chant "you can achieve anything" – and they are exhausted for most of that time. No wonder they're stressed!

With what I call the "Paris Hilton Effect," which seems to have exaggerated the focus on what young people look like and their "sex appeal", (hmmm, sorry, I don't want to be derogatory...) it's a growing trend that "being fabulous" is expected of them far too early. What happened to being a kid? We know that their frontal lobes aren't developing till later, particularly with boys.

These children were brought up watching 9/11 on the television and playing desensitizing video games for hours, and we wonder why they act strangely! To balance this, I have read studies that say that anxiety is *not* on the rise, so it's hard to tell.

My opinion is that they are not allowed to be kids for long enough. Not allowed to discover their own surroundings in their own time, and to work out their place in the world in their own way. It's all dictated to them by their parents and social media, the news, the internet, trends etc.

And I believe there's far too much external stimulation instead of self discovery, working it out, being left alone, being allowed to try and fail, and be bored (mentally healthy kids rarely are – they don't rely on external stimuli to figure out things).

The solutions aren't easy, and they certainly require going against the trends.

I'd be encouraging any hobby that kids have that they want to do, that isn't dictated to them. Get them away for camping holidays and something near nature, beach time. Find some country friends and sit by the fire and talk, even better around a camp fire.

Recently a very small study speculated that camping might be able to alter our circadian rhythm and bring it forward an hour, which would be great for adolescents?[17] Let your kids be immersed in the rhythm of nature as often as you can. It will allow them to physically and mentally re-attune to the way things are naturally. If this can be achieved they will know how to naturally find their place and inner peace without too much hullabaloo. We shouldn't really have to meditate to bring ourselves "down", it should be reasonably easy to just "go there". Nature will help us do that. (This study was really small, admittedly, and I'm pretty sure that running around in the fresh air makes most people and children fall asleep pretty easily. But I like where it's heading.)

Exercise as a side effect of being outdoors, not the main game, and not competitive. Maybe you have to walk to the river to put the kayak in... all that.

We used to go camping when I lived in the bush, down in the back paddock of a sheep grazing property, and I often had to convince my friends whose kids were apparently "addicted to video games" that they would be OK to come. Generally it was the parents who had the problem – because the kids would arrive, stick a stick in the fire until the stick lit up, and they would then wave it around for hours mesmerised by the smoke and burning tip. This nothingness in some random paddock out in the middle of nowhere was enough. 1200 acres of trees, a creek, birds, warm fire and great food cooked in camp ovens or over the coals.

They were the best times.

And the kids totally loved it. Never, and I mean never, did any of them come up and want us to give them something to do. Playing near the creek, or picking up rocks, or steaming down a hill on bikes was all they wanted to do, and they slept well at night in spite of the adults' noisy conversation around the fire.

There was something magic happening there, and I'm sure it made a lasting impression on the children.

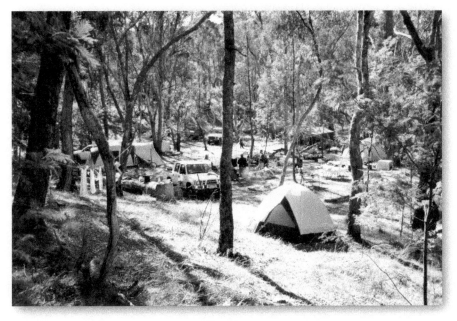

Camping

No mention of who was wearing certain brands of clothes, who was hot (OMG!), how totally dirty their clothes ended up being after a couple of days, who was cool and who wasn't...

Just exhaustion at the end of the day, and fun around the fire doing basically nothing. Scratching a stick into the dirt, finding a good rock to sit on, helping turn over the food, making a cup of tea.

Smelling the eucalyptus, watching the smoke rise, wishing there were more corn fritters.

Not too complicated really. Just let them be and give them time.

These kids, now grown up, did not achieved 99.99 in their HSC but they are all well rounded, conversational, creative and inspiring kids – making their way in the world in the way they choose to do it.

It hasn't all been smooth sailing, but they all have a great sense of self, which is priceless. That includes making mistakes, and permission to do that.

Fact: Teenagers and Delayed Sleep Phase

Teens can have a delayed sleep phase. Their circadian rhythm changes during these years to delay the time they feel like sleeping. They're *not* lazy, just more likely to be exhausted, because they are going to bed later and getting up at the same time to go to school.

They produce melatonin in the night (like everyone), and some of them are still producing melatonin as late as mid-morning the next day! Wherever possible, *let them sleep in.*

Teenagers and adolescents might be hitting the high-octane (and caffeine-loaded) drinks to make them alert when they are probably very tired. We are critical of them doing that, but we are still getting them out of bed early on Saturday mornings to play competitive sports!

Fact: Children grow while they are asleep. Are we stunting their growth by getting them up early, too?

If your child's delayed sleep phase means they go to bed at midnight, be mindful of the activities that you encourage on the weekends!

I'm aware of only one school where the seniors (years 11 and 12) started school at 11.00 am for years. It was Edmund Rice College in Wollongong, Australia, but I think they have changed the system in the last couple of years. It would have been amazing for someone to have done a full study on the effect this late start had on the attentiveness, alertness, growth, academic achievement and general attitude of these children. From what I understand, the timetable is about "efficient use of school resources," not better sleep, but I expect the benefits went way beyond their "resources."

A missed opportunity, because it sounded amazing.

Is acne an independent risk factor for suicidal ideation (thoughts about suicide)?

There appears to be some discussion about this, so I am including this in this book for you to be aware of the possible problem. It is outside the scope of this book, but I'll just mention it, because I know the kids get pretty thingy about what they look like.

There have been reports of suicidal thoughts and suicides from acne medications. Please do further research before you allow your children to be prescribed these medications.

Although one study I looked at in Cochrane[6] (covering just one medication) seemed not to confirm an increased risk. Further investigation might be appropriate.

Problems

Lastly, if you do have an aggressive, totally unhelpful and weird kid (and you're prepared to see it!), then you have to address the problems. I can't see what your child is like, that's your responsibility – I'm not letting them all off the hook here!

There is latitude without total permission, if you get my drift.

At some point in your children's lives (and in your own), you take on the consequences of all your activities and attitudes.

SLEEP DOJO - Teenagers & Adolescents

1. For heaven's sake, if you get to sleep in, take it! If you are a parent, don't make your kids feel that they are lazy or unmotivated if they are tired or grumpy. They ARE tired! Give them a break. When adults do the right thing and change the school hours so that adolescents and teenagers start school at 11.00 am in the morning, then we might have the right to complain if they still grunt!

2. Don't push them in your direction, support their dreams and enthusiasms - and *listen to them* even if you think their language is 'grunt' (or text messages)! Be there to support them through this trying and tiring period.

3. If you see behavioural and mental problems beginning to emerge, deal with them supportively and with subtlety – you don't want your children to be overly anxious about problems that might be surfacing at this time in their lives (it could just make them a lot worse). Help teens by putting things into perspective and by guiding them, not by putting them down. They may not appear to be

listening to you, but they generally are (you might not realize that for another few years).

4. One of my great friends says that "it takes a village to bring up a child," (which I love, because she has been part of my village). Ensure that you have great friends around you that your children can feel good about talking to. Create the village for your child by observing which of your friends has a natural connection with each of your children. This should happen naturally in great family environments, but a bit of encouragement might be necessary to bring it along. It is vitally important that it is your child's choice, not yours or your friends'. And don't wait for any problem to arise; that is too late. You may never find out there was a problem (apart from observing some unusual behaviour and attitudes around that time). For example, if your daughter becomes pregnant and you have been totally hard-nosed about anything like that, she is going to have much bigger problems to deal with than just the pregnancy if she has no one supportive to tell and to talk to. If she is not talking to you, who is she talking to? Ethical and loving extended families are very important. Be part of other people's villages, too! Are there children apart from your own that you like to encourage and talk to?

5. Talk therapy. Valid. Very valid. People need to feel safe to tell you stuff without being judged. The world is weird and random, chaos is normal. Listen up and help.

Menopause

I believe menopause is a transitionary period in a woman's life that is both physical and philosophical.

It is often associated with hot flushes, anxiety, mood swings and night sweats. And it is also often associated with women reassessing their careers and life paths, and looking to redefine their identities as they recognise their maturity and talents. For some this is also accompanied by the recognition that their other role as mothers and family makers is taking a back step.

Many choose this time as a reawakening and reinvention, which I think is excellent. Many women have already reinvented themselves a number of times, and I think they might find it easier to cope with. But I have no evidence, and I don't think anyone has bothered to study it.

With life spans reaching out towards 100, menopause is well named as "mid-life" – in spite of younger people thinking that you are getting old.

To be honest, I have not found quality solutions for the problems experienced by women during menopause. And certainly not ones that I believe are universal to all women, apart from continuing to look after your physical and mental health well by eating clean and enriching foods, exercising, meditation, nurturing constructive and expansive relationships and having a happy and fulfilling life.

By all means look into specialty doctors who deal with menopausal problems – I've heard excellent reports for a few of them. And I've also heard excellent reports from women who have used over the counter herbal supplements. I'm not going to be making specific recommendations, except to recommend doing thorough research into the side effects and possible problems with any supplements you might take.

Some people benefit from meditation and yoga, but my research into the clinical trials gives very varied reports – so you need to discover for yourself whether they work for you. They may not stop the hot flushes (though some reports I have heard say that meditation helps), but you will probably feel better by involving yourself in these practices anyway.

I personally recommend less strenuous physical and mental exercises such as walking, meditation, yoga, tai chi because they are kinder to us: and because I think we are more likely to keep the ritual up if it is gentle and supportive. "Me time" is important for most of the women I know, who seem to overreach for most of the hours in a day. Still.

I've seen studies that support yoga to improve menopausal symptoms generally[7], and others who say yoga is beneficial for insomnia during menopause but not vasomotor symptoms (hot flushes/flashes etc)[8]. Other trials say that aerobic exercise, yoga or omega-3 supplements had no effect on vasomotor symptom frequency or bother[9]; and yet another said that yoga was better than exercise[10]. Sorting that lot out would keep you up at night! So you're going to have to figure it out yourself, but I believe that it is worth the effort to try some new things to move you forward if you are feeling quite uncomfortable about this stage of life.

If you are interested in female sleeping patterns including the sleeping patterns during pregnancy and after giving birth, you may be interested in a detailed study performed by the US National Sleep Foundation in 2007[11].

It was not encouraging seeing how many women choose to use antidepressants and sleeping medications to help them sleep better – given what we now know.

I'll recommend *The Wisdom of Menopause* by Dr. Christiane Northrup.

This book covers a lot of areas, both physical and psychological and I think you will find it helpful and detailed to guide you through this time.

It includes information on a wide range of issues from supplements, bioidenticals, libido, diet, role changes, sexual function, skin care to Siberian ginseng.

She has a very positive approach to menopause and the transitions you might choose when you look around and realise "you're over folding the towels".

Northrup will get you motivated. She has been on Oprah and has pretty broad appeal for intelligent and open minded women I think.

SLEEP DOJO - Menopause

1. Attempts to randomly pull out information from Dr. Northrup's book would not do the work justice. She has a philosophy around menopause that adds to the solutions. Treat yourself to some "me time," and read the book. You will find out more than solutions to hot flushes/flashes and sleeping better – and gain new insights in what she regards as the great and pleasurable rebirthing into the last stage of our lives.

2. Have more fun.

3. What are you going to be for the rest of your life? Now's the time to sign up to something great.

Mature Age

One of the biggest changes in sleep patterns for mature-age people is the blurring of the circadian rhythm[12].

This means that your motivation to go to bed at a particular time every night, for example, is no longer so motivating. There is less sleep pressure at the end of the day.

As we get older, it makes sense that napping might become more a part of our lives, and that broken sleep at night might not be so detrimental to our attitude, relaxation, or learning.

Here's a great study *Sleep Disorders in Older Adults*[13] that covers a number of topics that relate to older age including:

- The decrease in the amount of deep sleep (stages 3 and 4),
- The slight decrease in the amount of REM sleep,
- The changes in sleep for older adults that include sleep fragmentation, sleep disordered breathing (SDB), behavioural and lifestyle factors (more time in bed),
- Other physical and medical conditions effecting sleep e.g. arthritis, restless leg syndrome (RLS), nocturia (urination frequency), prescription medications, periodic limb movement (PLM), psychiatric disorders, and neurological disorders,
- Advanced Sleep Phase Syndrome's effect on circadian rhythm. The timing of sleep shifts to an earlier time from adulthood to old age (the opposite of teenagers' Delayed Sleep Phase),
- A table of psychiatric and medical conditions that impact sleep and contribute to insomnia (including obesity),
- A table of medications and substances that may disrupt sleep,
- Solutions including napping (the pros and cons), keeping a sleep diary and daytime activity,
- Discussion of falls in older people, with consideration to daytime napping (short irregular naps seem to be preferred over longer, habitual napping), pharmacotherapy, and the perhaps more-preferred regularizing the sleep schedule and spending more time outdoors, and
- Discussion of medications, complementary and alternative therapies, herbal supplements, valerian and melatonin.

In the study *Secondary Insomnia: Diagnostic challenges and intervention opportunities* it is stated that "true primary insomnia (i.e. insomnia that is not attributable to a medical or environmental cause) is fairly rare among older adults, accounting for only 5-20% of cases"[14]

As this book is focused on natural solutions the following comments need to be highlighted from this study (which is specifically about mature age sleep):

- "A review of the literature on valerian and melatonin suggests that research does not support the use of these agents and, in the case of valerian, can cause adverse interactions with other prescription medications." Here is the original study reference where the conclusion states "The majority of studies of herbal agents to treat sleep disorders did not include elderly subjects in long-term care, the total number of available studies was small and most studies had small sample sizes. It appears, however, that valerian and melatonin may have some utility in the long-term care setting. Nonetheless, more research is needed. It is not yet clear whether these agents would be any more effective than current therapies or whether they may negatively interact with prescription medications. Overall, evaluation of CAM interventions in the long-term care setting needs further research before recommendations can be made regarding their use." It becomes complicated when older people are on a medication, or a number of them. Please note that polypharmacy – the use of four or more medications at a time – is generally not safe or recommended – but is incredibly common, particularly in older patients. They should not be taking four or more medications, with or without alternative nutritional supplements etc. How medications mix is not studied at all, generally – and will be an area of increased review in the next few years (it should *already be* the source of alarm, with increased falls and mortality being some of the adverse effects).
- Recent studies do suggest that T'ai Chi Chih can be helpful for older adults with moderate sleep complaints[15].
- "There is a growing body of evidence for the use of cognitive-behavioural therapy for insomnia (CBT-I) which is a multi-component approach designed to address multiple sleep issues concurrently"[16]. There is a table specifically outlining this CBT-I approach on page 28. I think this CBT-I list is relevant for all insomnia, not just

mature age insomnia, as there is no mention of 'age' on the table. Download the document and have a look at Table IV on page 28 if you want to use CBT. Don't get turned off by what I regard as the non-sexy brand "Cognitive Behavioural Therapy". Instead think of it as being "conscious of how you think" ... like "mindfulness" – a more successful branding of the similar idea.

The study also cites these additional medical conditions that impact sleep: dyspnea (shortness of breath or uncomfortable breathing) of cardiac or pulmonary origin, gastro oesophageal reflux, obesity, incontinence and neurodegenerative diseases (e.g. Alzheimer's disease and Parkinson's disease.

SLEEP DOJO - Mature Age

It appears that mature-age sleep might be of a lesser quality than "normal" sleep. But who really knows, we just might need to know more about how our brains work.

As a mature ager:

1. Implement the suggestions from the *Cognitive Behaviour Therapy for Insomnia (Table IV)*, as outlined in the document above,
2. Go to bed earlier to leverage your Advanced Sleep Phase Syndrome,
3. If you nap, make them short and irregular,
4. Be aware that your medications and medical and psychological conditions are probably the major factors in your insomnia,
5. Sit in the sun to help with your attitude and circadian rhythm and general health,
6. Concentrate on general health and lifestyle components,
7. Use Tai Chi and gentle exercise routines that do not increase falls and slipping dangers,
8. Have a full review done of your medications, especially if you are a victim of polypharmacy. If they justify you being on more than 4 medications, get a second opinion. My family had this problem with my mother later in her life, and it is very difficult to persuade the "experts" that polypharmacy is not good – even though all the evidence is against it. Polypharmacy increases your risks of falls, and

if you fall you increase your chance of dying significantly. Revisit Professor Peter Gøtzsche information from his *Mental Health - Overdiagnosed and Overmedicated* YouTube video – which I'm assuming you have watched by now.

9. For more complicated mature age conditions, including harmful night-time behaviours, seizures, or medical conditions, refer to the full document and your medical doctor or supervisor – these go beyond the scope of this book.

CHAPTER 35

More Strategies for Better Sleep and Improved Mental Health

I'm guessing some of you are very sick of people blaming sleep problems on the coffee, the pillow, the mattress, the position you sleep in, etc. – when you know of plenty of people who drink heaps of coffee, don't necessarily look after themselves and could sleep on the concrete pavement (some do).

You aren't alone if you feel this way—if I read one more time that if you don't drink coffee you'll sleep like a baby, I'll scream!

It's also easy to walk around the hard decisions, and not print the sometimes brutal facts: unless your life changes *substantially* things will remain the same.

Moreover, if you ignore problems they are inclined to get worse.

You are the only person who can really make decisions for yourself. Of course you can ask your friends and people whose life skills you respect. But the bottom line is that you alone can sort your problems out. It's not the fault of your parents, your family, your doctor, the TGA, the system – you need to decide what is best for you.

And take action to change.

I've put this chapter well towards the back of the book—for most of you, that's where it should be. If you skipped here as soon as you hit the "Decisions, Decisions" chapter, go back to the Decisions, Decisions chapter now – this chapter is NOT for you.

Avoidance doesn't work.

NOW we can recognize that there ARE benefits to be derived from other sources, some of them very powerful. I'm not denigrating them by putting them towards the end of the book, but I wanted you to go through the other processes, **first**.

And to learn about how the system works. Or doesn't.

Remember our first idea, that insomnia is ALWAYS a symptom of something else? Well, what is **your** something else? There is no point getting to this chapter if you haven't found out one or more good reasons why you are not sleeping! And what is causing your mental angst.

And before I get into the detail of this chapter, which includes some alternative and possibly contentious subject matter – I'll say this:

Most people who denigrate alternative health and the different complementary modalities fail to recognise the significant contribution that they make to real medicine (the stuff that works).

Some people denigrate alternative health because they don't understand it, some because they don't want to understand it, and some because it interferes with their business model and income.

For example:

- Meditation was knocked for years, and is still being knocked by dinosaurs. Seen as hippyish and alternative and nothing to do with medicine.
- The link between mind/brain and body – which has been talked about in alternative circles for at least 40 years that I know of – is now the new new thing. Called neuroscience. Oh dear, you mean our thoughts do have impact on our health and mental health? Duh. The other hijacking of this concept is into "Cognitive Behavioural Therapy", which is a backward step from mind management and positive thinking – because who the hell would want to do "Cognitive Behavioural Therapy", even if they bothered to find out what it is? Epic fail.
- The value of nutrition and diet to health. Health food "nuts" (yes, "nuts", remember that?) and vegetarians were regarded as wacky for decades. Now the best advice is to have 4-5 vegetables and 2-3 fruit per day. Oh, dear – so all that talk was valid after all?
- Napping – proved useful decades ago and still being downplayed as 'falling asleep on the job' and the like. No, duh.

- Manufactured food has been suspect for years, and continues. Our labelling laws are draconian, with laws to protect the manufacturers so that they do not have to say what a particular flavouring is actually made of, and they do not have to declare contents that are less than 5 percent of the ingredients etc. So if you put a toxin into a biscuit, but it is only 2 percent of the ingredients it doesn't have to be declared. Yeah, sure, that makes sense.

Here are health discussions that were started in alternative circles which are now proving true, and becoming mainstream:

- Countries are beginning to ban genetically modified foods for various reasons, links to cancer and other downsides are being investigated and proven at the moment.
- Sugar is seen as a problem.
- The environment has become an issue, what we have consumed, how we have consumed it, and how we dispose of it.
- Gut health is being respected as an important part of overall health.
- How you think, and what you think of has a direct relationship to your overall health.
- The importance of relationships and open discussion, love and support are directly related to mental health outcomes. Talk therapies and psychotherapy are evidence based.

Funnily enough if you dance naked under the fronds of the whacky whacky tree in Byron Bay on the third Monday of every month you would probably have a better result than taking an antidepressant. At least it won't kill you. And it won't bring on suicidal thoughts.

Far too much time is spent knocking fringe health experiments, when mainstream is a far bigger problem.

At least you'll be getting some time in nature and exercise - away from your screen.

In fact one of my friends said the other day, that's it's funny that most hippy things are actually turning out to be for real... and mostly going mainstream.

So for the forward thinking readers who have been yawning through most of this book because you already know, here are some more ideas and technologies that you might want to watch now and in the future (I've left many options off here, because I don't want to bring on a witch hunt):

- Get a Life!
- Kinesiology, Muscle Testing and Chinese Meridians
- Emotional Freedom Technique (EFT) and Thought Field Therapy (TFT), Tapping
- Music and Sound
- Supplements & Herbal Remedies (including herbal teas)
- Bach Flower Remedies and Homeopathy
- Healthy and Sedating Food
- Other

Get a Life!
Pleasure and fun are linked to good health and great attitudes.

We need to play more, laugh more and spend more time with our friends. Have decent conversations which include open conversations about what might be troubling us and how the wheels might even be off at certain times of our lives.

Because everyone has the wheels off at certain times of their lives.

Checking into Facebook 3 times a day is not included in having fun. If you do that often enough you start feeling inadequate that you don't spend 3 months of your year travelling overseas and buying expensive shoes. Travel is not therapy. Wherever you go, you take yourself with you.

What are you contributing to the world?

The lack of meaningful contribution is a problem. Having a job where you are doing what you are told, and not necessarily what you would like to do, is not your greatest contribution. Is your job aligned to your passions and talents? Does it excite you and challenge you?

What hobbies and fun activities do you do outside of work to relax – apart from going to the pub and drinking with your mates?

Do you do anything that requires you to work with your hands, such as old-school knitting or painting? Fixing up an old car, or doing woodwork? These occupations are incredibly valuable, even if they don't seem to make sense and might not be 'respected' by your peers.

Go on, get the enjoyment you felt as a child by making something with your hands that takes even months to complete. It is great for your mind, and incredibly relaxing. And also reduces stress and anxiety.

Kinesiology and Muscle Testing

The ultimate healing technique would be to ask *our bodies* what they wanted, and what they saw as the problem at any given time.

And to act on the answer that is being received.

Instead of administering what we think is the problem, and what we think is the solution.

Which is a fanciful idea really. As if our bodies could speak?

Or is it?

The premise of muscle testing is that the body can indicate to a practitioner that a question or premise is negative or positive. Advanced practitioners can learn more about a presenting problem through asking the body via muscle testing techniques.

The acknowledged founder of Kinesiology is Dr. George Goodheart (1964), and recognises the Chinese meridian system as an integral part of the modality.

I was introduced to muscle testing around 1985, and was pretty amazed with what our bodies could tell us, and the results. Notable contributors and researchers around 'muscle testing' that I was made aware of back then, apart from Dr. Goodheart, were Dr. John Thie (Touch for Health), Dr. Roger Callaghan (Thought Field Therapy), and Dr. John Diamond (Behavioural Kinesiology).

I don't pretend to know much about these disciplines, but I have seen them work very effectively. Being a practical person, that's the thing I want to see:

results! I have personally observed that the modalities don't involve the pain and intrusions that come with some healing, particularly emotional healing.

As I understand it, the testing process is based on the neurological system, and recognizes that the neurological system is integrated with our energy systems, emotions, muscles, meridians etc.

I have used kinesiology instead of a "personal coach" for years now, and have found the methods effective, painless and revealing. In fact, it has been quite creative.

Recently I told someone that I had been going to a kinesiologist for help for years, and they said "I wouldn't admit that if I were you," which I thought was *very* funny. Just shows that there is still that stigma about "getting help."

Too bad!

With neuroplasticity being the next big thing, I'm up for all of it! This stuff is ahead of the wave!

I've gotten well and truly used to these "new" ideas since 1985.

Cooks Hookup

There's a simple movement and breathing exercise to help you relax if you

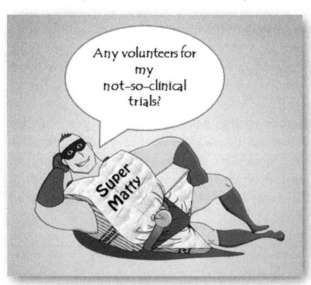

are too revved to go to sleep. With the name Cook's Hookup you might think it's about sex, but it isn't. (That works too, of course.)

In reference 2 for this chapter you will find details of a video by Dr Tracy Latz on how to do the Cooks Hookup breathing exercise[2]. Looking at it, it probably balances your left and right hemispherical activity in the brain. I'm not sure, but it works to calm you down when you are stressed and anxious.

Here's the thing, if something works, it's not really necessary to know exactly how and why it works. For example, we know that if you go for a 45 minute walk each day you will be less prone to depression and anxiety and sleep better, but why it works is not really that relevant.

Micro Movements

Micro movements are a concept from Neuro-Training™ learned during *Sleep with the Experts* to help people fall asleep. This is a really good idea if you wake up, and don't want to wake your partner by making a noise or moving too much. It involves moving parts of your body millimetres in order to "inform" the larger muscles to relax. It goes like this (you are in bed): move your right hand one millimetre (1 mm) to the left, then move your left hand 1 mm to the left. Then move your right hand another millimetre to the left, followed by your left hand another millimetre to the left. Keep doing this until you fall asleep (yes, you can go to the right too, just do the same direction with left hand and right hand – not mirroring). It is like a physical meditation, boring your body and mind to sleep perhaps?

Again, I don't know why this works, just try it.

My recommendation with Kinesiology and alternative health care practitioners (as with all healthcare professionals) is that you seek out expert and experienced practitioners that have a great reputation. And then do your due diligence on their track record to arrive at a preferred practitioner.

Emotional Freedom Technique (EFT), Thought Field Therapy (TFT) and Tapping.

Sometimes known simply as "tapping" or "energy tapping," EFT and TFT use the Chinese meridian systems and energy as part of their structured discipline. These methodologies recognize that emotions are stored in the body in energy systems, and they can be flushed by tapping certain meridian points.

There are a number of great books on the subject, including

Energy Tapping: How to Rapidly Eliminate Anxiety, Depression, Cravings and More Using Energy Psychology by Fred P Gallo PHD and Harry Vincenzi Ed. D.[3]

Tapping can be used to relieve anxiety and stress (again, relating back to the Chinese meridian system and the relationship to emotions), and other issues including more deep-seated unresolved issues. If you don't know much about EFT and TFT, go to an expert practitioner to get some work done (especially if your issue is unresolved childhood stuff, etc.).

Sometimes, when you "tap out" an issue, there can be underlying problems that surface. That's why I recommend working with a professional, qualified to help.

There is a collarbone breathing exercise on YouTube by Dr. Franzi Ng[4] that you might like to investigate if you are feeling out of sorts. You can try it now if you like, by following her video instructions. Dr. Ng shows you exactly which points to tap, and walks you through the whole process.

Tapping can be used if you feel anxious, or stressed before you go to sleep. What's more, as explained by Rod Sherwin in *Sleep with the Experts*, there are certain points on the body that you can just hold rather than tap (while saying statements silently to yourself) if you wake in the middle of the night, get anxious and you can't go back to sleep.

Have a few sessions with an expert before you commence doing the tapping yourself. They will probably recommend special points and words for you to use that are unique to you. That's the great advantage of having expert help.

Music and Sound

Music and sound can be very effective for a number of sleeping difficulties, and even to distract from pain (another reason people aren't sleeping well).

The documentary *The Music Instinct – Science: Song*[5] aired on ABC (Australia) in August, 2010 was very revealing, as it traced back scientific and cultural music links from the ancient Greeks to the latest scientific links between sound and string theory. The conclusion began to make me think that sound had a closer link than anything to the basic structure of the universe (the DVD set is available on the internet).

Angela Sciberras, our special therapeutic musician in *Sleep with the Experts*, shared the following ways that she uses music in palliative care and general healing:

- To distract people from pain in order to allow them to sleep,
- To bring people down and through depression (cathartic release), rather than attempting to "jolly them up" as a cure,
- For relaxation and feeling calm, relieving anxiety, and
- Even helping people die in peace.

Apart from the brain's natural inclination to mimic the sounds being heard (called 'brain entrainment') other characteristics of music and sound can be used to calm us down, make us feel better, lift our spirits, etc.

There are lots of options to experiment with, and each person (and generation?) will have a different reaction and interpretation to different music and sounds. Here are some ideas for you to think about:

- Melody, rhythm modes, harmony, beat and texture,
- Simple music (such as one person playing the harp) versus orchestral or group music,
- Different strains of music, weeping, slumber and merry,
- Which instrument(s) would you prefer (violin, piano, pan flutes, African drums, etc.)?
- Sounds that have nothing to do with music. Nature sounds (rain, streams, ocean roars, lapping waves), white noise (helpful with tinnitus etc.),
- Using your body in sync with the music,
- Metronome sounds that match the different cycles of sleep (e.g. alpha rhythm/metronome, theta rhythm/metronome),
- Humming, and
- Sighing (ahhh sounds, while breathing out).

During the music episode of *Sleep with the Experts*, Sciberras said that nine times out of ten, people would go to sleep to the Irish song Foggy Dew[6]. You might like to try that. You can hear Sinead O'Connor and the Chieftains perform it by following reference 6.

Of course, there are endless fantastic pieces of music, from all different instruments and voices. They don't have to be labelled as "healing music" for them to relax you, make you feel complete, or take you away from your day to day problems.

Music therapy is a growing modality, for good reason.

One of the greatest advantages is that if you find the right music you don't have to verbalise the problem and relive the experience, you can just absorb yourself in the catharsis and the music and feel released/healed/cleansed/relaxed.

Finally, sounds can be combined with slow movement (yoga, tai chi, etc) to great effect, as well.

Here's my take on it: It's like exercise. Make it very simple so you do it. Just download some great tracks into a special playlist in your mp3 player, call them "peace" or "meditation" so, when you get time at the end of the day (or anytime), you can just go there and chill out. Don't make it difficult, or it won't happen. After a while of doing this, the process will become a very enjoyable habit and part of your life. An enhanced, more relaxed life!

Stressed, anxious? Try these, do it now.

Here are some suggested music videos from YouTube:

Buddhist Meditation. Music. Zen Garden. Kokin Gumi.[7]
Crown of Creation by Jonathan Goldman. Daily Meditation.[8]
Gregorian Chants.[9]

Here are some other ideas that use different rhythm, tone and pitch. What is relaxing and uplifting to one person is not necessarily melodious to another.

Vaughan Williams, A Sea Symphony. [10]
Ave Maria[11]
Claire de Lune by Claude Debussy.[12]
Elvira Madigan, Wolfgang Amadeus Mozart - Piano Concerto No. 21 – Andante.[13]
The Most Relaxing Music: Ambiology. Barry Goldstein.[14]

Glen Velez frame drum.[15]
Snatam Kaur, Ek Ong Kaar.[16]
Snatam Kaur - Long Time Sun.[17]

(No belief/religious intentions meant. These are some random samples, I'm sure you have some of your own – or are about to.)

Brain Entrainment Using Alpha and Theta Sounds and Metronomes.

There are metronome sounds like a heartbeat (alpha rhythm), and the faster theta metronome, that you can purchase as simple sounds to listen to. According to brain entrainment theory, after listening to the sounds for a while, our minds will try to reflect the beat. That's the meaning of "brain entrainment."

Your mind starts to match the rhythm of the sound.

You can purchase audio programs (CDs and mp3 downloads) to use in this way. Just load them into your mp3 player to play whenever you want to (not in vehicles of course, as they are intended to help you fall asleep)!

I recommend these to people who have difficulty falling asleep at night, or who have difficulty trying to meditate.

Even in stubborn cases, with concerted repetition your mind will learn that you are serious and learn to surrender to the metronome/tone/rhythm/music.

Some other sounds and music will have a beat in the background, embedded into the music. If you can hear or feel that beat, you know what is happening.

Of course there are subliminal programs too, where you cannot consciously recognise what is going on in the background, and what messages are being "spoken" directly to your mind.

Examples of such a program is Dr Jeffrey Thomson's Theta Meditation System: Let Go of Stress, Renew Your Spirit, Gain Insight and Intuition.[18]

There are a number of these types of programs available, just have a look around on the internet.

Hypnotherapy

Hypnotherapy is a technique that has been used extensively for a number of different purposes, including sleeping better, going to sleep, etc.

There are a number of people who sell hypnotherapy audios, they are freely available.

I will repeat my mantra here: insomnia and mental health problems are symptoms of underlying problems. While I won't tell you not to use hypnotherapy – I'd prefer you addressed the underlying issues.

If, for example, you had a traumatic childhood that has plagued you for years, I would be looking at getting some counselling help, through talk therapies or other methods, rather than hypnotising yourself to sleep each night.

Hypnotherapy can help when it is used to identify the underlying problem.

Supplements and Herbal Remedies (Including Herbal Teas)

EXERCISE - I'm listing EXERCISE as a supplement? Why?

- So you don't forget it.
- Because it's possibly better than most of the stuff in this chapter anyway.
- It's free.
- It will improve your general health, weight and attitude.
- Just do it!

Omega-3

Previously something I was watching, but Cochrane is of the opinion that the studies supporting the use of Omega-3/PUFA with depression and mental health are inconclusive and further evidence is required.[19]

(That doesn't mean no, it just means that more studies need to be done to prove the case for or against.)

Supplements for Depression

I have not been able to find conclusive evidence supporting supplements to improve depression.

There appears to be some evidence that supports St. John's Wort for Major Depressive Disorder (MDD) in that "hypericum extracts tested in the included trials a) are superior to placebo in patients with major depression; b) are similarly effective as standard antidepressants; c) and have fewer side effects than standard antidepressants. The association of country of origin and precision with effects sizes complicates the interpretation."[20]

I personally encourage a good diet rich in fruit and vegetables, free of chemicals and food additives, daily exercise and regular, predictable sleep every night as the best safeguard against mental health problems. These basic preventative measures should be accompanied by a meaningful life, good friends and happy associations.

Herbal Remedies

There is a large list of herbal remedies and teas that are supposed to help you sleep better, and they might, if your problem is not severe. The list includes (but is not limited to) chamomile, valerian, passiflora, St. John's Wort, limeflowers, hawthorn berries, yarrow, fennel, Scutellaria lateriflora (skullcap), Zizyphus sativa seed, Melissa officinalis (Lemon Balm), Humuluslupulus flower (Hops), Verbena officinallis leaf (Vervain), Smilax officinalis root (Sarsaparilla), Bupleurumfalcatum root (Bupleurum), Aquilegia, Anethum Grav, Avena Sativa, Lupulinum, Ignatia, Coffea, Gelsemium, Hyoscyamus, Capsicum, Viscum album leaf (mistletoe) and Aesculus hipposastanum flower (white chestnut) – and we haven't even included the Chinese Herbs!

There is very little wonder that there seems to be a thousand mixed herbal remedies on the market, because the computations and permutations of that list would go on forever. If you're going to do "trial and error" on the list, make sure you live long enough to finish the study!

It appears to me that very few, if any, "real" clinical trials have been performed in this area.

Sadly.

I think that the 'milk and honey' examples that people quote largely work like the placebo effect... so if you think your warm milk and honey nightcap is working – keep doing it.

But remember that herbal teas and supplements can have adverse effects if taken with certain drugs, etc. Just because something is herbal doesn't mean it is harmless.

And if you are taking other drugs, recreational substances etc... the jury is out.

Herbal Teas

If you are going to use them, and I would definitely suggest that they are a good alternative to caffeinated drinks and sugary and stimulating beverages - make sure they are the best quality you can find.

This is a growing area, with many organic teas now marketed as well.

Homeopathy, Bach Flower Remedies, etc

The thing that makes me most interested in homeopathy (as I don't know a lot about it) is the extent to which mainstream medicine is trying to wipe it out totally.

Founded by Dr Samuel Hahnemann (1755-1843) homeopathy has been around since the 1700s which is a great achievement if it's doing nothing and/or harmful.

If it is so weak and useless, and basically water, why all the fuss?

And why all the bad press?

I'm not convinced it's about the waste of money, as we already know the situation with mainstream medicine.

And it's not killing anyone, or causing permanent brain damage, or permanent sexual dysfunction or akathisia...

I'll avoid the questions of energy and nanotechnology patches, as they are too obscure for me to understand.

Clinical Trials and Meta Analyses

The basic issues aren't being honoured by clinical trials – like the testing of about 50 food additives, chemicals, flavourings and colourings that are suspected to be bad for your health, and mental health and sleep patterns.

There is a lot of work to be done by a totally independent body in Australia and/or Cochrane.

It is a matter of making our sleep and mental health a priority when deciding what evidence reviews should be conducted and financed, and by whom.

Organic Foods

Yes, they have to be better than the ones produced with chemicals. That's pretty obvious.

And genetically modified? I'm avoiding that where I can. Call me old-school, that's fine.

Especially where the food item is genetically modified to react in a certain way to the patented chemicals that are supplied to the farmer to produce the crop.

And the recommended chemicals are effecting bee populations and polinization of our food supply – across the board.

Then the harvested crop is sold to "designated companies" to manufacture and market the food, that may or may not be good for our health.

Who knows, because our labelling laws are hopeless and no-one is conducting clinical trials on food consumption.

Yoga, Meditation, Breathing Exercises, Guided Relaxation, Tai Chi, Qi Gong

I'm pretty sure they're all good, and proven to be so for health, reduced anxiety, stress, sleep etc.

CHAPTER 36

Survival Skills During A 'Tired Day'

We all know that not sleeping well affects our attitude, accuracy, and enthusiasm, fogs our brain, and dulls our life. This chapter contains suggestions on how to cope when you are overtired, anxious, stressed, or making mistakes.

Some "conventional wisdom" appears to be that napping during the day is inadvisable if you are having trouble sleeping. Generally, this advice is based on correcting bad sleeping habits like going to bed at different times every day.

I think by now we know that insomnia can have a myriad of underlying issues beyond just bad sleeping habits.

I started napping in 1978 when I first learned about different brain wave patterns, the work that NASA had done, and the benefits of meditation.

Back then it was fringe dweller stuff apparently – I didn't care what the rest of the world thought.

It was the beginning of personal development, performance training and the self help movement, so some of the gurus were bound to be dodgy, and some still are.

In 2017 who would guess how slow the information uptake would actually be!

More recently I've read a valuable book about napping by Dr. Sara Mednick and Mark Ehrman, called *Take a Nap! Change your Life,* which I highly recommend to you[1]. Mednick is a Harvard-trained research scientist at the Salk Institute in La Jolla, California, and a consultant with both the military (one of the most sleep deprived and traumatised cultures in the world), and private businesses. The great news from her research is that napping can bring you well beyond just surviving the next day after a bad night's sleep!

Mednick's book illustrates that napping can be used strategically to stay alert, clear your mind, reduce your stress and anxiety levels – even improve your verbal memory, learn better, improve motor skills, and help find creative solutions to problems.

Does Napping Hurt Your Night Time Sleep?

Luckily the naysayers on napping are finally quietening down. They are being silenced by the scientific evidence, neuroscience and mindfulness meditation studies.

Here are some very positive statistics quoted by Sara Mednick in her presentation at the Beckman Centre that you can watch on YouTube:

- Napping decreased the time to fall asleep at night by 14%,
- Napping increased the ability to stay asleep through the night by 12%,
- Napping increased night-time sleep by about 20 minutes, and
- Napping increased the refreshed feeling upon waking by 5%[2].

These figures are very interesting and valuable when compared with the figures on sleeping pills that we talked about in Chapter 9. Who would bother taking a benzo when you can have a nap and get a better result with no adverse side effects?

Benefits have been shown from as little as 6 minutes of napping during the day, with research now studying the differences between a 20-minute nap, a 60-minute nap, a 90-minute nap, etc.

Here are some more statistics from her book and lecture that might motivate you to have a nap if you aren't already (40% of Americans that say they nap already – Australians are behind the game!):

- Siesta cultures have a lower rate of **coronary heart disease** (CHD). A 2007 study of about 24,000 Greek people showed that those who napped twice a week reduced their CHD by 12%. What is really amazing is that if they napped three times a week, their CHD reduced by a whopping 37%. That alone would be enough for me to start catching some zeds during the day, but there is more!

- Statistics support that a nap can be the equivalent of a whole night's sleep in terms of **improving learning** during the day! Learning from a nap is EQUAL to learning from a full night of sleep.
- Taking a nap improves your creative problem solving ability by almost 40%.
- Napping **decreased daytime sleepiness** by 10%.
- With napping it is 38% less likely that **sleepiness** will interfere with daytime activities. That is HUGE! Show it to your boss. Tell her/him you will be more accurate, more creative, and be in a better mood in the office if she/he provides some napping time, and possibly a quiet room for people to go during their lunchtime or breaks.
- Napping **elevated mood** by 11%.
- Napping improved the **quality of interactions** by 10%.
- Napping elevated **alertness** by 11%.
- Napping enhanced **mental abilities** by 9%.[3]

Strategically Choose the Time of Day that you take your Nap

Using the excellent research from this book, it is possible to tailor your nap depending on your desired outcome. According to Dr. Mednick and Ehrman, by using the nap wheel on the front of the book, you can dial up your ideal nap depending on the result you want to achieve. The book also helps you decide the best time of day to take a nap, and the duration of the nap in order to get the results you want. The time you wake up in the morning is also a very important factor in this tailoring process.

The results you may want from your nap vary from keeping your alertness high (with Stage 2 sleep) to repairing your body (requiring slow wave sleep, SWS), or to receive a boost of creativity or help with your memory (using rapid eye movement REM sleep). Learning advantages require both slow wave sleep (SWS) and rapid eye movement (REM) sleep, which can be managed by some efficient nappers in a 60-minute nap (other nappers require longer).

Interestingly,

- REM sleep peaks for everyone at basically the same time: 9 AM.
- Stage 2 sleep is linked to the REM sleep cycle (not occurring at the same time, but surrounding the REM times). It is always constant in the equation, so assume that the first 20 minutes of a nap are almost exclusively Stage 2 sleep.
- Slow Wave Sleep (SWS) occurs at the opposite time of the 24-hour clock to your wake-up time. If you wake up at 7 AM, your tendency for slow-wave sleep will occur at 7 PM. Obviously, if you take your nap at 7 PM, it will be naturally rich in SWS.
- Mednick considers 'the ultimate nap' to be a 90-minute nap (which will include stage 2 sleep, SWS and REM sleep), and the best time of the day to take that nap is shown in her Nap Wheel where the blue "REM sleep circle" crosses the yellow slow-wave sleep circle. I highly recommend purchasing her book to manipulate the Nap Wheel to suit your individual circumstance. Refer to *Recommended Reading*.

Other strategies have been isolated by Dr. Mednick, Ehrman and researchers for increased memory, better motor skills at the end of the day, and better learning.

The Length or Duration of your Nap is Important.
The longer you are napping, the more of certain sleep cycles you are likely to experience in your nap. Different lengths of nap are suitable for different benefits.

I'm sure watching Dr Mednick's presentation at the Beckman Centre, University of Irvine, California would be most helpful to you. It's on YouTube[4].

In this video you will learn:

1. There are **shadow sleep stages** during the day that you may not have been aware of. After reading the explanation it makes sense that towards the end of the day (as you get more tired) your body

will be more likely to slip into more slow-wave sleep (SWS) napping than early in the morning. I appreciated the details of the research, because it means that there are different times of day that are more appropriate for different types of napping – and the nap wheel allows you to get very specific. For instance, your natural circadian rhythm at 9-10 AM generates a more REM-rich nap, great for creative problem solving.

2. How to use the nap wheel on the front of her book to calculate your best nap time, depending on the time you wake in the morning.
3. A perfectly-timed nap can consolidate the benefits of a full night of sleep into a single cycle.
4. The different stages of a nap, and the relevance of the length of your nap. The Power Nap (20 minutes or less) is very good for improving alertness. SWS during your nap will be very restorative, clear your mind of useless information, and improve your declarative and spatial memory. REM in your nap will help with creativity, visual memory and dreaming.

Did you know that pilots are napping on the job, too? It is not generally publicized, says Mednick, because people are more freaked out by that than they are by knowing that pilots are working too-long shifts. After hearing her presentation, I'm very pleased they are. Let's hope they have an alarm clock!

Biphasic Sleep

The book discusses **biphasic sleepers** – people who wake up very alert in the middle of the night, do things, and then go back to bed for another phase of sleep. This used to be quite common, apparently. She doesn't think that's a huge problem – especially if you combine your biphasic pattern with a nap during the day. Interesting.

This information is very helpful; I'm a great believer in dealing with your lack of sleep *kindly*, so that you are not adding more stress and anxiety to the problem.

Knowing that we can catch up some sleep during the day will help us relax about having broken sleep, which is a good thing.

Can a Nap Replace your Night-time Sleep?

There are some people who like playing around with their sleep, wanting to stay up longer and experiment with sleep deprivation and sleep minimization. Strategies for this are outside the scope of this book, because I'm focused on helping readers get *more* sleep and reducing their stress and anxiety.

Dr. Mednick does mention certain "macho attitudes" around lack of sleep in some professions, and that one study indicated that doctors who did 30-hour shifts were 700% more likely to make errors than when they worked a 10-hour shift. Some of those situations are problems with the industries themselves being understaffed, expecting employees to work too-long hours.

I am NOT advocating skipping sleep at night. Napping should be used to enhance your sleep, not replace it.

Coffee, Anyone?

The video[5] contains some great information about using coffee and whether or not it works when we are tired to help us concentrate and stay focused and accurate. The results aren't too pretty! Coffee is addictive, we know that, but there are very few times when it has much worth. It just makes us feel better because we have had our fix!

Placebo results were quite high for a number of trials, but only once (in the studies featured) did caffeine beat the placebo, and it never beat having a nap[6].

Sleep Inertia

Sleep Inertia (when you wake up feeling groggy) is generally because you have come out of slow wave sleep (SWS, sometimes known as deep sleep) with a jolt, and it takes a bit of time to readjust.

This is some of the reasoning behind the power nap (or shorter periods of napping). Mednick's research has indicated that up to half an hour will generally be Stage 2 sleep (not deep sleep), and anything from as little as 6 minutes can be beneficial to help us stay alert and feeling good.

For many years, I napped at lunchtime for between 15 and 23 minutes, and I found it very beneficial to reduce stress, freshen up, clear my head and help re-plan the rest of the day. You can do this sitting up, and after a while the discipline will be established to the point where you will wake up automatically after the particular time, without an alarm.

So, in order to avoid sleep inertia: either nap for less than half an hour or nap for longer (60-90 minutes, depending on your pattern and personal experiments), so that you are not waking in the middle of slow wave sleep (SWS) feeling groggy. Generally, the 90-minute nap will take you through all the sleep cycles, ending in REM sleep, which will be refreshing.

Establishing the Habit

In the first few days of napping, you may not feel you are getting a lot of benefit.

Persist! Generally we resist change. The discipline will confirm to your mind that you are serious about establishing a new habit. Within days you will feel really good about it. After a while you will actually miss your nap if you don't get it, because it makes you feel better, more relaxed and happier.

It will be a bit like an early-morning walk habit. It might feel hard the first few days while you set up the new habit. Then with persistence you will feel more relaxed, more flexible, clearer in the head, feeling good again, and getting back out of your head and into the present moment.

Should I Nap if I'm Not Tired?

Yes, there are many benefits to napping, so do it even on your "good days"! Establishing the habit is very beneficial, and makes it easier to slip into your nap when you didn't sleep so well the night before.

Practice will also make you a more efficient napper. Dr. Mednick indicates that some people can cycle through all the sleep phases in 60 minutes rather than 90 minutes – you could become an expert napper, too!

Business Owners/Entrepreneurs

Take note! Your employees will feel happier, be more productive, remember more, keep up their motor skills, get along better with each other, and think more creatively if you establish a napping room and a napping culture at work.

Some businesses and governments have been encouraging napping for years: it's not new news.

Should I Eat Lunch Before or After my Lunchtime Nap?

My opinion here is to eat lunch after your (lunchtime) nap for a number of beneficial reasons.

- You will achieve your relaxed brain wave patterns easier if you're not digesting food at the same time (especially if you just ate a burger and your body is working overtime to digest it!),
- If you relax first, you will probably eat less, and need fewer sugary and/or fatty foods,
- Your digestion will probably work better in your post-nap relaxed state, and
- You will probably take a little bit longer chewing and eating properly if you're not feeling rushed and stressed.

Avoid coffee, if you want to sleep better and perform better.

Sleep Restriction Programs

We are not advocating napping if you are on a "sleep restriction" program with your doctor, or are within 3 hours of going to bed. It is up to you to formulate your best program.

Is Napping the Same as Meditation?

Napping and meditation are different things. When you nap, certainly for longer periods (like 30 – 90 minutes) you actually fall asleep. Depending on the nap, different types of sleep are experienced such as slow wave sleep, stage 2 sleep and REM sleep.

During meditation you are actually consciously aware of what is going on, although the feeling is different to full consciousness. Most people who meditate are meditating in the higher brain wave frequencies (REM and stage 1). More experienced meditators are able to meditate in theta brain wave pattern frequencies, and there are rare people, I've heard, who can maintain the delta brain wave pattern.

Metronome Sounds

If you want to experiment with the slower theta brain-wave pattern meditations, there are metronome sounds in these patterns, some containing guided meditations. These audios are freely available on the internet.

Of course, when experimenting with theta brain-wave meditations, take great care not to play these frequencies while in the car or operating machinery. Ever.

To start, I would be lying down in every case, somewhere you will not be disturbed.

It is quite difficult to maintain the theta brainwave pattern without falling asleep; it takes practice.

(Hint: This is why theta sounds are so good for people who can't sleep.)

There are also delta brain-wave metronome audios available. I *would not* be using these without expert guidance. I've heard that there are very few people in the world who can keep consciousness with the delta brain-wave pattern, and until you can find a good reason to do that, I don't see the point.

Many guided meditation cycles involve taking you to a peaceful place or an imaginary place (floating in a boat, a crystal cave, walking down stairs, flying music, lying in a feather bed, swimming in warm water, etc.) to help you relax but stay focused. Some are very creative and pleasing; you will find your own favourites.

If you haven't meditated before, don't expect great results the first few times. Continue to meditate, as the benefits can be significant for everyone. It can take some time to "train your brain" to think this way and to relax.

You may even find the metronome sounds quite aggravating at first; it is a normal reaction (especially the theta metronome sound, which actually sounds fast, not slow).

Start with the alpha brain-wave pattern (which is all most people ever use), and later do some theta cycles if you like the idea.

Finally, if some of the cycles in alpha and theta seem a bit crazy, don't get upset about it! Some cycles in deeper brain wave states are seen by some as "spiritual," and have certainly been used by many spiritual leaders and yogis. Some people might "see" symbols and experience different things in meditation. Just keep doing it and see how you go.

Everyone has a spiritual aspect if we think of *developing our spirit.* Having been brought up in a very restrictive religious environment as a child (which turned me off religion totally), I put perspective on it by thinking of it as "Spirit-You-Will".

I can relate to great people having great spirits, and I don't see it as having much to do with religion. (The Dalai Lama might be an exception.)

Some readers of this book might be having problems sleeping because they haven't recognized a contribution bigger-than-themselves that enthuses them and makes their life fun and enriching. What you do with your life should be enriching and contributory - not just focused on making heaps of money for the heck of it – for example.

It's a reason some people can't sleep, but is not often spoken about. Most people yearn to be great at something, and to contribute in their unique, creative way to make the world a better place. Going to work every day to a job that you don't particularly like (or for an unethical company, for example) is soul destroying, and eventually will affect your health and vitality – no doubt about it.

Lightening up (enlightenment) is part of a fun and full life. The opposite, spiritual pain, is sometimes why people:

- lack self esteem, confidence and passion,
- don't have stimulating and meaningful relationships,
- are confused and procrastinate about life's priorities,
- feel low and depressed, and/or
- don't sleep properly.

Your waking up pattern is just that. Your spirit telling you to wake up.

Don't get the word "spiritual" confused with "religious" – we are talking about a unique experience for <u>you</u>, not an organized group belief system. We are trying to free-up here, not sign-up!!

Remember, the napping times are NOT meditation cycle naps. Mednick's naps are sleeps that involve cycling through (or in) the different brain-wave cycles to receive the benefits described. If you play a theta metronome sound for an hour, you will most likely NOT be cycling through the different sleep cycles described in her research, so don't get your information confused.

Try meditation (as well as napping) see whether or not it is for you.

Other Alternatives to the Basic Nap

Apart from meditation, you might like to listen to music, guided relaxation cycles, hypnosis, or paraliminal cycles during your nap time, which is fine.

You can use timed hypnosis cycles or timed music tracks loaded into your mp3 player if that helps, and I'm pretty sure it will.

One of my favourite hypnosis cycles, and one that a lot of my clients have enjoyed over the years, is called A Chakra Meditation by Glenn Harrold[7]. Yes, it's a bit "new age" with chakra talk and all, but it's great to listen to, and irresistibly relaxing for those who are having trouble switching off. I bought the CD years ago and put it in my phone. It has a long version of the 'cycle' (42.40 minutes) and a short version (28.17 minutes).

The good part about this cycle is that Glenn will actually wake you up at the end, so there is no danger that someone will walk into your office after lunch and find you asleep, or that you'll be late for a meeting.

While we are talking about that, you don't have to do this in your office. You can sit in your car in the parking station – where no one has a clue that you are "refreshing" during your lunch break.

10-Minute Supercharger Paraliminal[8]

I'm putting this suggested CD/audio in for people who might want to experiment with this short 10-minute cycle, or who have very restricted times that they want to maximize. This audio has been used very effectively by a number of clients, and you might enjoy it too.

I personally prefer longer than 10 minutes, but that choice is up to you.

Other Relaxation Mp3s

Look around the internet for numerous examples of relaxation cycles, and look specifically for cycles that might suit your specific purposes. Here are some more examples that I have been recommending to clients for years:

Letting Go of Anxiety, Dr Sarah Edelman.
Guided Body Mind Relaxation, James Wild, Quiet Earth Publishing.
Sleep Peacefully, Subliminal, Quiet Earth Publishing.
Feeling Relaxed, Say Goodbye to Stress. Subliminal. Quiet Earth Publishing.
Deep Sleep Every Night, Glenn Harrold.
Complete Relaxation, Glenn Harrold.
Music for the Healing Arts, James Wild, Quiet Earth Publishing.
Alpha Metronome, James Wild, Quiet Earth Publishing.
Theta Metronome, James Wild, Quiet Earth Publishing.

Quiet Earth Publishing has a range of awesome meditations from mindfulness meditation to the verging-on-wacky and arrived at wacky. I love this site as it pushes the envelope! Have a poke around in the website www. QuietEarth.org.

I just listened to James Wild's recording *Songs of the Forest with the Grey Shrike-thrush*[9], for example, if you want to be transported to the Australian bush of Mount Macedon in Victoria.

There is a range of metaphysical audios in this website, for those into esoterics and future trends. (None of it is futuristic, it just looks that way if you haven't been tracking this stuff for decades.) Have fun, but don't get turned off if you are just a beginner. Each audio has a short sample you can listen to before you buy.

Or you could just Google up 100 relaxation cycles! There are heaps up there you can listen to now. E.g. Chris Brown's *Guided Meditation for Full*

Body Relaxation[10]. I'm nearly falling asleep just referencing this while it plays in the background!

What did we do before the internet?

SLEEP DOJO – Surviving When You Are Tired

1. Whether or not you feel tired during the day, there is significant evidence that napping during the day can help you feel better, think more creatively, learn more, perform better, enhance relationships, improve your health and rejuvenate.
2. Experiment with the timing and duration of your nap.
3. If you are experimenting with meditation, try different audios to enhance your meditation time.
4. Persist through the first few meditation and/or napping sessions when you feel you may not have received a lot of benefit. The habit is easy to establish and the benefits are felt after only a few days. The discipline is well worth the effort.
5. Become a napping expert by buying Sara Mednick's book *Take a Nap! Change Your Life* and strategise your best napping tactics.

Part Four: Where to From Here? Healthy, Happy and Smart.

CHAPTER 37

Who to Believe, Who to Watch and What to Read

As I've mentioned before, I have deliberately limited the number of key people who I am referencing in this book because I want my readers to get the real story.

Really get it.

As I have previously mentioned, one of the ways *real evidence-based medicine* is being thwarted is through **confusion**: I have no intention of adding more confusion in this book.

If you're wondering why I have neglected to quote from other leading experts, or "supposed leading experts" it is because I do not want to add to the confusion.

There are businesses and individuals that are making millions out of misinformation masquerading as evidence-based-medicine and costing lives every day.

Another way that real evidence based medicine is being kept from the general public is by not having effective governance in Australia to ensure that our health and medical systems are really evidence-based – not just claiming to be.

One of those facilities would be a **federal ombudsman** where you could complain when you could see a problem. And that that federal ombudsman would be correctly staffed and financed to get to the bottom of problems.

For example, how does Australia have an unqualified doctor Shyam Acharya (aka Dr. Sarang Chitale) practice medicine in our hospital system for over 11 years without detection?[1]

Furthermore, "Dr Chitale" was not actually reported by any government authority or hospital he had worked in, nor any medical registry or government instrumentality. It took him to work in the medical research company Novotech before anyone sounded the alarm[2]. OMG.

Furthermore, why, when they are actually 'found out' (March 7, 2017) can our system not know whether or not they performed surgeries during that time? Or are they just covering up the extent of the problem (at March 27, 2017 as I write this)?

If it wasn't private enterprise that exposed this fraud, would the public know about it at all?

If we had a federal government ombudsman I doubt it would take over 11 years to resolve problems like these. Participatory members of the public are smart, sometimes very smart.

I've got very little doubt that a Federal Health Ombudsman would help upgrade our medical system and that it would be cost effective, as the reporting is always done by member of the public, at no cost to the government. (Make no mistake about federal, separate state ombudsmen would be a nightmare.)

Personally my efforts to bring the issues outlined in this book to the attention of federal and state health and mental health ministers in Australia has resulted in nothing. Comments such as "sleep has got nothing to do with mental health" have been common and the attitude towards my reports has been derogatory at best.

On one phone call to a ministerial office I was asked if I was a doctor, but when I asked the name of the person in the ministerial office that I was speaking to she replied "you don't need to know that".

It has been a wild ride.

And a very disappointing one.

But it did manifest this book.

When you build up a head of steam, you'd better do something about it.

The federal minister for health should establish a federal ombudsman in order to help them perform their complex job correctly.

There is no other way that federal health ministers could possibly know the problems in the system without a federal ombudsman.

Clearly the present system is severely broken.

So, as at the end of March 2017 what's in the pipeline?

The Antidepressants Class Action in Australia

A class action is being prepared at the moment by Drayton Sher Lawyers in Sydney because of the lack of adequate warnings and information about antidepressant problems.

These medications are being given to children under 18 years of age.

For more information visit the Facebook page "Australian Antidepressants Class Action"[3], register your complaint, and/or make a donation to the crowd funding initiative[4] in order to get this case running in Australia.

You can join the class action by sending your complaint to tony@draytonsherlawyers.com.au.

Our Part in the Problem.

I've spent a fair bit of time in this book 'pointing the finger' at organisations, systems, the government... but let's look in the mirror now.

Do you have shares in the offending drug companies?

Have you figured out who the offending drug companies are?

Do you have shares in the offending listed medical centre management organisations?

Now I know most of you just said no.

But I bet you don't really know.... because I don't either.

You see, you and I have superannuation policies, probably, which have a certain percentage of their investments in listed company shares.

We have investments in ASX/S&P bundled indexed stocks, and other investments that include these companies that are behaving badly.

And none of the super funds have rulings on evidence-based medicine, how they report their clinical trials, total disclosure, etc.

Australian Ethical Super is the only one I see in Australia that is making an effort to select ethically based investment, but I don't see any mention of a number of companies which I would regard as unethical. There may be others, I'm just not aware of them, and they certainly aren't common.

I won't list them here as that is far too much information for this book – but let's just consider pharmaceutical companies that are killing thousands of people each year (even hundreds of thousands), technology companies that are exploiting minors, slave labour, unsafe workplaces, illegal workers, paying their female staff members less than the men – as a start.

So we now know that if our super funds invest in shares then we are very likely to own shares indirectly in the companies and listed organisations mentioned in this book.

We are part of the system that finances and supports the ongoing inadequacy and unethical behaviours outlined in this book.

As a shareholder (and therefore owner) of companies we are invited and encouraged to go to the annual general meetings and voice our opinions.

But how many of us do this?

And if it is our superannuation fund that owns shares in these companies, we have an indirect responsibility to pass on our grievances to the super funds to express our dissatisfaction at the annual general meetings of the companies that we own.

Yes, this is a little extreme. And a bit purist.

But unless someone takes responsibility we can't just blame all this on everyone else.

We can't just point the finger and say that the pharmaceutical companies are acting unethically in some cases. No-one is holding them to account.

I personally believe that if everyone just did something to improve the world, the world would be a completely different place.

My responsibility this year is to write this book.

I'd like to make a documentary next.

So, what are YOU doing? What's your thing?

It doesn't have to be huge, but it does have to be something.

And posting up your opinion on social media is not counted... you need to be taking action of some description or nothing changes.

It's hard enough to bring about change even when we're working our butts off.

And unfortunately most people chose not to notice what's happening.

"Another chardy darling?"

Where to from here?

I've included a recommended reading list and resources from world leaders in sleep and mental health at the back of the book, so that you can subscribe to their blogs, read their books, watch their YouTube presentations and become an expert in this area too.

You don't have to be a medical doctor or psychiatrist to learn this stuff. Don't fall for superior put-downs. You understand this now.

And you're now in a position to help other people by explaining to them the basis of how and why things got so out of hand that young kids are now being prescribed deadly drugs instead of being told to get some good sleep, listening to them (however weird it might get sometimes), giving them some kind and helpful counselling, providing them with a loving and stable family environment, sitting with them in non-judgement, encouraging them to do some exercise, eat well and find supportive and nice friends.

And making people feel that they are OK if they have emotional problems.

Because we all do at different times in our lives.

It's called having a life! Duh.

So plug into Gøtzsche, Whitaker, Healy, Mednick, Dengate, Jureidini, Mohnihan, and all the other awesome, courageous people who are telling the truth.

And watch out for your loved ones, friends and family to make sure they are getting the right advice, and not being harmed by incorrect strategies.

Popping pills is not the answer, we know that.

And keep away from hot horses.

I'm making a documentary

That's my next mission.

Preferably funny. Definitely disruptive.

Let's make a difference and get broad reach.

Please email me at elizabeth@SleeplessNoMore.com with your proposal.

It will be heaps of fun, and I'm ready to start.

Finally, Would You Help By Reviewing this Book on Amazon.com?

Did you benefit from the information in this book *Alarming Sleep Secrets?*

Do you think that other people would benefit from the information too?

Do you think that this book might save a young person's life? Or someone else's?

If so, would you mind going over to Amazon.com and giving *Alarming Sleep Secrets* a five star ranking making a short comment to indicate how you think readers of the book would **benefit** from reading it?

For example, I'm very concerned that children at school are getting the correct counselling, support and sleep instead of being given drugs that double their suicide rate. They need to be listened to.

If you think that this book would help others understand this problem, or any other, it would be highly beneficial if you were to write a good review of the book on Amazon.

And it would help me continue my work in educating people about sleep and mental health issues.

Thank you in advance for doing that.

Love and Peace

Elizabeth

Appendices

APPENDIX 1 FATIGUE AND MENTAL HEALTH: BEDROOM TO BOARDROOM. DO THE NUMBERS.

This spreadsheet is supplied to help you calculate your organisation's exposure to sleep and mental health issues.

The spreadsheet goes beyond the question "what has sleep got to do with fatigue?" and includes the costs of inappropriate coping mechanisms, the side effects of medications, and how management and staff's mood and performance is hindered by incorrect strategies.

It enables you to look at your duty of care and what is considered to be culpable behaviour by experts.

Hopefully after reviewing Appendix 1 you will proactively participate in policy and staffing decisions where you know your employees and the organisation are being adversely affected by the present outdated policies.

Fatigue and Mental Health: Bedroom to Boardroom.

COST FACTOR	Factors that Affect your Bottom Line, your Duty of Care, Employee Performance and Wellbeing.		Yearly Cost to Your Organisation	
	DESCRIPTION	Source	$ Per 100 Employees	Total Cost $
HOW MUCH ARE FATIGUE AND MENTAL HEALTH PROBLEMS COSTING YOUR ORGANISATION?	Base your calculations on the daily average salary of your staff members.	1		
	Daily average salary in Australia was $ 269.20, full time adult average weekly ordinary time earnings at the end of November 2016 was $ 1,533.10.	121		
DO THE MATHS …	*Insert your organisation's daily average salary here: $*			
	Insert the number of your employees here:			
AVERAGE AMOUNT OF SLEEP PEOPLE ARE GETTING. The figures vary…				
United States of America	6 hours 40 minutes/work night	26		
Australia	Half of Australians say they don't get enough sleep.	130		
	35-44 year olds get 6.4 hours of sleep	130		
	44 percent say they come home exhausted from work	130		
	6.8 hours (mean hours of sleep). Those who worked full-time and those who are dissatisfied with their levels of stress sleep the least. Average: 6.5 hours a night.	61		
	6 hours	5		
	7 hours and 18 minutes of sleep on average, with 66% saying their sleep was disturbed.	123	66	
	8 hours and 1 minute	60		
Conflicting statistics…	8 hours 30 minutes (2006), 8 hours 20 minutes in 1992.	107		
Historically in Australia	*Notes*	29, 30		

SLEEP HOURS WE NEED?	Generally accepted as 8 hours for adults of working age, though evidence exists that performance is enhanced with 10 hours.	86	
CONTRIBUTING FACTORS TO LACK OF SLEEP REPORTED:	Long hours, work related stress, and job insecurity were among the top factors contributing to Australians becoming 'semi-insomniacs'.		
HOW MANY STAFF ARE AFFECTED BY SLEEP DISORDERS?	65% of Americans report experiencing a sleep problem	10	65 people
	61% of Australians would like more sleep	5	
	51% of Australians say they are not getting enough sleep	61	
	80% of Australians are experiencing some issue with sleeping	62	
	28% say they experience a sleep problem almost every night	10	
	8.9% consist of 3 disorders: Obstructive Sleep Apnea 4.7%, Primary Insomnia 3%, Restless Legs Syndrome 1.2%.	23	
	"95% of people with sleep disorders are undiagnosed and untreated, and must struggle through the day feeling unmotivated and exhausted."	84	
Sleep less than 7 hours a night?	40% have a higher rate of coronary artery disease or heart attack.	56	
Primary Insomnia	Estimated prevalence of insomnia 3%	70	3 people
	The economic cost of 'insomnia' in 2002 dollars, annual total (not just work related):	68	$ 5,867 pp.
Restless Legs Syndrome	Estimated prevalence of Restless Legs Syndrome (RLS) 1.2%	70	1.2 people
	The economic cost of RLS in 2004 dollars, total (not just work related):	67	$ 5,000 pp.

COST FACTOR	DESCRIPTION	Source	$ Per 100 Employees	Total Cost $
Obstructive Sleep Apnea	Estimated prevalence of Obstructive Sleep Apnea (OSA) 4.7%.	70	4.7 people	
	The economic cost of OSA in 2006 dollars, total (not just work related):	69	$ 6,433 pp.	
ABSENTEEISM				
Taking a sick day	Police study showed more likely to take a sick day if they have a sleep disorder. 26.0% vs 20.9%.	53	5.1 people	
Arrive late to work	12% were late to work in the past month because of sleepiness. Assume 15 minutes, once a month.	42	12 people	
Gone to work sick	14%, citing concerns about how it might be perceived by the employer or work colleagues.	64		
Due to primary insomnia	5.5 days per person employed per year	71		
Due to RLS	5.5 days per person employed per year	71		
Due to OSA	5.5 days per person employed per year	71		
PRESENTEEISM				
Lower productivity at work	Lost work performance equal to 7.8 days/year/insomniac	23	8.9 people	
		22	18,687.86	
Loss of 'work performance'	$ 2,280 per person per year	24		
FALLING ASLEEP AT WORK				
Generally	29% of people have been very sleepy or fallen asleep at work in the past month.	12	29 people	
	56% of shiftworkers fall asleep on the job at least once a week.	82		

LOSS OF PERFORMANCE AND PRODUCTIVITY	Apart from daytime sleepiness etc, sleep deprivation is associated with microsleeps, sleep seizures, mood shifts, lack of interest in socializing, loss of coping skills and loss of sense of humour.		
REDUCED EXECUTIVE FUNCTIONING OF THE BRAIN	Reduced ability to concentrate, reduced memory function (particularly short term), unable to handle complex tasks, reduced decision making ability, impaired motor skills and coordination, inability to think logically, assimilate and analyse new information and think critically.	87	
	Reduced vocabulary and communication skills, creativity, reduced perceptual skills.	87	
Making Errors at Work:			
6 hours sleep over a period of 14 days?	11 times more likely to demonstrate performance lapses.	78	
Less than 5 hours sleep?	Impaired performance comparable to being legally drunk.	19	
Important Administrative Errors	Of the police who had sleep disorders 17.9% reported having made these errors, compared to 12.7% without disorders.	53	
The Cost of Making Errors	Your company/organisation must decide the cost of these errors:		5.2 people
	Are your staff dealing with high value transactions?		
	Valuable equipment?		
	Are errors reversible? Which errors are reversible?		
	At what cost?		
GENERAL BEHAVIOUR AND ATTITUDE AT WORK			
Impatient and/or irritable	40% say they have become impatient with others at least a few times that month (during the survey).	8	40 people

COST FACTOR	DESCRIPTION	Source	Employees	Total $
Bad mood at work	44% likely to be in a bad mood at work as a result of poor sleep.	65	44 people	
Uncontrolled anger towards a citizen or suspect	The police study showed 34.1% compared with 28.5% of the non-sleep deprived group.	53		
Difficult to Concentrate	27% find it hard to concentrate	9	27 people	
Productivity reduces with length of hours worked	A 10% increase in overtime in manufacturing operations results in a 2.4% decrease in productivity; in white-collar jobs performance can decrease by as much as 25% when workers put in 60 or more hours per week for prolonged periods of time.	59		
	One study showed that working more than sixty hours a week and failing to get regular sleep can double the risk of having a heart attack.	111		
Productivity	20% said their productivity at work was often lower than they had expected.	10	20 people	
Job Satisfaction?	The 49% of respondents that were less than "very satisfied" with their job, were also more likely to report their sleep needs were not being met, less than 6 hours sleep typically, and report symptoms of insomnia at least a few nights a week in the past month.	11		
Diminished Motivation	"Studies commissioned by the Department of Defense and the Defense Advanced Research Projects Agency found that lack of sleep degrades not only the ability of combat soldiers to identify and locate the enemy, but also - and even more disturbingly - *their capacity to care whether they succeed or not.*"	57		

PSYCHOLOGICAL CONDITIONS ASSOCIATED WITH LACK OF ADEQUATE SLEEP	*Do you think the previous exposure is relevant for the police force, with longer shifts and increasing firepower?*		
SLEEP	1 in 5 suffer from a mental health problem in a 12 month period.	25, 54	20 people
	22 per cent of women and 18 per cent of men in the 12 months prior to an ABS study showed symptoms of a mental health disorder.	117	22 or 18
	Over a lifetime 45 per cent of people show symptoms of a mental health disorder.	118	45 people
Depression			
Percentage of population who are depressed.	4.5% experienced symptoms of major depression in the last 12 months.	17	4.5 people
	In 2006-7 there were 12 million scripts written for antidepressants in Australia. This represented 7.62% of the population of Australia.	33, 41	7.62 people - old figure
	This figure more than doubled by 2016, with 1 in 6 Australians now taking antidepressants - or 16.6 percent of the population/your employees.	Ch. 1	16.6 people
Cost of each depressed person to an employer per year.	$ 9,665 per year/person	13	160,439.00
"At risk" industries and careers?	**Police officers** in the US and Canada reported rates of depression and burnout roughly double those of the general population.	53	
	A study of **paediatricians**: residents rate of depression range between 7% and 56%.	55	7 to 56 people

COST FACTOR	DESCRIPTION	Source	Employees	Total $
Errors when depressed	Depressed resident doctors made 6.2 times as many errors per resident month as residents who were not depressed. (Some of these errors are in life and death situations.)	55		
	Nurses doing shift work, and depression…			
	14% of night shift workers had symptoms of shift work disorder and nearly one third of those were depressed.	76	14 people	
	SBS Insight quoted nurses as having triple the suicide rate of the normal population.			
Anxiety and panic disorders	Percent of population - any anxiety	17	4.7 people	
	14 per cent of the population	116	14 people	
	2.72% prescribed for anxiety and panic in 2006-7	35, 41	2.7 people	
The majority of people suffering mental disorders do not seek professional help.	68% of those that had feeling and symptoms associated with the surveyed mental disorders or substance dependencies did not talk to, or see a health professional in the last year.	79		
SIDE EFFECTS OF MEDICATIONS				
Sleeping Pills	6.95 percent reported taking a sleeping pill last night	123	6.95 people	
Refer to Chapter 9 for the list of 32 side effects.	Last night:			
	Prescription medication 1.71 percent	123		
	Over the counter medications 2.86 percent	123		
	Herbal remedies 2.38 percent	123		
	"Some sort of sleep medication"			
	Men: 3.76 percent	123	3.8	
	Women: 8.34 percent	123	8.3	
	If you present to your doctor in Australia with insomnia you will be prescribed in 95.2 percent of cases.	124		

	Nearly 7 million benzodiazepine prescriptions are written in Australia each year. The most common being Valium and Temazepam. Ref. Medical body report.	125	
	35,513,140 psycho scripts were written in Australia 2015-16, consisting of 25,845,076 psychoanaleptics and 9,668,064 psycholeptics.	126	
	When people present to their doctor:		
	3.9 percent present with insomnia	128	
	2.2 percent present with sleep apnea	128	
Sleeping Pill use	6-10% of people took pills in the US in 2010.	2	
	Using the 10% figure, if we assume they take them evenly throughout a week, then: M-F is 5/7 = 7.14% of staff are taking them the night before a working day.		7.14
	Times those that were prescribed took a tablet that year (low end of statistics) - 18 times.	3	
	2.71% of Australians prescribed hypnotics/sedatives in 2006-7	33	
	10% of Australians take sleeping pills. A third of these admit to taking them every night.	62	2.7 people
	Sleeping pills should not be used if you have sleep apnea.	90	
	The half-life of sleeping pills vary from about 1 hour to as long as 24 hours, so the effect of the one sleeping tablet can, in some cases, last for days (without taking one the next night).	39	
	"All hypnotics at some doses produce decrements in performance the next day."	18,21	11,417.20
	Hypnotics associated with mortality or cancer	2	

COST FACTOR	DESCRIPTION	Source	Employees	Total $
	Professor Malcolm Lader, whose research in the 1980s suggested a link between long-term tranquilliser use and brain damage, said he now gives legal advice about negligent prescribing and dangerous detoxifications "at least every three months".		115	
	A report by the All Party Parliamentary Group on Drug Misuse (UK) estimated in 2009 that there were 1.5 million involuntary tranquilliser addicts in the UK.		115	
Side Effects of Sleeping Pills/Benzodiazepines	Sleeping pills mask the symptoms, delay correct diagnosis, and often worsen the problem.		122	
	Akathisia, which predisposes suicide and homicide		122	
	Hangover effect felt the next day and subsequent days		122	
	Congential abnormalities/ birth defects including oral cleft, floppy infant syndrome, dependence in babies, marked neonatal withdrawal, sucking difficulties and vigorous sucking.		122	
	Benzodiazepines are in FDA Pregnancy Category D which recommends against their use during pregnancy.		122	
	Drowsiness		119	
	Light-headedness		119	
	Hospitalisation		119	
	Cognitive impairment		122	
	Pain in the limbs, back and neck, teeth and jaw.		122	
	Stabbing pins and needles in the limbs and face.		122	
	Dizziness		122	
	Tinnitus		122	

346

(side effects continued…)	
Hypersensitivity to sound, light, touch and taste	122
Muscle pain and twitches	122
Tremor	122
Hallucinations	122
Anxiety	122
Disorientation	122
Difficulty walking	122
Drugged feeling	122
Poor memory and concentration	122
Nausea, vomiting	122
Abdominal pain, diarrhoea and constipation	122
Agoraphobia and other phobias	122
Panic attacks and palpatations	122
Pills make the problem worse, not better, in the long term	122
Bizarre behaviours	122
Driving while asleep, with no memory of it	122
Increased risk of depression	122
Four-fold risk of death with overuse	122
Cancer risk increased with overuse	122
Memory impairment and anterograde amnesia	122
Overdose deaths	122
Restless sleep and insomnia	122
Other sleep disorders	122
Higher risk taking and more impetuous behaviour	120
Reduced alertness	120
Coordination effected	120
Reaction times effected	120

COST FACTOR	DESCRIPTION	Source	Employees	Total $
(side effects continued...)	It takes longer to complete tasks	120		
	Increased risks of falls or accidents	120		
	Lowered inhibitions	120		
	50% increased risk of alzheimers	122		
	Greater risks when combined with alcohol or drugs	120		
	Sleeping pills are addictive.	122		
	Sleeping pills are abused and used for recreation	122		
	Unresolved health, mental health and underlying emotional disorders not addressed before medicating.	122		
	Treating the symptom not the cause, delaying any solution.	122		
	Rebound insomnia	122		
Side Effects of withdrawal and tapering from sleeping pills:	Suicidal ideation	122		
	Completed suicide	122		
	Akathisia, which predisposes suicide and homicide	122		
	Unusual depressed or anxious mood	122		
	Persistent withdrawal syndrome	122		
	Sweating, shakiness, anxiety	122		
	Fatigue	122		
	Irritability	122		
	(Can be any of the side effects from going ON the drug, but tapering is considered by many to be the most dangerous stage.)	122		
Anti-depressants, SSRIs	1 in 6 are taking antidepressants	122	16.66 people	
	1 in 6 babies in the United States is born to a mother who took a psychiatric drug during pregnancy.	127		

(antidepressants/SSRIs continued...)		
When people present to their doctor:		
16.6 percent present with depression	128	
12.0 percent present with anxiety	128	
Side Effects of antidepressants/SSRIs:		
Depression!	122	
Suicidal ideation	122	
Increased risk of suicide	122	
Akathisia, which predisposes suicide and homicide	122	
Violence and aggression	122	
Homicide	122	
Addiction	122	
Murder and suicide combined	122	
Produces multiple chemical imbalances in the brain	122	
SSRIs increase alcohol use and addictions	122	
SSRIs increase obesity risk	122	
Temporary sexual dysfunction	122	
Close to 100 percent experience sexual side effects	122	16.6
Post-SSRI Sexual Dysfunction(PSSD) can persist for months, years or indefinitely. There is no known cure.	122	
Permanent sexual dysfunction	122	
Increased interest in consuming alcohol.	122	
Boosted respiratory failure risk in patients with COPD (respiratory problems).	122	
1 in 6 babies in America is born to a mother who has taken antidepressants while pregnant.		
Link to autistic babies	122	
Emotional burden of babies being born with birth defects	122	

COST FACTOR	DESCRIPTION	Source	Employees	Total $
(withdrawal symptoms, continued...)	Antidepressant use in the third trimester of pregnancy is associated with problems feeding, respiratory difficulties, jitteriness.	122		
	Increased risk of falls in older people, followed by death in 1 in 28 of them.	122		
	Adverse outcomes for diagnosed people, in the areas of employment and incapacitation.	122		
	Shortened life span.	122		
	Serious adverse effects on the basal ganglia of the brain.	122		
Withdrawal and Tapering Symptoms:	Depression!	122		
(similar to "symptoms" above)	Suicidal ideation	122		
	Suicide	122		
	Akathisia, which predisposes suicide and homicide	122		
	Violence and Aggression	122		
	Homicide	122		
	As a general rule, if there is a side effect going on the drug, the same effect will be experienced coming off the drug. Sometimes the tapering effect is more severe.	122		
ALCOHOL USE	33.5 percent of people consumed alcohol yesterday.	123	33.5	
	People with psychological problems have an increased risk of alcohol use and abuse. If they are taking SSRIs that risk increases.			
	The overall proportion of employed recent drinkers who usually drink at work is 10.2%. (Averaged over low risk 7.1% and high risk 16.0%).	80	10.2	

(alcohol at work, continued…)	The percentage of these workers who missed one or more days of work due to illness/injury in the last 3 months? Average 40.5% (low risk 35.1%, high risk 54.6%).	80
	The industries listed on the 'proportion of employed recent drinkers, by risk category and industry' classification Australia 2001 are (risky and high risk combined): mining, wholesale, manufacturing, transport, services, administration and defence, financial, construction, education, agriculture, hospitality and retail.	80
"AT RISK" INDUSTRIES	Included in at-risk industries are the police, emergency workers, first responders, medical (doctors, nurses, ambulance, etc.), transport industry, mining, international financial traders, travelers, security personnel, overnight shift workers. This list is not conclusive.	
GLOBAL-FINANCIAL-CRISIS-AFFECTED INDUSTRIES	The newest at-risk industries are all those affected by the GFC, still being felt internationally. Particularly Wall-Street-related (financial, investment, trading, etc.) and Main Street industries where the effects have been felt as well - though not as dramatically.	
	In industries such as these anxiety, stress and sleep are definitely being affected.	
	Following the GFC, the American evidence, specifically on Wall Street, where employees describe feeling 'paralysed' (74%), 'demoralized' (73%), and 'demotivated' (64%).	88

COST FACTOR	DESCRIPTION	Source	Employees	Total $
(At risk industries, continued...)	Survivors of the RIFs (reductions in force), reported extremely high levels of stress, more than twice the number as one year earlier, with symptoms ranging from ulcers and migraine headaches to a new dependence on sleep medication.	108		
	Negative coping strategies are outweighing the positive. They include taking sleeping pills, drinking (23% which increased to 30% one year later), smoking, overeating (30% to 41%), and losing one's temper.	108		
	After the GFC 22% of high-echelon workers were working an extra nine hours a week.	109		
	Flight Risk? 78% of high-echelon workers reported experiencing high levels of stress, more than twice as high as one year earlier.	110		
	64% of Wall Street and 41% of Main Street employees were considering leaving their current companies.	110		
	"Merrill Lynch found that health care costs at the company shot up in 2008, a year of great turmoil, as many employees leaned heavily on medical services. Stress, it turns out, costs money."	111		
POLICE	40.4% screened positive for at least one sleep disorder.	53	40.4 people	
	28.5% experienced excessive sleepiness.	53	28.5 people	
	33.6% screened positive for Obstructive Sleep Apnea (OSA)	53	33.6 people	
	10.7 percent with sleep disorders reported having depression, compared with 4.4% who did not have a sleep disorder.	53		

(Police, continued…)

34.1% (of the sleep disorder group) showed burnout/emotional exhaustion compared with 17.9% without a sleep disorder.	53	
14.5% of those working night shift had shift work disorder.	53	
80% of Police reported having fallen asleep once a week while working the night shift.	95	
ACCIDENTS AND INJURIES		
Work-related injury or illness		
6.4% of workers experienced a work-related injury or illness.	16	6.4 people
More accidents occur between 2 and 4 pm than any other daytime hours.	92	
Workplace injury		
Population Attributable Fraction (PAF) of a workplace injury due to OSA is 0.6%	73	
PAF of a workplace injury due to insomnia is 3.90%.	73	
How many drove drowsy in the last year?		
27% report having driven drowsy less than once/month	11	
17% drive drowsy 1-2 times/m	11	
6% drive drowsy 1-2 times/week	11	
5% drive drowsy 3 + times/week	11	
28% have nodded off or fallen asleep while driving in the past year.	11	
26% drove drowsy during the workday in the past year.	42	
The number of hours worked has a relationship with the risk of falling asleep at the wheel.	112	
Less than or equal to 35 hours, 20%; 36-40 hours 25% had dozed off; and 50 hours plus - 50% falling asleep at the wheel.	104	

COST FACTOR	DESCRIPTION	Source	Employees	Total $
MOTOR VEHICLE ACCIDENTS	Sleepiness is estimated to be a factor in 20% of motor vehicle accidents.	6		
	30% of highway vehicle accidents are caused by drivers falling asleep at the wheel.	98		
	1% have had an accident or near accident due to drowsiness while driving in the past year.	11		
	At least 1 in every 20 Americans has caused an accident by falling asleep at the wheel.	97		
	Having one less hour of sleep can increase the number of road accidents by 8%, with the opposite happening at the other change of daylight saving time.	66		
	9.3% of those with severe daytime sleepiness had experienced a motor vehicle accident in the past 12 months compared to 4.7% who did not suffer from daytime sleepiness.	81		
	People with sleep apnea (OSA) are two to seven times more likely to have a motor vehicle accident than people without OSA.	81		
	People with undiagnosed OSA are 7 times more likely to have multiple accidents.	101		
TRANSPORT/TRUCKING AT RISK	Sleepiness/fatigue is the number one cause of heavy trucking accidents.	99		
	1 in every 5 victims is in the cab of a truck, the remaining four victims are innocent pedestrians or motorists.	100		
	In one major trucking company 75% of its drivers were found to have sleep apnea.	102		

NEW PARENTS AT RISK	
On average a parent of a new baby loses 400-750 hours of sleep during the first year.	105
About 30% of young children (1-4 y.o.) demand parental intervention at least once nightly.	106
SHIFT WORKERS AT RISK	
Shift workers account for 16% or one sixth of all people who work.	15
25% of Americans are shift workers.	93
Shift workers report more sick days, have more heart attacks and cardiovascular diseases, and suffer more mood disorders, depression and psychiatric problems than their counterparts on regular day shifts.	31
70% of shift workers have trouble falling asleep.	29
Shift workers average one to two hours less sleep than their daytime counterparts during the week, and three to four hours less on weekends.	29, 30
INJURIES - SHIFT WORKERS	
19% said they have injured themselves or had an accident on the job in the past year.	10
The work-related injury rate of shift workers was 113 per 1000 employed people - almost twice the rate of those who worked regular hours (60 per 1000 people employed).	15
Shift workers are 40 times more likely than day workers to be involved in accidents - at work, on the highway, and at home.	94
31% of the injuries of shift workers were a sprain or strain, 20% were a chronic joint or muscle condition.	15
Of the shift workers who experienced a work-related injury:	

COST FACTOR	DESCRIPTION	Source	Employees	Total $
(Shiftworker injuries continued...)	19% were intermediate clerical sales and service workers, 17% were labourers and related workers, 64% other.	15		
	Shift workers who miss three or more hours of sleep decrease their resistance to viral infections by as much as 50%.	96		
	Research indicates that in the 4 days after we lose one hour of sleep (following the start of daylight savings), there is a 7% increase in accidental deaths, a pattern that is reversed in autumn when it is reversed.	85		
Professionals and shift work	Are 3 times more likely to experience work-related injury compared to those who do not undertake shiftwork. 97 per 1000 vs 35 per 1000 employed.	15		
Intermediate clerical, sales and service shift workers.	Are more than twice as likely to report an injury than those who did not (109 and 46 per 1000 employed).	15		
OVERNIGHT FLIGHTS AND RED-EYES	Should never be followed by driving. Ever.	45		
INJURIES - AT RISK INDUSTRIES	"Medical residents and interns are among the most severely sleep-deprived individuals".	83		
MEDICAL PROFESSIONALS AND HOSPITAL WORKERS AT RISK	A study of interns who had been scheduled to work at least 24 hours increased their odds of stabbing themselves with a needle or scalpel by 61%, crashing a motor vehicle by 168%, risk of a near miss by 460%.	44		
	Psychiatrists have the highest rate of suicide. Male doctor suicide rate is one and a quarter times the rate of the general population, and female doctors two and a half times the general population.	74		

Category	Description		
(Medical workers continued…)	As compared to when working 16-hour shifts, on-call residents have twice as many attention failures when working overnight, and commit 36% more serious medical errors. They also report making 300% more fatigue-related medical errors that lead to a patient's death.		44
	Nearly half of interns reported falling asleep at the wheel on the way home.		75
MINING INDUSTRY	The use of sleeping pills increased from 3.5% use to 13% in the most extreme shifts.		49
	Difficulty sleeping between night shifts when workers have a say about their hours and shifts 22.12%. When they have no say, 29%.		50
	Use of antidepressants ranges from 6% to 10.6% of workers.		51
POLICE	26.1% of police reported falling asleep while driving at least 1 to 2 times a month.		53
	6.2% reported falling asleep while driving at least 1 to 2 times a week.		53
HIGHER INCIDENCE OF RISK-TAKING BEHAVIOUR	Police study showed 23.7% vs 15.5% reported making errors or committing safety violations due to fatigue.		53
LITIGATION EXPOSURE	Accidents at work	8.2 people	53
	Motor vehicle accidents at work		
	Long-term shift workers and proven illnesses.		7
	Depression was recognized as a disability in the Disability Discrimination Act 1992.		
REHABILITATION AND DETOX	Benzodiazepines, sleeping pills, antidepressants and SSRIs are all addictive. The problems coming off them are well documented, but not well known in the community.		Ch. 10

COST FACTOR	DESCRIPTION	Source	Employees	Total $
(Rehabilitation and Detox continued....)	According to Prof. Peter Gotzsche we do not have the facilities to deal with the numbers of people who should be tapering down from their antidepressant medications under strict supervision.	129		
	This problem is already a crisis, and will surface as a costly national crisis as soon as people wake up to the extent of the problem.			
JAIL AND INCARCERATION	Yet to be costed?			
COUNSELLING FOR THE BERIEVED AFTER SUICIDE AND/OR HOMICIDE.	Yet to be costed?			
COPING MECHANISMS	*What Strategies are Insomniacs Using to Help Them Sleep Better?*			
	10 percent use sleep aids.			
	7% use over-the-counter/store bought sleep aids.			
	3% use sleep medications prescribed by a doctor.			
Alcohol used to sleep "better"	8% use alcohol which they perceive as a sleep aid, at least a few nights a week	42		
	30% of people with persistent insomnia reported using alcohol to help them sleep in the past year, 67% of those reporting that it was effective.	43, 47		
	One drink on six hours of sleep is the equivalent of six drinks on eight hours of sleep.	103		
	You should never use alcohol to help you fall asleep.	89		
Over-The-Counter sleep aids and/or alcohol.	20% reported trying untested over-the-counter substances or alcohol.	4		
	Over-the-counter drugs should be taken with the same caution as prescription drugs.	91		

Illicit/illegal	Cannibis/marijuana	52
	Other, 'downers' etc.	?
	What Strategies are People Using to Stay Awake and Alert?	
Alerting medications	5% are taking alerting medications	10
	"No drug has yet been invented that is a substitute for sleep."	58
Caffeine and Energy Drinks	58% consume caffeinated beverages.	10, 47
	88.67 percent consumed caffeine, with the average consumption 147.29 mg.	113
Nicotine, cigarettes	People who smoke at least one cigarette a day are more likely to use caffeine and nicotine to get through the day. And less likely to work efficiently because of being too sleepy.	123
High sugar & carbohydrates	38% will choose these food	11
Napping	37% will take a nap later, of approximately 1 hour	10
	13 percent said they had at least one nap yesterday	27, 28
Other Health Conditions Associated with sleep disorders, medication side effects, and permanent health problems.	Cardio-vascular disease, reduced immunity to disease and viral infections, weight gain and obesity, elevated blood pressure, feelings of being chilled, premature death, cancer, brain damage, the list goes on....	123

APPENDIX 2 THE CASE FOR SLEEP EDUCATION

My investigations to find a cohesive body or organisation that teaches people how to sleep better in NSW or Australia have resulted in nothing.

Many people insist that sleep is taught by doctors and sleep clinics. This is not the truth.

If you present to your doctor with insomnia you will be prescribed in 95.2 percent of cases. Therefore this educational body would have to be independent.

Sometimes, if your doctor believes you have sleep apnea, or a snoring problem, you will be referred to a sleep clinic. Sleep clinics will generally recommend that you stay overnight for a sleep and respiratory examination. They will teach you about sleep apnea and how to use your sleep apnea mask, of course.

But their purpose is not to educate about sleep.

Sleep clinics do not teach about sleep. I have found one that gives sleep classes to young people, but I'm not sure how people find it nor how children get referred there.

Community health groups do not teach about sleep, and NSW schools cover the topic inadequately.

There is clearly a lot to know about all aspects of sleep that is not being taught – particularly to school children and other vulnerable citizens.

I have managed to find less than 5 places that teach about sleep, and most very inadequately.

After reading this book it is clear that *early and correct intervention* when a person presents with sleeping problems, stress, anxiety and early mental health symptoms is vital to the health of the nation.

Early and correct intervention requires getting to the bottom of the problem. Such as finding the underlying issues that are resulting in the problem – however difficult that might seem, and however time consuming that process might be.

The present system is not working, and needs to be significantly disrupted.

Federal and State Health and Mental Health Ministers

Disappointed with these findings, in 2015 I telephoned the Australian Federal Health Minister's office, the NSW Health and Mental Health Minister's office and the NSW Deputy Health and Mental Health Minister's office wishing to talk about the issues raised in this book.

When introducing my interest as sleep and sleep education I was variously told that "sleep has got nothing to do with mental health", "patients learn about sleep in consultations with their GP", "this is the health department" (!), "I'm not sure what you mean by that", that I had the wrong department, was I a general practitioner? etc.

It was not inspiring.

Following that, I prepared *The Case for Sleep Education* and sent it to their respective offices, as well as to the highest management of a NSW Local Area Health District, and NSW education (public, private and independent schools).

I'm including *The Case for Sleep Education* (2015) here, knowing that it doesn't include my most recent mental health research.

The report was recognised as being received in most cases, by I was fobbed off in all ministerial cases.

After a number of determined contact attempts to a number of non-ministerial employees I managed to gain 2 meetings. One resulted in being fobbed off again, and the schools representative encouraged me to create a free online resource for schools (at my own considerable expense).

Here is the argument, a little outdated and changed a bit – but you'll get the point. (A lot has changed in just 2 years.)

The Case for Sleep Education (2015)
Introduction

The Australian government, schools and medical professionals wrongly believe that the public knows about sleep. They also believe that the public knows how to sleep; and that it's important.

The reality is very different.

This report illustrates that sleep education is just about non-existent in Australia.

Incorrect information, inappropriate policies and subsidized medications are fortifying sleep misinformation and management - causing accidents, errors, illness, suicides and death every single day.

The simple solution of sleep education could save billions each year, and make Australia a smarter, happier and more productive country.

Costs to Australian Economy

Dr Charles Czeisler of Harvard's Medical School says
70 percent of people say they frequently don't get enough sleep,
with 30 percent saying they don't get enough sleep every single night. [1]

I'm reluctant to quote some of the Australian studies quantifying the cost of sleep disorders and fatigue to the Australian economy, because I believe the figures are grossly understated.

We as a nation spend about $ 155 billion a year on health.
And about a third of that, $46 billion, each year is being squandered. [2]

According to Deloitte's *Reawakening Australia* report, sleep disorders cost the Australian economy $ 5.1 billion a year, $ 53 million in work accidents and $ 3.1 billion in lost productivity.

The Lancet in 2012 revealed that sleep disorders contribute to 5.3% of strokes, 10.1% of depression, 4.3 % of motor vehicle accidents and 4.5% of workplace injuries.

An employee with depression will cost their employer $ 9,665 per year; and fatigued worker's loss of productivity is equivalent to 7.8 days/year or $ 2,280 per person.

One example of why these figures are understated would be that, for example, anyone who is taking a sleeping medication with a half life of say 20 hours, will have their work performance impaired for at least the next full day at work, possibly two. That's from one sleeping pill, once a year. (This is not a recommendation for short half-life sleeping pills.)

The studies differ greatly on how many motor accidents relate to fatigue, and the definition of 'fatigue related accidents' differs in Australia from state to state, so it is difficult to make sense of it.

1 in 5 motor accidents are fatigue related.

Here are **some** of the cost that don't seem to be added into the figures I've seen:

- Errors at work caused by fatigue – such as placing incorrect trades, incorrect financial information, bad strategic decisions, etc;
- Ineffectual grumpy and short tempered management, with the resultant lack of work productivity in their departments and organisations;
- Relationship problems, divorce, lack of self esteem, abuse, domestic violence – medicated and not medicated;
- The cost of listing ineffectual drugs on the PBS, and the cost of those prescriptions to the patient (e.g. over 7 million benzodiazepine prescriptions written each year, part of 35 million psycho scripts);
- The cost of undiagnosed physical and mental health problems that are being overlooked because the root cause of insomnia is not being thoroughly investigated up front;
- Wasted time not knowing what the cause of sleeplessness is, and never addressing the actual problems;
- The cost of suicides and homicides;
- Opportunity cost of Australian citizens' days spent in a dopey daze because they are sleepy; and
- Drug rehabilitation processes to get people off the addictive and sometimes dangerous medications, which many of them should not have been prescribed in the first place.

The Medical Benefits Scheme is not Evidence Based

Very little of the Medical Benefits Scheme (MBS) has evidence attached to it. Of the 5,769 services listed on the MBS about 269 are evidence-based. 5500 items do not have that evidence base. Robyn Ward.[3]

Why was this review left to *Four Corners*?

Who will similarly review the Pharmaceutical Benefits Scheme (PBS) and the National Prescribing Service's (NPS's) evidence base?

Why Bother Sleeping?

Lack of sleep:

- Has been associated with the following **physical health problems**: obesity, coronary heart disease, diabetes, impaired immune function, reduced grey matter in the brain and inflammation,
- Exacerbates **mental health problems** such as depression, all anxieties (including OCD etc), and stress, and
- Increases the likelihood of **accidents and errors** and involuntarily falling asleep – at work, in cars, working machinery, doing school exams, playing sport, competing in the Olympics and elite sports, etc.
- **Increases risk taking** behaviours, the probability of eating junk food, and **substance abuse** (nicotine, drugs and alcohol).

What Happens While We Sleep?

Our brains use more oxygen at certain stages of sleep than when we are awake. While we sleep we dream vividly and deeply, integrate spatial and long term memories, break down fats, make sense of the day, connect memory pathways, heal, recover, get restorative sleep, rest our bodies and parts of our brain, release hormones including growth hormones, grow, anabolically build tissue, clear toxins, regulate our immune system and regulate reproduction and sexual arousal.

The organ of the body most affected by lack of sleep is the brain, specifically what is called the "executive function". The brain is regarded as the most important organ of the body because that's where the instructions are controlled. Executive function includes working memory, task switching, planning, the ability to focus, attention span, decision making ability, verbal reasoning, mental flexibility, and making sense of things.

Frankly, if we don't sleep we become uncoordinated, anxious and stupid. Our mental health is challenged and we're prone to risk taking behaviours and substance abuse. Also we're more likely to become fat and die earlier of one of a number of serious diseases such as heart disease or cancer.[4]

The government has a duty of care - especially to its employees, and people in its care.

Therapeutic Goods Administration (TGA)
Benzodiazepines
The TGA recently attempted to move all benzodiazepines from Schedule 4 to Schedule 8, which was unsuccessful (except for Alprazolam).

They obviously have serious concerns. But no power to act?

Energy Drinks, Caffeinated Drinks, Oxedrine, Stimulants, etc.

- A full and scoping investigation should be conducted into how and why some "energy drinks" were registered as therapeutic goods, and/or dietary supplements by the TGA - thereby avoiding food regulations. "Energy drinks" have been the subject of medical complaints in Australia and to the Food and Drug Administration (FDA) in America (including pancreatitis and death); have been found to contain caffeine quantities outside approved guidelines; are known to impair sleep if used inappropriately; and their advertisers have been successfully sued in the US for false advertising.
- Although warnings have been posted on their website, the TGA appears reluctant to show exactly which branded products are those which they are concerned about. So which products are we talking about exactly?[5]
- Of course it's not just the TGA involved here – but the NSW Food Authority and the FSANZ agreements. None of these organisations seems to be making any new rulings. Complaints continue to be made and documented (including to the FDA). What progress has been made?

Mental Health Drugs

Lack of sleep is a mental health issue.

The international debate about the efficacy and appropriateness of anti-psychotic and antidepressant medications has passed the tipping point.[6,7,8] Refer "Sleep Is a Mental Health Issue" section below.

Trans Pacific Partnership (TPP)

Unfortunately the contents of the TPP have been suppressed.

How will the TPP effect Australia's sovereign decisions, the availability of solutions, food quality, labelling laws, the Australian public's ability to research their own health options, the cost of insurance, and health information?

Pharmaceutical Benefits Scheme (PBS) and National Prescribing Service (NPS)

These government run services should have their evidence bases reviewed. The Australian public are subsidising dangerous drugs. For example "If you use medicines for a long time your sleep problems may become worse or you may become dependent on pills to sleep. Long-term use can also increase the risk of accidents and falls."[9,10]

Falls in elderly patients are increased with the use of certain drugs, and falls are followed by death within 12 months for some.[11]

Doctors Don't Teach About Sleep, They Prescribe Medications

Often the best medicine is no medicine at all – or the best intervention is no intervention at all. But these conversations with patients that take time to explain that the evidence simply doesn't support doing a test, or prescribing a drug, are long conversations. And it's much easier in clinical practice to do things quickly and prescribe or order a test. Robyn Ward.[14]

- When someone presents to their doctor with insomnia they are pre-scribed medications in 95.2 percent of the cases.[12]

- When the TGA recently attempted to move all benzodiazepines from Schedule 4 to schedule 8 the move was objected to by the AMA and the RACP among others. Many problems were exposed with this back down.
- Apart from never addressing the underlying issues, sleeping pills have, at least, some of the following side effects: suicidal ideation, addiction, cognitive impairment, bizarre behaviours (such as sleep driving and sleep eating), withdrawal symptoms, hallucinations, disorientation, falling risks, muscle weakness, change in hormone levels, decrements in performance (can be over the whole next day), a four-fold risk of death and increased rates of cancer - for those who take a lot of tablets per year[13], anterograde amnesia, and more.
- Viewed as a group, sleeping pills increase your sleep time by 11.4 minutes and reduce the time it takes to fall asleep by 12.8 minutes compared with fake pills.[15]
- One sleeping pill was the most complained about medication to the *Australian Medicines Event Line* run by the NPS and Brisbane's Mater Hospital between September 2007 and February 2009. This pill had 670 percent more complaint calls than the second on the list.[16]
- Insomnia and sleep disorders are the known side effect of many prescription and non-prescription drugs. What *monitoring systems* convince us that best practice prescribing guidelines are being followed? Where are the guidelines?
- Health problems that are left untreated become a more costly problem for the patient, the government and health insurance companies.
- Furthermore, because of the ignorance of addiction and withdrawal symptoms, many patients think that rebound insomnia (for example) is an indication that their medication is working: rather than a manifesting withdrawal symptom.
- Procedures should be put in place to flag addicts, long term users, mental health patients, and other underlying physical health issues that are not being detected or addressed in sleep disorder consultations.
- Where do medical professionals learn about sleep? Either universities don't cover the topic adequately, or doctors aren't practicing what they learned at university. They can and do earn professional

development points by attending sleep courses run by pharmaceutical companies.

- From what I understand Australia's health infrastructure is inadequate if we were to adopt world's best practice around prescription drug withdrawal. We simply don't have enough suitable facilities.[17]

My concern is that sleep disorders, an early physical and mental health warning symptom, are being over-treated, ignored, complicated and worsened by medication and/or interpreted abysmally in the present medical model. In many cases without first addressing really obvious questions about stressors, grievances, diet, exercise, side effects of existing medications, life experiences etc.

"Chronic benzo use .... produces stupid people."
Professor Gavin Andrews.[18]

Sleep Disorders are not Limited to Sleep Apnea and Snoring

Bear with me on this one.

It's becoming very common that health care professionals and individuals think that sleeping problems begin and end with sleep apnea and snoring – that going to a sleep clinic and being tested is the only strategy to solve sleep problems, and the ultimate solution (along with sleeping pills).

While recognising the marketing reach of sleep apnea clinics, snoring devices, and respiratory research, medical and dental surgical procedures (and the like) it is very important that the basics of sleep education still be covered for all individuals, as early as possible, and hopefully before these problems arise. E.g. The link between obesity and sleep apnea is proven. Wouldn't it be better to discuss this in schools rather than to have the cost and complexity of addressing it later?

The underlying problems manifesting as sleep disorder symptoms go far beyond these issues (and industries).

Insomnia is a **symptom** of something else. "Insomnia" is not the problem. Not now, not ever.

The underlying problems include everyday stress; unresolved emotional issues (grief, depression, anxiety, PTSD, trauma, violence, sexual abuse etc);

food allergies and intolerances; substance, drug and alcohol abuse; the side effects of medications (including withdrawal from sleeping medications); physical pain or illness; anaemia; financial, relationship and work stresses; hormonal imbalance; lighting issues; lifestyle imbalances; shift work; circadian imbalances; inappropriate life choices; poverty; inappropriate diet; lack of exercise; age related challenges; self esteem issues; bad sleep hygiene and environmental factors – to name some.

We need to wake up about the broad ranging issues that result in insomnia and sleep disorders.

And we certainly need to be educated to recognise and manage them, up front, before taking symptom-masking and addictive medications.

To shift doctors' behaviour, physicians need hard data
to tell them about how well or badly their patients have fared.
And in Australia we're truly lousy at that. Dr Norman Swan.[19]

Who Teaches Sleep Education?

- There is no Australian institution, public or private, that covers sleep education adequately.
- I have personally contacted Federal and State Health Minister's, the State Minister for Mental Health's office, Sleep Clinics, Federal and State Education Ministers, Local Area Health groups, Community Health, local councils, Medicare Locals, hospitals, the Police Human Resources and Police Safety Control, universities, sporting associations, Sydney medical centres, listed ASX companies, corporate Employee Assistance Programs (EAPs), fatigue RTOs, and special health bodies etc.

    The problem never seems to be about sleep. In every case the institution has "got it under control" with no need for improvement. Well, no.

- A *very small* percentage of sleep clinics teach about sleep as part of their sleep apnea testing and other functions. However, all sleep clinics require a referral from a medical professional, and generally they are referred because of the possibility of having sleep apnea or snoring problems – not for sleep education. Doctors may give sleep tips while they write a prescription, but this is clearly not enough.

Schools Teach Sleep Inadequately
The George Institute on Global Health
found that young adults who get less than 5 hours sleep on average
are 3 times more likely to develop mental health problems
than those who slept 8-9 hours regularly.

Sleep is included in the NSW school's PDHPE syllabus for years 7-10, strand 4 under "Lifelong Physical Activity". It can also be included in well-ness and pastoral care and holistic health discussions.

Sleep is not <u>sold</u> to the students adequately, given its importance.

The following connections are not being made adequately in the school curriculums:

- How lack of sleep effects the brain, executive function, memory, cognitive processes, learning, coordination, sporting ability, motor skills, focus, attention span, decision making etc.,
- How sleep is directly connected to performance – mental, physical and emotional intelligence,
- The connection to mental health issues, depression, anxiety and stress, mood,
- How sleep can affect relationships, family relationships and resilience,
- How sleep affects eating, weight management, the ability and enthusiasm for exercising and movement,
- What happens while we sleep (see above),
- How computers and blue light are rewiring our brains,
- How you can sleep your way to look better, stay slim, eat correct food etc.,
- How to read food labels, specifically in relation to what foods and additives prevent adequate sleep,
- Delayed sleep phase, melatonin production, circadian rhythm – all very important to teenagers and young adults. Some young adults

are still producing melatonin (the sleep inducing hormone) in the morning. Little wonder they seem dull!

- How energy drinks and high octane drinks effect your sleep and health,
- How to reduce accidents and risk taking behaviour,
- How napping and meditation improve emotional intelligence, alertness and memory,
- How to do better in exams using sleep techniques,
- The link between lack of sleep and psychological problems and substance abuse, and
- How to manage the dark hours for success and safety.

Half of all lifetime cases of mental illness begin by age 14.
75 percent of all severe mental illness begins before the age of 24 years.[20]

A recent study by the division of Sleep Medicine Harvard Medical School showed that restricting the hours that teenagers can drive in the night time hours resulted in a 40 percent reduction in fatal and incapacitating injury crashes observed for teen drivers.[21]

Sleep is a Mental Health Issue
The underlying problems with sleep disorders are not necessarily physical. The mental health issues can include anxieties, depression, stress, unresolved emotional issues, PTSD, abuse, grief, etc.

The psychiatry profession's diagnosing and medicating practices are now being questioned by international research leaders including Professor Peter C. Gøtzsche of the Nordic Cochrane Collaborative[22], Robert Whitaker[23], and many others.

The results of Study 329 into paroxetine (an SSRI) has recently been overturned, showing that it performed no better than placebo, but has serious adverse effects such as suicide and suicidal ideation.[24] (The original study was the subject of fraud charges.[25])

Interestingly and alarmingly, the National Prescribing Service lists 34 side effects of paroxetine on its website, with no mention of suicide or suicidal ideation.[26]

Medical and psychiatric practices raise obvious duty of care exposure questions now and into the future, including (but not limited to) government departments responsible for the mental health of people in their care (e.g. the military, prisoners, etc).

The Definition of Fatigue in the Workplace

"Top executives now have a critical responsibility to take sleeplessness seriously."
Professor Charles Czeisler, Harvard Sleep Medicine.[27]

Beyond the scope of this paper for practical reasons, but I believe organisations are attempting to limit fatigue-related exposure by disconnecting sleep from their definition of "fatigue".

When I was first asked by a fatigue registered training organisation (RTO) "what has sleep got to do with fatigue?" I thought they were joking. It isn't funny when the same question is being asked many times to other experts and by many organisations. It is common.

"Every important mistake I've made in my life, I've made because I was too tired." Bill Clinton

Fatigue management in all organisations should include sleep education, showing its *direct connection* to fatigue.

Organisations should recognise that workers can *arrive to work* fatigued ... because that happens.

The proven quantifiable benefits of quality sleep should be part of employee education to ensure that organisations understand the direct relationship to reduced accidents and deaths; improved performance; sharper mental acuity; elevated mood; reduced absenteeism and presenteeism; better executive functions of the brain; and the long term reduction of mental and physical illnesses etc.

Alert, happy and emotionally intelligent employees improve profitability.

By avoiding sleep education and policies, organisations are breaching their duty of care.

How are Government Departments Fulfilling Their Duty of Care?

Our research indicates that it is government departments that are often the most exposed, and continue with draconian sleep, fatigue and mental health practices. They include the police, military, ambulance workers, shift working hospital staff and nurses, interns and doctors, prison personnel and prisoners, mental institutions, fire brigade and emergency services workers.

One large US/Canada study found that about 40 percent of the police force have a sleep disorder.[28]

I have no doubt that adding trauma, stress, violence, long hours, night time shift work, desensitizing and stress to their jobs increases their sleeping problems as well as other mental health issues such as anxiety, depression and post traumatic stress disorder (PTSD).

Litigation Exposure

Here are some other possible exposures:

- The Danish Government began paying compensation in 2009 to long term night shift workers because of a link to breast cancer. Night shift work is linked with a number of cancer types.[29]
- Studies show interns making 700 percent more errors in their long shifts, with some of those errors being life threatening to patients. (Medical professionals have above average suicide rates – with women doctors having over twice the average rates of the population.)

Food and Cosmetics Labelling Laws

Food, cosmetics and other ingested products can affect sleeping patterns, but the labelling laws make it nearly impossible to isolate the offending substances for the people affected.[30]

"Labelling is a massive problem." Jamie Oliver[31]

The Benefits of Sleep Education

The benefits of sleep education include:

- Sleep disorders will be recognised as a major preventative medicine signal to allow early detection and solutions to physical and mental health problems.
- A population that sleeps better is healthier, less likely to be obese, happier and more productive at work.
- With adequate sleep, less road and work accidents will occur.
- An alert workforce will make fewer errors, requiring less fixes.
- Less major catastrophes will occur because of fatigue (Chernobyl, Exxon Valdez, Challenger, etc)
- School students will relax more and perform better when they get more sleep.
- Sporting results will improve, with improved hand-eye coordination, response times, healing and recovery times. This can include elite sports and the Olympics.
- Patients with sleep disorders can avoid medical fees by working out what their underlying sleep problems are and taking responsibility for them up front.
- People will be encouraged to move more and exercise more when they see the benefit it has on their sleep patterns.
- People will eat healthier foods when they see the sleep benefits they receive.
- With adequate sleep there will be less mental health problems.
- People will relax about their sleep instead of worrying unnecessarily when they occasionally don't sleep well.
- Organisations and employers will better understand how to get the most out of their workers, and how to keep them safe.
- Workplaces will become more cheerful and have less conflict.
- The practice of using uppers and downers, alcohol, drugs and stimulants to sleep better (or stay awake) will be reduced when people understand how to manage their own sleep patterns.

- More attention will be paid to shift workers and their mental and physical health and alertness during critical functions and dangerous situations.
- Savings will be made because the population will become healthier and take responsibility for their health earlier.
- The government will cut billions of dollars from PBS and MBS subsidies, insurance fees, Medicare claims and litigation.
- There will be less people addicted to sleeping and mental health medications.
- Personnel in our police, emergency services and difficult careers will learn how to manage their pressure situations better, and will ask for help earlier because of the known benefits of early intervention and action.
- Australia becomes a smarter, more productive, cooperative and happier country.
- The cost of sleep education could be minimised using state of the art technologies.

Proposal

I would like to contribute to sleep policy and education in Australia.
The problems are large and systemic.

Lives are being lost every single day,
Health problems are going undiagnosed every single day,
Work productivity and brain function are compromised every single day,
Health care costs are escalating every single day, and
Relationships are being strained every single day.

I have many practical, cost-effective strategies for how this could be done, working within existing structures.
Can I collaborate with you to solve this most important problem?
Can we discuss the possibilities?

The problems outlined in this book are so widespread and entrenched it's laughable!

I'm interested in making a documentary to reach a wider audience. And preferably a funny one. Because it really is a joke.

Contact me if you want to play.

Here's the information, mostly put together in 2015, presented in a different way.

Refer to Chapter 19, The Seventh Dwarf for the characters.

How Government, Medical Policy and Laws are Keeping Us Sleepy, Grumpy and Dopey

Fatigue and sleeping problems are an increasingly important mental and physical health issue. They are costing Australia billions of dollars each year by reducing our work and sporting performance, causing road and work accidents, and compromising family and work relationships. Left ignored, they accelerate health issues such as obesity, heart disease, substance abuse, immune suppression and even cancer. And lack of sleep causes and/or exacerbates all mental health issues.

Outmoded and inappropriate government, laws, organisations and medical professionals have now *institutionalised the problem.*

Many current policies actively discourage wellbeing. Appropriate policies are simply being ignored.

It has become a human rights issue.

POLICY is a major part of the problem.

Specifically, the problems include, but are not limited to:

- the gross (and subsidized) overmedication of insomnia and mental health patients by medical practitioners and psychiatrists;
- increased suicides, homicides, akathisia, addictions, unemployment and permanent health issues caused by wrongly prescribed pharmaceuticals;
- the degradation of food quality and deceptive food labelling laws;

- the limited definition of fatigue in the workplace which alienates sleep deprivation discussions, and does not recognise inappropriate medication use;
- the decades-long lag between scientific and neuroscientific research and policy;
- governments' preference to fund drugs and medical interventions after-the-fact rather than allocate budgets to preventative health initiatives;
- inappropriate sleep education at schools, tertiary institutions and in the community;
- increasing pressure on school students during their sensitive final years that has a disturbingly high correlation to psychological problems then and soon after;
- the growing ignorance of common sense approaches to mental and physical health - like exercise, good nutrition, adequate sleep, weight loss, mental discipline and personal responsibility;
- the barrage of pharmaceutical and medical advertising directly to consumers in the Australian media, with no evidence-based review of the information prior to approval;
- an increasing number of distressing news stories that are followed by community announcements that encourage people to contact mental health bodies that have misleading information on their websites. This occurs during prime time television and during 'the news'; and
- the community's addiction to *quick and easy solutions* which in many cases translates into popping a pill: which often becomes the *long and protracted non-solution* and worsening of the condition.

Why is Sleep so Important?

Thankfully neuroscience has proven what many suspected for decades - that improved sleep quality directly improves the brain's executive functions – enhancing memory integration, problem solving and planning ability, focus and attention span, task switching, decision making ability, elevated mood, clearer thinking and spontaneity, and reduces errors and accidents. For sports people this includes integrating and memorizing complicated play sequences, improved motor skills, faster reaction times and quicker recovery.

Health problems associated with lack of sleep include attitude and mood disorders, anxiety, stress, depression, mental health problems, obesity, diabetes, cancer, elevated blood pressure, drug and alcohol addictions (including sleeping tablets and antidepressants), shortened life span, motor vehicle and other accidents, exhausted adrenals, inflammation, stunted growth, sexual dysfunction, relationship problems, learning difficulties, compromised immune function, increased chance of heart disease, misdiagnoses of ADHD - even reduced grey matter in the brain – yes, literally!

Energy Drinks, Highly Caffeinated Drinks and other Stimulants

The marketing of energy drinks is highly contentious throughout the world, with documented evidence suggesting they are both inappropriate and even dangerous.

Certainly these stimulants compromise a good night's sleep.

A number of bodies regulate energy drinks. Therapeutic goods are regulated by the Therapeutic Goods Administration (TGA) where some of these drinks have been registered. Dietary supplements are regulated under New Zealand law, and because of FSANZ Australia does not have sovereignty over how drinks are governed in Australia.

Similar problems exist in the USA, where "energy drinks" are not regulated by the FDA.

The number of emergency department (ED) visits in the US involving energy drinks doubled from 10,068 visits in 2007 to 20,783 visits in 2011.[1] As reported by the FDA and the *Medical Journal of Australia*, problems associated with energy drinks include heart palpitations, pancreatitis, life threatening acute myocardial infarction, intracardiac thrombus, chest pain, dizziness, increased blood pressure, anxiety, convulsion[2,3] and sudden cardiac deaths[4].

- **Energy Drinks should be deregistered**. The TGA should not allow certain drinks to be registered as energy drinks, thereby avoiding regulations set up for food standards. E.g. Highly caffeinated energy drinks marketing mainly to adolescents and young adults. Why have the problems recognised by the TGA in its product register and the problems documented in other countries (such as the US) not been addressed after problems were discussed as early as 2009.[5]

- **Food Standards of Australia and New Zealand (FSANZ) should be disbanded.** We should have sovereignty over our own food standards. Some adverse foods and drinks are entering Australia simply because they are allowed in New Zealand. If this system doesn't work, then we need to change it.
- A special enquiry should be established to fully investigate the documented and suspected adverse health effects of energy drinks and other beverages.
- That enquiry should include how, given the existence of numerous food monitoring bodies (or because of that), we still have major problems with our food quality, labelling, advertising etc.

Food Labelling Laws

- **The 5% Loophole.** There should not be a ruling that the contents of a food do not have to be labelled if the content ingredient constitutes less than 5% of the quantity of that item. E.g. 282 calcium propionate is contained in breads and very adversely affects some people's sleep patterns. Please note "intolerance" *is not* "allergy".
- **Natural Glutamates to be labelled correctly.** People intolerant to glutamates have no way of knowing they are eating them from food labels. And there are a number of ways to add glutamates to food which look innocuous e.g. hydrolysed wheat (gluten free).
- **"All natural", "natural", "pure", "original", "fresh", "wholesome", "goodness", and "preservative free" labels to be stopped** because there are inadequate legal definitions, and are therefore deceptive. These words mean nothing and can include sleep depriving substances including salicylates, amines, glutamates etc. This is relevant for all people who suffer these food intolerances.
- **Flavourings – regarded as trade secrets - don't have to be revealed/ labelled.** We need to know what we are eating. At the very least, there should be a special label for undisclosed ingredients.

Recently in Australia we have had major focus on the county of origin of food and the percentage of that food that is processed in Australia. Having been a farmer for years I agree with this initiative, which has taken decades to establish.

But, even though I care about the origin of my food, and Australian industry – I care more about whether a food item or ingredient is *injurious to my health*.

NSW Food Authority

The fate of Minister Ian Macdonald is dubious as I write this in May 2017, and so has the lack of action on his promise to investigate taking energy drinks off the shelf around September 2009[6].

Why has apparently no action been taken on highly caffeinated energy drinks since his undertaking reported in the Sydney Morning Herald in 2009?

Food Complaints

There is no national complaint facility where consumers can complain about labelling laws, food quality standards, manufacturer's compliance etc.

If the system is so complicated that government bodies themselves are found negligent in exercising their duties, how can members of the public deal with a complaint about a food health issue?

Important complaints of national interest apparently have to be dealt with at local council level or through a very limited system set up by NSW Food Authority or NSW Health Service (for example). And to expect the average person to make an official complaint to FSANZ is unworkable.

If you want to make a food complaint in NSW, here is a link to investigate, but the authority would be limited. https://nswfoodauthority. transactcentral.com/contactcentre/landing.htm?formCode=Complaint

Cosmetics and Beauty Products Regulators

Cosmetic companies can put almost anything into their products even though the ingredients are ingested into the body or inhaled. And they do – including known carcinogens. The industry is largely unregulated.

There are toxic and unhealthy substances in cosmetics, body products, hairsprays, sunscreens etc. Compulsory labelling should show all their contents. Toxic contents prevent people from sleeping properly, are associated with cancer, and other health problems.[7] E.g. inhaled salicylates from hairsprays. Salicylates are associated with difficulty getting to sleep and night terrors in children[8].

Benzodiazepines/Sleeping Pills

Please refer to chapter 9, which shows all reference sources for statements made in this appendix.

Benzodiazepines are known to be addictive, have many adverse side effects including bizarre and dangerous behaviours (including sleep driving), memory loss, and are not suitable for long term use.

One sleeping pill was the most complained about medication to the *Australian Medicines Event Line* run by the National Prescribing Service and Brisbane's Mater Hospital between September 2007 and February 2009. Of 1669 calls, 196 (or 12%) related to just one sleeping pill.

The National Prescribing Service (NPS) states on its website that "Sleeping tablets usually make sleep problems worse, not better, in the long term."

The TGA and NPS both have issues with sleeping pills.

However, sleeping pills are prescribed in 95.2 percent of cases by doctors when patients present with sleeping problems!

In Australia, over seven million prescriptions, both Pharmaceutical Benefits Schedule (PBS) and private prescriptions, for both short and long-acting benzodiazepines are written annually.[9]

Their use continues to be subsidized by the PBS.

The TGA recently wanted to move all benzodiazepines from schedule 4 to schedule 8. After a number of submissions to the contrary from the industry (including the Australian Medical Association[10] and Royal Australian College of Physicians) only one benzodiazepine, Alprazolam, was moved to schedule 8.

The three main policy questions to be fully investigated are:

1. Why weren't all benzodiazepines moved from Schedule 4 to Schedule 8 as recently suggested by the TGA? Why did the "administration costs and challenges" put forward by the AMA and RACP cause the TGA to back down on the rescheduling?
2. What are the powers of the TGA so that it could not act in this case?
3. Why are sleeping pills prescribed in 95.2 percent of cases?
4. Why does the PBS still subsidise sleeping pills, and how much is it costing Australians every year?

Summary

The cost of the present system of prescribing sleeping pills to the Australian community, knowing that this is not the solution, includes: the PBS subsidy of the medications, the ineffectual doctor's appointments and wasted time taken to get to these appointments, the addiction issues, the side effects of the medications, the negative coping strategies of drugs and alcohol, the continuance of undetected mental and physical health issues, suicide, etc.

For more information on benzodiazepines visit the work of Professor Heather Ashton, www.benzo.org.uk, and http://www.benzo.org.uk/profash.htm, and chapter 9.

Antidepressants/SSRIs

Please refer to Chapter 10 for information about Antidepressants/SSRIs.

To get up to date on antidepressants over the last couple of years I recommend you follow the following leads and links:

- Dolin vs. GSK. In April 2017 GSK was successfully sued by Dolin after the suicide death of her husband Stewart Dolin.[11] https://www.baumhedlundlaw.com/prescription-drugs/paxil-injuries/gsk-paxil-trial-transcripts/
- Professor Peter Gøtzsche's YouTube presentation *Mental Health, Overprescribed and Overmedicated*.[12]

- Joanna Le Noury et al. *Restoring Study 329: efficacy and harms of paroxetine and imipramine in treatment of major depression in adolescence.*[13]
- A notable and award winning study on psychiatric drugs and mental illness by Robert Whitaker and published in his book *Anatomy of an Epidemic: Magic Bullets, Psychiatric Drugs, and the Astonishing Rise of Mental Illness in America.* This book is still the most definitive book I can find outlining the long term effects of mental health drugs, and the inadequacies of our mental health support services. Published in 2010, it traces problems back to the 1950s!

These 4 studies cover a fair bit of territory. If you do nothing else, I'd review them.

The Definition of "Fatigue"

"Fatigue" is not all about work health and safety (WHS).

It just appears that WHS is attempting to hijack the word and bend its meaning to affect legal liability and financial exposure.

"Fatigue" has also been redefined in relation to car accidents and deaths.

In the transport industry road fatigue and fatigue deaths have different rules again. E.g. In some cases (or states) a road accident is not called fatigue-related unless it is a single vehicle accident, sometimes a fatigue death is limited by how many kilometres the accident happened from a post office. Sometimes it is not called fatigue if the driver is killed! And it's not counted as fatigue if an accident happens at 10 a.m.[14]

It's the *definition of fatigue* that varies between states that makes the figures vary significantly – e.g. from 5 percent to 30 percent for fatigue related accidents.

In my research I have not found a definition of fatigue that would indicate that a worker could EVER arrive at work at 9 o'clock on Monday morning, actually fatigued.

And who doesn't know, just someone (maybe once), who partied hard on a weekend, dropped a recreational drug, had very little sleep, got lucky, and came to work Monday morning "wasted"?

But not *fatigued*, of course.

Fatigue Management Registered Training Organisations (Fatigue RTOs)

When contacting Fatigue RTOs in Australia I often get asked "What has sleep got to do with fatigue?"

You probably don't believe me. I thought they were joking.

I've spoken to human resource professionals who either think that way, or are amazed at how common the question is within the industry.

This disconnect has very serious, even fatal ramifications.

Safe Work Australia

In my review and submission to the Safe Work Australia *Preventing and Managing Fatigue in the Workplace Draft Code of Practice* I found similar problems with the definition of fatigue.

The draft code of practice was very inadequate, and has improved after the review process.

Shift Workers

Not enough attention is being paid to the adverse affects of shift work, which is very prevalent in Government e.g. intern doctors in hospitals, other hospital staff (nurses, night surgery staff, security, etc), ambulance drivers and officers, police, fire brigade officers, etc.

Readiband, one of the latest technologies used by the US military, shows that people who work on the midnight till 9 am shift are working for 71 percent of the time with a performance level equivalent (or worse) than if they were legally drunk (0.05 percent alcohol level).[15]

Long term shift work can seriously affect the circadian rhythm, melatonin production and mental and physical health. The Danish government paid compensation to nurses and flight attendants in 2009 as a result of the adverse affects linked to breast cancer.[16]

Australia denies a proven connection between long term shift work and some sorts of cancers (e.g. breast cancer). Australian governments continue to allow long-term shift work, in spite of the Danish case.

My personal concern is that most of these environments are high stress, which adds to the problems. See the following discussion on high stress jobs.

There has been work done on genetic predispositions to shiftwork health issues, but it's early days.

Summary: The rulings on fatigue are not harsh enough for night time workers and shift workers – especially in stressed environments and in long term employment situations.

High Stress Jobs

A study of police officers in the US and Canada showed that generally they have twice as many sleep disorders as the normal population.[17]

I'm guessing that stress, trauma, anxiety, and shock are all factors.

Apart from the military, I'm expecting that other high stress jobs such as emergency medical operators, first responders, ambulance drivers, SES personnel etc would fall into this high-sleep-disordered group.

These issues are not being properly reflected in work and other policies around these types of personnel – in and outside work hours.

The Great Divide Between Alopathic and Natural Health Models

In spite of the evidence supporting both allopathic and natural health models the movement towards integrating the two is moving at a glacial pace, if at all.

This is not the forum to go into drug patenting laws and the reasons why so few clinical trials are conducted to prove the efficacy of certain natural health remedies. But these issues are severely impairing health outcomes.

We appear to be moving away from common sense, and moving towards the population wanting a "quick fix". That often results in them "popping a pill" – whether that is good for their health or not.

And with very little regard to drug side effects and drug combinations.

Schools and Students

- School curriculums should improve their sleep education – particularly in years 9-12 when lack of sleep coupled with exam stress is causing and exaggerating psychological and physical problems (e.g. anxiety, substance abuse, weight problems, inappropriate eating, the use of caffeinated drinks, etc).
- The George Institute for global health studied 20,000 17-24 year olds and found those sleeping fewer than five hours a night are three times more likely to become mentally ill than those sleeping for eight or nine hours.[18]
- The common "delayed sleep phase" that teenagers experience (where they can even be producing melatonin mid morning the next day) explains why they appear so listless and unmotivated. It's a bit like sleep walking, as they are not totally awake. Is it surprising that 'energy drink' companies are having a lot of success marketing to this age group?
- School students and tertiary students are not adequately trained on how to sleep, food labelling and additives, sleep nutrition, exercise for sleep and how to use sleep technologies for memory enhancement, brain skills, cognitive improvement and better motor skills.
- An overhaul of the curriculum needs to occur to train children on how to sleep and the importance of sleep, its inverse relationship to obesity and poor school grades etc. Who establishes the curriculum is a big question, as many so-called-experts appear to be clueless.

- This review should include student culture, school canteen food, nutrition and its affect on weight, health, sleep, attitude, results and sporting success. The present system is clearly not working as Australia is now the most obese country in the world. Jamie Oliver's work to educate children on nutrition is excellent, but there needs to be an accelerated effort, which includes education through the media and media law changes.

- Another strategy that some students use is Ritalin – most common among law and medical students – which doesn't auger well for future prescribing habits.[19]

Advertising Drugs in The Media

One study found that while 33 percent of prescription and non-prescription drug advertisements were objectively true, 57 percent were potentially misleading and 10% were false.[20]

A 2007 study published in the Annals of Family Medicine "found that no drug advertisements touted lifestyle changes as part of therapy, but 95 percent of the ads studied used emotional appeals" – which of course, is the way to sell.[21]

All drugs have side effects, which are rarely mentioned.

Interestingly the US federal law does not even ban drug ads that have serious risks:

"Federal law does not bar drug companies from advertising any kind of prescription drugs, even ones that can cause severe injury, addiction, or withdrawal effects. However, companies cannot use reminder ads for drugs with certain serious risks (drugs with "boxed warnings")."[22]

The truthfulness of claims of over the counter medications appears to be worse.

It should be illegal to advertise drugs directly to the patient, including sponsorship of major sporting events and the like.

All counselling sites mentioned at the end of disturbing media stories should be thoroughly reviewed and vetted for up to date evidence-based information, as this is not happening.

Mental health websites should show clearly every donation that is being made to them from all sources, using strict and transparent criteria.

Some information contained on these websites is misleading and incorrect, some information could be fatal.

Listed Companies and Organisations

- Have very few policies related to peak performance, health, sleep and nutrition, often with canteens selling junk foods and sleep-inhibiting foods.
- Have policies which are commonly 4 decades out of date with the latest peak performance, health and neuroscience research.
- Commonly do not understand the connection between sleep and fatigue.
- By excluding sleep discussions in their WHS and fatigue policies means they are allowing behaviours and procedures to continue which international experts believe to be culpable. E.g. No worker should catch a red-eye flight and then drive a car. Ever.
- Are overlooking negative coping mechanisms used by employees to deal with stress, anxiety, night-time shifts and lack of sleep. E.g. the use of stimulants (caffeinated drugs, cocaine etc), alcohol, prescription and non-prescription medications, etc.
- In some high status, highly paid jobs they are happy to burn out employees by having them work late nights for a number of "profitable years".
- Are exposed because of their antiquated policies.

Pharmaceutical Companies

- Their reputation as a group is increasingly being eroded due to known conflicts of interests, proven off-label marketing, undeclared payments for expert medical endorsements, various "incentives" to medical professionals, government lobbying, questionable PBS subsidies, the registration of medications that have later been withdrawn, the downplaying of side effects, lack of long term studies, information suppression, etc.
- The backlash that is happening may or may not be in the best interest of the patient. Certainly in some cases the patient does not know who to believe.
- Unfortunately because the lack of trust is so large and the systems so entrenched there may not be a solution.

- It is much more informed and realistic for the general public to assume profit is the major goal of all listed medical companies.

Medical Professionals

- In cases of insomnia doctors are prescribing in 95.2 percent of the cases against the recommendations of the National Prescribing Service (NPS) and best practice. In the case of insomnia problems – there is always an underlying problem that shows up as the *symptom* of insomnia. "Insomnia" is never the problem. It is the medical practitioners' responsibility to attempt to isolate the underlying problem, not to prescribe. Taking medications can mask the symptom, which is not helpful, and can be harmful.
- Supply sleeping medications and antidepressants/SSRIs long term. This means they are supplying to addicts and facilitating the misuse of medications.
- Some medical practices are part of ASX listed companies (e.g. Sonic Health Care & Primary Health Care).

  Questions have been raised if this puts pressure on the medical professionals to see a certain number of patients each day; limiting appointment durations and sometimes the level of care, or pressure to refer to extra services (e.g. aligned imaging services, etc).

  In 2015 the federal government was investigating one case where bonuses were allegedly being offered to doctors to see extra patients and overservice – putting profits before patients.[23]

  When some medical practices joined listed health companies the doctors bought, or received shares in those listed companies, which have not always had increasing stock values. In some cases this has resulted in financial pressure to the doctors involved.
- Doctors can receive their professional development training points by attending training from drug companies. That may or may not be in the best interest of the patients, and certainly can present a conflict of interest. E.g. exercise, nutrition and other alternatives may not be thoroughly explained as possible

solutions when a drug company derives profits from the sale of their own drugs.

- Have a difficult time keeping up with all the drug information, and rely on information supplied by the drug companies, their marketing, clinical trials etc. This has resulted in off label prescribing in some cases – knowingly or unknowingly.

- Are increasingly moving away from common sense approaches and preventative health, with alarmingly few medical practices adequately training their patients on nutrition, exercise, sleep and mental health disciplines.

- Although integrative/nutritional/dietary/natural/organic strategies are proven to be beneficial to health outcomes (and are often supported by peer-reviewed scientific research), they are only given 'lip service' in most cases, sometimes even derision.

- The prescribing of antidepressants/SSRIs continues, in spite of the significant evidence against them.

- Medical professionals do not independently self regulate their profession to ensure that only evidence-based practice is performed. If they do, it is clearly failing, as 95 percent of listed MBS items are not evidence based, and there has been no adequate study of the PBS.

- Clinical governance is failing… *Has failed.*

It's no wonder many people "Doctor Google".

Why wouldn't we?

Well now we know to doctor "*Cochrane Library*" to get the really juicy stuff.

The Commercialisation of "Best Practice"

After considering the facts, it is disturbing to see the increasing trend towards commercialising the information that is taught in universities and schools – whether it is through scholarships, sponsorships, promotions, gifts, grants and research material.

Knowing that some doctors and professors are on corporate payrolls (directly and/or indirectly), and that agreeing with the opinion of your lecturers is often part of getting good academic results, the trends are questionable.

While corporate involvement can be both positive and negative, who is to know one way or the other?

Who decides what is best for the student and the future of citizens' health?

Any Hope for the Sleepy, Grumpy and Dopey?
Australians

- Are grossly under-informed. It's complicated even for the knowledgeable to get to the bottom of why we find it hard to sleep, and why we have mental health challenges from time to time;
- Typically limit thoughts of "sleep issues" to sleep apnea, snoring and pills, because that is where the marketing and profits are focused;
- Have very little hope of a solution. When they finally visit their general practitioner for a solution they are prescribed in 95.2 percent of the cases, which masks the underlying problems;
- Do not address sleeping problems until a subsequent, sleep-related problem arises. Such problems include: obesity, diabetes, anxiety or depression, stress, elevated blood pressure, heart conditions, impaired immune function, cognitive impairment, Alzheimer's, etc
- Do not connect their sleeping problems to poor diet, lack of exercise, being overweight or an unresolved emotional issue (to name a few);
- Think antidepressants/SSRIs and sleeping pills work;
- Believe what their doctors tell them – even when it is wrong;
- Do not respect sleeping problems as the powerful early warning symptoms they are. This is where preventative health should start!
- Buy foods for themselves and their children that are causing harm – knowingly or unknowingly;
- Find it very difficult to lobby for change; and/or
- Take no political action and put no pressure to bring about change.

The Cost of Fatigue and Lack of Sleep

There have been a lot of reports quantifying the cost of lack of sleep and fatigue, none of them are conclusive, so I've compiled a list to give more details on the extent of the costs.

Fatigue and sleeping problems are costing Australia tens of billions of dollars each year in:

- Health costs; doctors visits, scripts, apnea masks, sleep clinic costs, snoring options, dental visits and fees, over the counter medicines, general research;
- road accidents; deaths, injury, funeral expenses, insurance costs of vehicle smashes, counsellors, medical services, ambulance services, road signage, tow trucks, vehicle repairs, other smashed property, paperwork time, Medicare rebate;
- work accidents and errors; medical fees, insurance costs, paperwork, management time, fixing errors, unfixable errors (e.g. trading losses on markets), administration;
- ineffectual PBS drug subsidies; the cost of PBS subsidies of part of the 7 million sleeping pills prescribed each year; and 35 million psycho scripts, paperwork involved in the PBS administration;
- mental health issues (recognised and overlooked) including anxiety, depression and suicide; abuse; medical/doctors fees, Medicare rebate on doctors visits, counsellors fees, administration, travelling time, family trauma and stress, generational cycles of family issues, mental health support hotlines, services and foundations;
- absenteeism and presenteeism; days off work 'coping' from the night before, the use of stimulants at work to stay focused (cigarette breaks, sugar and junk food breaks, coffee breaks), lost performance at work, falling asleep at work, impaired work performance, late to work, at work but can't concentrate, gone to work with the hangover effects of their sleeping pills, effected by alcohol or drugs;
- health insurance costs – both Medicare and private health insurance - medical visits, accident visits, counselling
- wasted medical appointments; time taken off work to go to the doctor, time filling scripts, cost of scripts, no resolution of the underlying problem causing insomnia, stress and anxiety;

- drug and alcohol abuse; to combat emotional problems, to get to sleep, to stay awake: drugs, alcohol, use of caffeine and energy drinks, use of caffeine tablets, cocaine to keep awake, other recreational drugs because of mental health problems;
- other negative coping strategies – other stimulants include cigarettes, junk food (obesity), high fat and sugary snacks, salty foods, energy drinks, anger and emotional release;
- addictions and rehabilitation; sleeping pills and antidepressants, sometimes followed with psychological disorder medications, rehab clinics, family emotional issues, sometimes trauma, counselling;
- death, suicide, self harm, suicide attempts;
- broken relationships; "grumpy and tired" leads to more stress, divorce, legal fees, property settlements, vicious cycle of unhappy children, domestic and other violence, business breakups, less joy and fun, less caring and support, loss of friends, social isolation;
- health problems caused by some degree of fatigue and lack of sleep – the cost of obesity, reduced immune function, elevated blood pressure, heart disease, cancer, reduced brain function, possible link to Alzheimer's disease;
- side effects of medications – mental and physical, short term and permanent;
- sporting underachievement – the cost of not winning, slower recovery times, slower reaction times, depleted memory, reduced executive function of the brain, etc
- the dumbing down of the national – the organ most effected by lack of sleep is the brain, specifically the executive functions including memory, task switching, sorting out what is important, strategising, decision making ability, emotional intelligence, less improvisation, less creative solutions, less inventions, bad management decisions, grumpy bosses etc.

Far Too Hard to Complain or Change?

To raise a query or make a complaint is fraught with challenges.

There are too many health and medical authorities and bodies.

There is no federal ombudsman for health.

For example: the following is a link to a code of conduct complaints index of sorts. Where on the following page of the Medical board of Australia can you complain about approved courses, medical practitioners, etc?

http://medicinesaustralia.com.au/code-of-conduct/lodging-responding-to-a-code-of-conduct-complaint/

Let me guess: very few complaints are ever being made?

And should policy making be complaints-driven?

I used to be a proud Australian because we would call out bullshit. What happened to our clear and bright spirit?

Waking Up to the Latest Trends and Technologies

Most organisations in Australia refuse to recognise the value of napping/meditation/mindfulness meditation as a means to improve physical and mental performance and/or to catch up on missed sleep.

Research has shown for over 4 decades that these activities are scientifically supported – yet many regard the idea as 'falling asleep on the job' or similar.

Leading companies that support napping and meditation include Google, siyli.org, BUPA, Virgin Active Health Clubs, Cisco, P&G, BMA, iSelect Insurance, Yarde Metals, The New York Times, the Huffington Post, NASA, KPMG, Nike and Deloite. The napping trend is most entrenched in Silicon Valley according to Dr Sarah Mednick of *Take a Nap! Change Your Life*.

The world's leading governments and cities that support napping include Danish hospitals, transportation departments and oil industries, all citizens in the town of Hillerod (north of Copenhagen), and Vechta, Germany.

APPENDIX 4. EXECUTIVE FUNCTION REPORT

Here is my *Executive Function Report* for organisations who are interested in improving their bottom line with low cost productivity-enhancing innovations.

This report was compiled some years ago, before I researched the huge impact of mental health problems and the inadequate treatment of mental health problems, so it's limited to sleep issues. Now that you have read the book, you'll be able to add many more pieces to this puzzle.

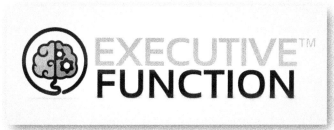

No single organ is affected by lack of sleep more than the brain. The areas affected are those associated with executive function.

Executive Function includes the cognitive processes of working memory, planning, the ability to focus, attention span, response initiation, problem solving, verbal reasoning, strategic thinking, mental flexibility, task switching, inhibitory control, and executive skills.

How Fatigue Affects Profitability

Fatigue and the related issues of anxiety, depression, stress, absenteeism and presenteeism, errors, uncontrolled emotions, productivity losses, accidents, litigation, medication use and substance abuse cost large companies millions of dollars every year.

- Around 1 in 3 workers have taken a sick day to catch up on sleep, about 43% have arrived late to work because of sleeping in or catching up on sleep, 19% admit to having fallen asleep in a meeting.
- 12 percent were late to work in the past month because of sleepiness.

- Fatigued workers' cost of loss of work performance is equivalent to 7.8 days/year or $2,280 per person.
- Fatigue and depression are linked. On average each employee with depression symptoms will cost their employer $9,665 per year.
- Staff are more likely to take a sick day if they have a sleep disorder 26.0% vs. 20.9%.
- A fatigued individual increases accident risk by up to 65 percent.
- Individuals that sleep less than 6 hours are eleven times more likely to make work related errors than those that get 8 hours sleep. Those that get less than 5 hours sleep have an impaired performance comparable to those who are legally drunk.
- Some sleeping pills have a half life of 20 hours. This means that for the full next day at work that person experiences 'hangover sedation', with 50-100% of the active components of those pills still affecting and sedating them.
- Shift workers, at-risk industries (such as the police, emergency workers, transport industry workers, etc) and sleep apnea sufferers show far worse patterns in all areas (including 19% of shift workers saying they have injured themselves or had an accident on the job in the past year).
- Fatigued workers are more willing to make hazardous and risky decisions.
- Rio Tinto used the findings of a fatigue study to implement new guidelines that no worker should operate equipment after being awake for 14 hours. Apparently the change has eliminated all fatigue related accidents, without reducing productivity.
- 1 in 5 motor vehicle accidents is fatigue related.
- A study performed using Readiband in one control centre of Queensland Rail increased employee sleep by an hour which translated to a 39 percent reduction in fatigue risk.
- Negative coping strategies for fatigue include overeating, junk foods, 'high octane' drinks, caffeine, alcohol, cocaine, sleeping pills, uppers, marijuana and losing one's temper.
- The 2003 US National Highway Traffic Safety Administration (NHTSA) shows the average motor vehicle crash costs the employer

$ 16,500. When a worker has on-the-job crash that results in an injury, the cost to their employer is $ 74,000, and can exceed $ 500,000 when a fatality is involved. Off-the-job crashes are costly to employers as well.

The Number of Your Staff Members Who are Fatigued is Significant

Dr Charles Czeisler of Harvard Medical School says 70 percent of people say they frequently don't get enough sleep, with 30 percent saying they don't get enough sleep every single night.

The American National Sleep Foundation 2008 survey found 65% of Americans experienced sleep problems, with 40% of respondents impatient with others at work, 27% finding it hard to concentrate, 20% admitting to having lower productivity than they expected and 29% having fallen asleep during work because of sleepiness or a sleep problem.

Three-quarters of respondents to a 2009 Career One survey said work stresses were keeping them awake.

The Most At-Risk Organisations

- Where staff are travelling overseas through time zones, catching red-eye flights, with limited recovery periods while travelling.
- Where staff are driving motor vehicles while under the responsibility of the company.
- Organisations employing heavy machinery operators.
- Organisations employing shift workers (especially long-term shift-workers and difficult shifts such as midnight till early morning). Shift workers have more than twice the injury rates.
- Organisations in high risk industries – agriculture, hospitality, heavy machinery, mining, etc.
- Emergency and trauma situations such as the police, fire and rescue, first responders, defence force personnel, ambulance, hospitals etc.

Litigation

- The Danish government has commenced paying compensation to long-term shift workers for their increased occurrences of cancer.
- The technology is now available that proves, for example, that a midnight to 9 am shift for 5 consecutive days means staff members are working at a fatigue level equivalent to being legally intoxicated (.08%) for 71 per cent of the time.
- Depression was recognized as a disability under the Disability Discrimination Act 1992, and has definite connections to lack of sleep.
- How are you scheduling your staff? The number of hours spent at work affects how much sleep they get. A British survey found that people working 55 hours a week rather than 35-40 are twice as likely to sleep less than six hours, nearly four times as likely to have trouble going to sleep and twice as likely not to feel refreshed the next day.
- Some reports indicate that banning napping in the workplace might become a legal liability sometime in the future.

"Our High End Employees are Doing Fine."

If you're struggling with the effects of the sluggish economy on profits, incentives and the reduced equity value of bonus stock offers, then we're guessing you're looking for new and economical ways to motivate and inspire your top performers?

Sylvia Ann Hewlett, founding president of the New York based Center for Work-Life Policy and author of *Top Talent* has the following observations to make about the post-GFC work environment for high end and long-hour employees:

- A reduction in force (RIF) is not the solution to your problems. In fact, in the wake of a RIF between June 2008 and January 2009 14 percent of college graduates lost their jobs in the US – of those 32 percent were fired, but another 68 percent voluntarily left their jobs.

- The words used by Wall Street employees in the financial sector were "paralyzed" (74%), "demoralized" (73%) and "demotivated" (64%).
- The survivors of RIF are having a hard time focusing on work with nearly eight out of ten participants reporting extremely high levels of stress, more than twice the number than a year earlier, with symptoms ranging from ulcers and migraine headaches to a new dependence on sleep medication.

Like few other times in history, this is the opportunity to implement meaningful non-monetary rewards and inexpensive cultural changes to our workplaces.

Would Workers Welcome the Changes?

A 2010 survey reported 89% of Australian workers are keen to improve their daily routine to achieve a healthier and more balanced lifestyle. The most common area workers would like to do this was more exercise (81%), followed by a healthier diet (66%) and more sleep (60%).

Encouraging findings, given that more exercise and a healthier diet are key components of a better night's sleep.

This same Australian study highlighted that as many as 62 percent of workers believe a regular 20 minute lunch time nap would make them more motivated and productive in the workplace.

Three Solutions that Increase Productivity and Reduce Fatigue (With A Number of Other Proven Benefits):

1. EXERCISE
   - Improves performance through better time management and improved mental alertness.
   - Improves mood, with greater tolerance of others and themselves.
   - Reduces stress, anxiety and depression.
   - Helps people sleep better at night. Good sleep is a factor in reducing depression, anxiety, stress and keeping weight under control.

Depression is nearly twice as common among those with obesity compared to those who are not obese. The incidence of diabetes is five times higher in people who are obese.

2. NAPPING AT WORK OR DURING BREAKS

Napping is NOT "falling asleep at work", is NOT a siesta, and is NOT permission to goof off – it is a highly scientific, disciplined and timed process.

Napping can be customized by individuals for specific purposes. E.g. Depending on the person's circadian rhythm there are different times of the day to nap to integrate memory (if a staff member is reading complicated new material, or memorizing a presentation), problem solving, improving motor skills, refresh from a concentration slump, etc. Commonly requiring a few days practice before feeling the benefits, it can be accompanied by guided relaxation audios, quiet music or other customized tracks heard through a simple mp3 player. Any quiet room or area at work could double as a napping zone.

Here is the scientifically-based evidence supporting napping:

- With napping it is 38% less likely that sleepiness interfered with daytime activities.
- Napping reduces absenteeism and increases the length of night-time sleep.
- It elevates mood, improves alertness, accuracy, stamina, motor performance and memory.
- Increases employee retention, satisfaction, morale and productivity.
- Learning from a nap is equal to learning from a full night's sleep.
- Napping can be strategically designed to achieve targeted outcomes.
- The only way to reduce sleep debt is by sleeping. 4-6 minutes or more delivers results.
- Reyner and Home have conducted studies showing that a 15 minute nap was as effective as 150 mg of caffeine, and that combining a nap and caffeine was particularly effective for driver fatigue, for up to 2 hours.

- One N.A.S.A. study found an increase in their pilot's productivity up 34% from a 26 minute nap.
- 35 percent of Americans say their workplace permits napping during breaks at work, and 16 percent say their employer provides a place for them to nap. Organisations have encouraged napping since 1969 and now include Google, Cisco, P&G, BUPA, BMA, Virgin Active Health Clubs, iSelect Insurance, Yarde Metals, The New York Times, Huffington Post, NASA, Nike, and Deloitte.

3. EDUCATION

Evidence-based information from leading research will change the way your executives, managers and staff members think about sleep, mental health, fatigue and their performance at work.

From the underlying reasons for sleep disorders, sleep's connection to mental health, the 50 food additives and chemicals that affect sleep (even naturally occurring substances in fresh fruit), the value of exercise, the link to physical health problems, the limitations of medicating the problems, sleep hygiene, the sleep environment - to proven solutions.

The other areas of life that are improved with reduced fatigue through better sleep include: mental health, reduced risk of heart disease; lower blood pressure; elevated immune function; longer life; a reduced use of medication; lower use of inappropriate coping strategies (addictions etc); reduced risk of cancer; and better relationships.

The National Cost of Fatigue and Mental Health

The cost of mental illness in Australia was reported to be $ 207 billion in 2016. Refer chapter 11.

Disasters Where Fatigue was Cited as a Major Factor

Chernobyl, Exxon Valdez, Challenger space shuttle, Union Carbide disasters.

APPENDIX 5. THE POISONS SCHEDULE/STANDARD.

Scheduling is a national classification system that controls how medicines and chemicals are made available to the public. Medicines and chemicals are classified into Schedules according to the level of regulatory control over the availability of the medicine or chemical, required to protect public health and safety[1].

The schedules are published in the Standard for the Uniform Scheduling of Medicines and Poisons (SUSMP) and are given legal effect through state and territory legislation. The SUSMP is legally referred to as the Poisons Standard.

This appendix is included to support the discussions about rescheduling sleeping pills and antidepressants/SSRIs.

The Poisons Standard[2]

Schedule 1	Not currently in use
Schedule 2	Pharmacy Medicine
Schedule 3	Pharmacist Only Medicine
Schedule 4	Prescription Only Medicine OR Prescription Animal Remedy
Schedule 5	Caution
Schedule 6	Poison
Schedule 7	Dangerous Poison
Schedule 8	Controlled Drug
Schedule 9	Prohibited Substance
Schedule 10	Substances of such danger to health as to warrant prohibition of sale, supply and use.

APPENDIX 6. SLEEP DIAGNOSIS QUESTIONNAIRE.

Available through consultation with Elizabeth. If you would like to develop an app with me, please send your proposal.

Part One. The Lights are Out and No-One's Home.
Chapter 1. Introduction.

1. Purcell, Andrew. *Antidepressants: How Drugs Got into Australia's System.* Sydney Morning Herald, October 10, 2015. http://www.smh.com.au/national/advance-antidepressants-fair-how-drugs-got-into-australias-system-20151006-gk2jjh.html. Accessed May 8, 2017.

2. Australian Government, Department of Health. The Pharmaceutical Benefits Scheme. Expenditure and Prescriptions Report 2015-16, Table 12. ATC Level 2 Drug Groups Sorted by Highest Script Volume, 2015-16. Includes subsidized and under co-payment scripts. Section 85 only; incl. Drs Bag. *http://www.pbs.gov.au/statistics/expenditure-prescriptions/2015-2016/expenditure-prescriptions-report-2015-16.pdf* Accessed May 8, 2017.

   35 million psycho scripts consisting of 25,845,076 psychoanaleptics: antidepressants (SSRIs, SNRIs (serotonin-norepinephrine reuptake inhibitors), TCAs (tricyclics antidepressants), tetracyclic antidepressants (TeCAs), monoamine oxidase inhibitors (MAOIs), etc), psychostimulants, nootropics, anti-dimentia drugs and combinations with psycholeptics. And 9,668,064 psycholeptics (antipsychotics, anxiolytics, hypnotics and sedatives)

3. Charles, J., Harrison, C., Britt, H., et al. *Bettering the Evaluation and Care of Health* (BEACH). April 2006 – March 2008. Australian GP Statistics and Classification Centre, the University of Sydney. The most commonly prescribed sleeping tablet in Australia, Temazepam (at 1.7 million prescriptions in 2011) has a half life of 8 - 20 hours.

4. Britt, H., Miller, C., Henderson, J., Bayram, C., et al. *General Practice Activity in Australia, BEACH Bettering the Evaluation and Care of Health 2013-14.* Family Medicine Research Centre, Sydney University. General Practice Series No. 36. https://ses.library.usyd.edu.au/bitstream/2123/11882/4/9781743324226_ONLINE.pdf Accessed April 19, 2017.

5. Swan, Dr N and Balendra, Jaya. *Wasted*. Four Corners. September 28, 2015. Presented by Dr Norman Swan. http://www.abc.net. au/4corners/stories/2015/09/28/4318883.htm. Accessed January 14, 2016. Full transcript available on the website.

6. The Australian Government. Pharmaceutical Benefits Scheme (PBS) Information Management Section, Pharmaceutical Policy Branch. *Expenditure and Prescriptions 12 Months to 30 June 2016*. Summary of Pharmaceutical Benefits Scheme 2015-2016 Total Pharmaceutical Benefits Scheme (PBS) government expenditure (both Section 85 and Section 100) on an accrual accounting basis for the 2015-2016 financial year was $10,838.0 million, compared with $9,072.1 million for the previous year. This is an increase of 19.5% in one year. https:// www.pbs.gov.au/statistics/expenditure-prescriptions/2015-2016/ expenditure-prescriptions-report-2015-16.pdf Accessed April 19, 2017.

7. Australian Government, Department of Employment, *Health Care and Social Assistance*. 1,523,000 employed at November 2015, projected to increase by 16.4 percent over the next 5 years. https://australianjobs. employment.gov.au/jobs-industry/health-care-and-social-assistance Accessed May 8, 2017.

8. Antidepressant Medication. Page 1 of 4. Beyond Blue downloadable factsheet. BL /0125 12/16 http://resources.beyondblue.org.au/prism/ file?token=BL/0125 Accessed May 8, 2017.

9. Raymond, Nate and Grzincic, Barbara. *GSK Must Pay $ 3 Million in Generic Paxil Suicide Lawsuit: US Jury*. Reuters Business News, April 20, 2017. http://www.reuters.com/article/us-gsk-lawsuit-idUSKBN17M2SH Accessed May 8, 2017.

10. Sterling, Greg. *Google Introduces Rich Medical Content Into Knowledge Graph. Users will soon see deeper health information for more than 400 conditions*. Search Engine Land blog. February 10, 2015. http://

searchengineland.com/google-introduces-rich-medical-content-knowledge-graph-214559 Accessed May 10, 2017.

11. Swan, Dr N and Balendra, Jaya. *Wasted*. Four Corners. September 28, 2015. Presented by Dr Norman Swan. http://www.abc.net.au/4corners/stories/2015/09/28/4318883.htm. Accessed January 14, 2016. Full transcript available on the website.

Chapter 2. History of a Problem.

1. Whitaker, Robert. *Anatomy of an Epidemic. Magic Bullets, Psychiatric Drugs, and the Astonishing Rise of Mental Illness in America.* Broadway Paperbacks, Random House, New York. 2010. Page 52.

2. Ibid, page 53.

3. Op. Cit.

4. Fintel, B., Samaras, AT., Carias, E., *The Thalidomide Tragedy, Lessons for Drug Safety and Regulation.* July 28, 2009. https://helix.northwestern.edu/article/thalidomide-tragedy-lessons-drug-safety-and-regulation Accessed November 28, 2016.

5. Wikipedia. *Thalidomide.* https://en.wikipedia.org/wiki/Thalidomide Accessed November 28, 2016.

6. Healy, David. *Austistic Spectrum Disorder and SSRIs.* http://rxisk.org/autistic-spectrum-disorder-and-ssris/ Accessed October 31, 2016

Chapter 3. Keeping us in the Dark with "Evidence Based Medicine".

1. Healy, David. *Pharmageddon is the Story of a Tragedy.* Changing Habits website. November 14, 2012. https://changinghabits.com.au/pharmageddon-is-the-story-of-a-tragedy-by-dr-david-healy/Accessed December 1, 2016.

2. Healy, David. David Healy Lecture, *Alcohol.* December 4, 2012. https://vimeo.com/59145379 Accessed November 28, 2016.

3. Healy, David. *Pharmageddon is the Story of a Tragedy.* Changing Habits website. November 14, 2012. https://changinghabits.com.au/pharmageddon-is-the-story-of-a-tragedy-by-dr-david-healy/Accessed December 1, 2016.

4. Ibid.

5. Gøtzsche, Peter, C. *Mental Health, Overdiagnosed and Overmedicated.* Australian tour 2014. Youtube video. https://youtu.be/ZMhsPnoIdy4. Minute 7.29. Accessed September 5, 2016.

6. Moynihan, R., Cassels, A., *Selling Sickness: How the World's Biggest Pharmaceutical Companies are Turning us All into Patients, 2005.*

Chapter 4. Cochrane: Who are They and Why do they Exist?

1. LaMattina, John. *Pharma Controls Clinical Trials of Their Drugs. Is this Hazardous to Your Health?* Forbes Magazine. October 2, 2013. http://www.forbes.com/sites/johnlamattina/2013/10/02/pharma-controls-clinical-trials-of-their-drugs-is-this-hazardous-to-your-health/#1becb053189d Accessed December 6, 2016.

2. Ibid.

3. Gøtzsche, Peter. *Our Prescription Drugs Kill Us in Large Numbers.* Pol Arch Med Wewn. 2014;124(11):628-34. Epub 2014 Oct 30. https://www.ncbi.nlm.nih.gov/pubmed/25355584 Accessed December 6, 2016.

4. Gøtzsche, Peter. *On Pharma, Corruption and Psychiatric Drugs.* Mad in America Website. http://www.madinamerica.com/2013/11/peter-Gøtzsche-2/ Accessed July 28 2016

Chapter 5. "Promote a Dickhead" and other Marketing and Public Relations Strategies.

1. Fugh-Burman, Adriane. *Prescription Tracking and Public Health.* US National Library of Medicine, National Institutes of Health. J Gen Intern Med. 2008 Aug; 23(8): 1277–1280. Published online 2008 May 13. doi: 10.1007/s11606-008-0630-0 PMCID: PMC2517975. https://www.ncbi.nlm.nih.gov/pmc/articles/PMC2517975/ Accessed June 18, 2017.

Chapter 6. The Trojan Horse. Lessons from Ancient Greece.

1. Fintel, B., Samaras, A., Carias, E. *The Thalidomide Tragedy: Lessons for Drug Safety and Regulation.* Helix, Connecting Science to You website. July 28, 2009 https://helix.northwestern.edu/article/thalidomide-tragedy-lessons-drug-safety-and-regulation Accessed March 1, 2017

2. McEwan, John. *A History of Therapeutic Goods Regulation in Australia,* September 2007. https://www.tga.gov.au/sites/default/files/history-tg-regulation.pdf Accessed December 12, 2016

3. Healy, David. *Pharmageddon is the Story of a Tragedy.* http://davidhealy.org/pharmageddon-is-the-story-of-a-tragedy/ Accessed March 2, 2017.

4. Gøtzsche, Peter. *Deadly Medicines and Organised Crime, How Big Pharma has Corrupted Healthcare,* back cover. Radcliffe publishing, London, 2013.

5. Healy, David. *Go Figure: A Geek Tragedy.* September 19, 2016. *http://davidhealy.org/go-figure-a-geek-tragedy/* Accessed November 14, 2016.

6. Dunlevy, Sue. *Vaccinations without the pain of a needle prick are on the way.* News.com.au. Technology, Science, Human Body section. http://www.news.com.au/technology/science/human-body/vaccinations-

without-the-pain-of-a-needle-prick-are-on-the-way/news-story/
bc6b109e0a1bef7fd21eee0abaae8e31 Accessed May 10, 2017.

Chapter 7. You are the Perfect Market. Ouch!
1. Davies, Julie-Anne. *Anxiety Nation.* Sydney Morning Herald Good
   Weekend Magazine. July 14, 2012. Full article available for download
   with permission from the Sydney Morning Herald, Good Weekend
   at: *https://www.sleeplessnomore.com/anxiety-nation-and-drug-addiction/*
   Accessed March 14, 2017.

Chapter 8. Sick and Tired of Medical Evidence Jet Lag?
1. ABC News, *Badgerys Creek: timeline of second Sydney airport.* http://
   www.abc.net.au/news/2014-04-15/badgerys-creek-timeline-of-second-
   sydney-airport/5390064 Accessed March 1 2017

2. NASA Science (Beta) *Space Travel is Sleepless Work.* NASA Naps, June
   3, 2005. https://science.nasa.gov/science-news/science-at-nasa/2005/
   03jun_naps Accessed March 14, 2017.

3. Mednick, Dr Sara, C. *Take a Nap! Change Your Life.* Workman
   Publishing, 2006.

Part Two. Deadly Sins: Brain Damage, Addiction, Suicide, Homicide, Lies, Manipulation, Fraud And Avarice.
Chapter 9. Sleeping Pills: 34 Dark Secrets.
1. Gøtzsche, Peter, C. *Mental Health, Overdiagnosed and Overmedicated.*
   Australian tour 2014. Youtube video. https://youtu.be/ZMhsPnoIdy4.
   Minute 55.03. Accessed September 5, 2016.

2. Charles, J., Harrison, C., Britt, H et al. *BEACH Bettering the Evaluation
   and Care of Health.* April 2006 – March 2008. Australian GP Statistics
   and Classification Centre, The University of Sydney.

3. Davies, J-A. *Anxiety Nation*, Sydney Morning Herald Good Weekend Magazine, July 14, 2012. Julie-Anne Davies. Full article available here: https://www.sleeplessnomore.com/anxiety-nation-and-drug-addiction/ Accessed November 18, 2011.

4. Australian National Prescribing Service. *Addressing hypnotic medicines use in primary care*. Published in *MedicineWise News* 01 February 2010. http://www.nps.org.au/publications/health-professional/nps-news/2010/nps-news-67 Accessed November 21, 2016.

5. Richardson G, Wang-Weigand S. *Effects of long-term exposure to ramelteon, a melatonin receptor agonist, on endocrine function in adults with chronic insomnia*. Hum Psychopharmacol. 2009 Mar; 24(2):103-11.

6. Benzo.org.uk website. *Benzodiazepine Equivalence Table*. Revised April 2007. http://www.benzo.org.uk/bzequiv.htm Accessed November 21, 2016.

7. Marcus, C., *Sleep Pill Blamed for Weird Actions*, The Sydney Morning Herald, May 10, 2009, viewed February 4, 2016, http://www.smh.com.au/national/sleep-pill-blamed-for-weird-actions-20090509-aykz.html

8. The Australian National Prescribing Service Limited (NPS). http://www.nps.org.au Accessed July 2012.

9. Charles, J., Harrison, C., Britt, H. et al., *BEACH (Bettering the Evaluation and Care of Health)*. April 2006 – March 2008. Australian GP Statistics and Classification Centre, The University of Sydney.

10. Saul, Stephanie, *Sleep Drugs Found Only Mildly Effective, but Wildly Popular*, New York Times, October 23, 2007. http://www.nytimes.com/2007/10/23/health/23drug.html Accessed August 2, 2012.

11. Ibid.

12. Saul, Stephanie, *F.D.A. Warns of Sleeping Pills' Strange Effects*, March 15, 2007. New York Times. http://www.nytimes.com/2007/03/15/business/15drug.ready.html Accessed August 23, 2017.

13. Gilmore, Heath. *Sleeping Pill Safety Under Federal Review*, The Sydney MorningHerald,March11,2007.http://www.smh.com.au/news/national/sleeping-pill-safety-under-federal-review/2007/03/10/1173478729115.html Accessed November 21, 2016.

14. Kripke Daniel F. *Greater incidence of depression with hypnotic use than with placebo.* US National Library of Medicine, National Institutes of Health. 2007. https://www.ncbi.nlm.nih.gov/pmc/articles/PMC1994947/BMC Psychiatry. 2007; 7: 42. Published online 2007 Aug 21. Doi: 10.1186/1471-244X-7-42 Accessed November 21, 2016.

15. Kripke, Daniel F, Langer, R.D., Kline, L.E., *Hypnotics' association with mortality or cancer: a matched cohort study.* BMJournal's Open 2012;2:e000850. Doi:10.1136/bmjopen-2012-000850 http://dx.doi.org/10.1136/bmjopen-2012-000850 Accessed July 28, 2016.

16. Saul, Stephanie, *Sleep Drugs Found Only Mildly Effective, but Wildly Popular*, New York Times, October 23, 2007. http://www.nytimes.com/2007/10/23/health/23drug.html Accessed August 2, 2012.

17. Ibid.

18. Saul, Stephanie. *Some Sleeping Pill Users Range Far Beyond Bed*, New York Times, March 8, 2006. http://www.nytimes.com/2006/03/08/business/08ambien.html Accessed August 2, 2012.

19. Saul, Stephanie, *F.D.A. Warns of Sleeping Pills' Strange Effects*, March 15, 2007. New York Times. http://www.nytimes.com/2007/03/15/business/15drug.ready.html Accessed August 23, 2017.

20. Op.cit.

21. Maas, James D, *Power Sleep*, page 91 and 117.

22. Wang P.S., Bohn R.L. et al., *Zolpidem use and hip fractures in older people*. US National Library of Medicine., National Institutes of Health. J Am Geriatr Soc. 2001 Dec;49(12):1685-90. https://www.ncbi.nlm.nih. gov/pubmed/11844004 Accessed July 27, 2012.

23. The Australian Government, National Prescribing Service of Australia (NPS) website. *The Sleep Cycle, Normal Sleep, How it Works.* http:// www.nps.org.au/conditions/mental-health-conditions/sleep- problems/insomnia/for-individuals/normal-sleep-how-it-works. Accessed November 21, 2016.

24. Mednick, Sara C., *Take a Nap! Change Your Life.* Workman Publishing Company, chapter 4.

25. Wikipedia, *Slow Wave Sleep.* http://en.wikipedia.org/wiki/Slow-wave_ sleep Accessed September 13, 2012.

26. Ibid.

27. Neutel, C.I., Patten S.B., *Risk of suicide attempts after benzodiazepine and/or antidepressant use.* US National Library of Medicine, National Institutes of Health. Ann Epidemiol. 1997 Nov;7(8):568-74. https:// www.ncbi.nlm.nih.gov/pubmed/9408553 Accessed November 18, 2016.

28. Rxisk.org website. http://rxisk.org/drug/2702/zolpidem/ Accessed August 11, 2016.

29. Mason, M., Cates C.J., Smith I., *Effects of opioids, hypnotic and sedating medications on sleep-disordered breathing in adults with obstructive sleep apnea.* Cochrane Database of Systematic Reviews 2015, Issue 7. Art. No.: CD011090. DOI: 10.1002/14651858. CD011090.pub2   http://www.cochrane.org/CD011090/

AIRWAYS_effects-opioid-hypnotic-and-sedating-medications-obstruc-tive-sleep-apnea-osa-adults-known-osa Accessed October 17, 2016.

30. Australian Government, Department of Health, Therapeutic Goods Administration. *Scheduling delegate's interim decisions and invitation for further comment: ACCS/ACMS, May 2013.* May 23, 2013. https://www.tga.gov.au/book/interim-decisions-proposal-referred-advisory-committee-acms-march-2013 Accessed November 18, 2016.

31. Australian Medical Association (AMA), *Rescheduling of Benzodiazepines,* 15 July, 2013. https://ama.com.au/ausmed/rescheduling-benzodiazepines Accessed November 18, 2016.

32. Miller, CH, Fleischhacker, WW. *Managing antipsychotic-induced acute and chronic akathisia.* US National Library of Medicine, National Institutes of Health. Drug Saf. 2000 Jan;22(1):73-81. https://www.ncbi.nlm.nih.gov/pubmed/10647977 Accessed November 18, 2016.

33. Gøtzsche, Peter, C. *Mental Health, Overdiagnosed and Overmedicated.* Australian tour 2014. Youtube video. https://youtu.be/ZMhsPnoIdy4. Minute 34.15. Accessed September 5, 2016.

34. Wikipedia. https://en.wikipedia.org/wiki/Alprazolam Accessed November 17 2016.

35. Davies, Julie-Anne, *Anxiety Nation*, Sydney Morning Herald Good Weekend Magazine. July 14, 2012.

36. Uzun S, Kozumplik O, Jakovljević M, Sedić B, *Side Effects of Treatment with Benzodiazepine,* US National Library of Medicine. Psychiatr Danub. 2010 Mar;22(1):90-3. https://www.ncbi.nlm.nih.gov/pubmed/20305598 Accessed November 17, 2016.

37. Anderson, L. *Benzodiazepines Overview and Use.* May 4, 2014. Drugs dot com website.
Benzodiazepine Use in Pregnancy and Breastfeeding. https://www.drugs.com/article/benzodiazepines.html#pregnancy-breastfeeding Accessed

November 17, 2016. The FDA classification https://www.drugs.com/pregnancy-categories.html#catd

38. The State Coroner's Court of New South Wales, Australia. The inquest into the deaths of Christopher SALIB, Nathan ATTARD and Shamsad AKHTAR by the State Coroner's Court of New South Wales http://www.coroners.justice.nsw.gov.au/Documents/doctor%20shopping%20amended%20finding.pdf Accessed November 18, 2016.

39. Ibid.

40. Kelly, Shane. *The Benzodiazepine Medical Disaster.* Leader Productions, October 20, 2016. https://vimeo.com/188181193 Accessed February 27, 2017.

41. Ibid.

42. Ibid.

43. Ibid.

44. Ibid.

45. Ibid.

46. Ibid.

47. Ibid.

48. Ibid.

49. Ibid.

50. Ibid.

51. Ibid.

52. Ibid.

53. Ibid.

54. Ibid.

55. Ibid.

56. Ibid.

57. Ibid.

58. Ibid.

59. Ibid.

60. Ibid.

61. Ibid.

62. Ibid.

63. Ibid.

64. Ibid.

65. Australian Government, Department of Health, Therapeutic Goods Administration. Medicines Safety Update, Volume 5, Number 4, August 2014. *Zolpidem and Next Day Impairment.* https://www.tga.gov.au/publication-issue/medicines-safety-update-volume-5-number-4-august-2014#zolpidem Accessed March 1, 2017.

66. Shannon, E. *Alarming Sleep Secrets.* Chapter 10, point 14.

67. The United States Food and Drug Administration (FDA), consumer updates. *Some Sleep Drugs Can Impair Driving.* January 10, 2013. https://www.fda.gov/ForConsumers/ConsumerUpdates/ucm322743.htm Accessed August 23, 2017.

68. Jones AW, Holmgren A, Kugelberg FC; Holmgren; Kugelberg (2007). *Concentrations of scheduled prescription drugs in blood of impaired drivers: considerations for interpreting the results.* US National Library of Medicine. National Institutes of Health. Ther Drug Monit. 2007 Apr;29(2):248-60. https://www.ncbi.nlm.nih.gov/pubmed/17417081 Accessed August 23, 2017.

Chapter 10. Antidepressants/SSRIs: Facts to Make You Mad and Sad.

1. Gøtzsche, Peter, C. *Deadly Medicines and Organised Crime: How big pharma has corrupted healthcare.* Radcliffe Publishing, London and New York. 2013. Chapter 18. *Pushing children into suicide with happy pills.* Page 233.

2. Breggin, Peter, MD. *Psychiatric Drugs Are More Dangerous than You Ever Imagined.* November 4, 2014. *http://*youtu.be/luKsQaj0hzs Accessed February 10, 2017. 9 minutes long.

3. Purcell, Andrew. *Antidepressants: How drugs got into Australia's system.* Sydney Morning Herald. October 11, 2015. 4.49 am. http://www.smh.com.au/national/advance-antidepressants-fair-how-drugs-got-into-australias-system-20151006-gk2jjh.html Accessed January 26, 2017.

4. Gøtzsche, Peter C. *Mental Health, Overdiagnosed and Overmedicated.* The Nordic Cochrane Centre, presentation given in Australia February 2015. YouTube video, Minute 29. https://youtu.be/ZMhsPnoIdy4 Accessed February 10, 2017.

5. Ibid. 29 minutes into the video.

6. Ibid. Minute 30:35

7. Ibid. Minute 31.

8. Ibid. Minute 32:36.

9. Ibid. Minute 32 – 35.

10. Ibid. Minute 22.

11. Australian Medical Association Website. *Continuing Professional Development.* https://ama.com.au/careers/co ntinuing-professional-development Accessed February 10, 2017.

12. Le Noury, J., Nardo, J.M., Healy, D., Jureidini, J., Raven, M., Tafanaru, C., Abi-Jaoude, E., 2015. *Restoring Study 329: efficacy and harms of paroxetine and imipramine in treatment of major depression in adolescence.* British Medical Journal BMJ 2015; 351 doi: http://dx.doi.orgt/10.1136/bmj.h4320, September 16, BMJ 2015;351:h4320, Viewed January 14, 2016. http://www.bmj.com/content/351/bmj.h4320

13. Le Noury, J., Nardo, J.M., Healy, D., Jureidini, J., Raven, M., Tafanaru, C., Abi-Jaoude, E. *Medicine's Most Infamous Clinical Trial.* https://study329.org/. Accessed February 1, 2017

14. Ibid.

15. Stiles, Laura. *Antidepressants may Double the Risk of Suicide, Aggression in Adolescents.* Psychiatry Advisor. February 11, 2016. http://www.psychiatryadvisor.com/mood-disorders/antidepressants-may-double-risk-suicide-aggression-children-adolescents-depression-akathisia/article/473591/ Accessed October 24, 2016.

16. Sharma, T., Guski, L.S., Freund, N., Gøtzsche, P.C. et al. *Suicidality and aggression during antidepressant treatment: systematic review and meta-analyses based on clinical study reports.* BMJ 2016; 352 doi: http://dx.doi.org/10.1136/bmj.i65 Published 27 January 2016, BMJ 2016;352:i65. Accessed October 24, 2016

17. Ibid. Accessed January 18, 2017.

18. Gøtzsche, Peter C. *Mental Health: Overdiagnosed and Overmedicated.* Presentation given in Australia, February 2015. YouTube video, 34:31 minutes. https://youtu.be/ZMhsPnoIdy4 Accessed February 10, 2017.

19. Ibid.

20. MISSD Foundation. *What is Akathisia* You Tube video. The Medication-Induced Suicide Prevention and Education Foundation in Memory of Stewart Dolin. Published October 26, 2016. https://youtu.be/x86aCDtvbT0 Accessed January 30, 2017.

21. Karter, Justin. *Legal Journal Says Antidepressants Can Cause Violence and Suicide.* April 18, 2016. https://www.madinamerica.com/2016/04/legal-journal-says-antidepressants-can-cause-violence-and-suicide/ Accessed January 23, 2017.

22. Gøtzsche, Peter C. *Mental Health: Overdiagnosed and Overmedicated.* Presentation given in Australia February 2015. YouTube video, 34:31. https://youtu.be/ZMhsPnoIdy4 Accessed February 10, 2017.

23. Ibid.

24. Ibid. You Tube 22:00.

25. Healy, David. Rxisk: Prescription Drugs Side Effects Website. *Post SSRI Sexual Dysfunction*: PSSD. http://rxisk.org/post-ssri-sexual-dysfunction-pssd/ Accessed August 11, 2016.

26. Gøtzsche, Peter C. *Mental Health, Overdiagnosed and Overmedicated.* Presentation given in Australia February 2015. YouTube video. https://youtu.be/ZMhsPnoIdy4 Accessed February 10, 2017.

27. Healy, David. *Liability.* Rxisk.org website. https://rxisk.org/drugs-liability. Accessed February 10, 2017.

28. Gøtzsche, Peter C. *Mental Health, Overdiagnosed and Overmedicated.* Presentation given in Australia February 2015. YouTube video. https://youtu.be/ZMhsPnoIdy4 Accessed February 10, 2017.

29. Healy, D. *Driven to Drink: Antidepressants and Cravings for Alcohol.* http://rxisk.org/driven-to-drink-antidepressants-and-cravings-for-alcohol/ Rxisk.org website, October 15, 2012. Accessed October 26, 2016.

30. Brookwell, L. et al. *Ninety-three cases of alcohol dependence following SSRI treatment.* International Journal of Risk & Safety in Medicine 26 (2014) 99-107 DOI 10.3233/JRS-140616 IOS Press Accepted March 9, 2014. http://rxisk.org/wp-content/uploads/2015/02/2014-Brookwell-SSRIs-and-Alcohol-JRS616.pdf Accessed October 26, 2016.

31. Healy, D. *Keeping an Eye on the Ball: Visual Problems on SSRIs.* Rxisk website. http://rxisk.org/keeping-an-eye-on-the-ball-visual-problems-on-ssris/ Accessed October 26, 2016.

32. S. Kalra, A. Einarson RN, Gideon Koren MD, FRCPC. *Taking Antidepressants during Late Pregnancy - How should we advise women.* August 2005. MotheRisk website. http://www.motherisk.org/women/updatesDetail.jsp?content_id=730 Accessed December 8, 2016.

33. Fiore, Kristina. MedPage Today website, CME/CE. *Antipsychotics May Boost Respiratory Failure Risk in COPD. Risk was dose-dependent; no safe dose found.* January 8, 2017. http://www.medpagetoday.com/Psychiatry/GeneralPsychiatry/62407 Accessed February 10, 2017.

34. Eikelenboom-Schieveld, Selma J. M., Lucire, Yolanda, Fogleman, James, C. *The Relevance of Cytochrome P450 Polymorphism in Forensic Medicine and Akathisia-Related Violence and Suicide.* Journal of Forensic and Legal Medicine. July 2016, Volume 41, pages 65-71. http://dx.doi.org/10.1016/j.jflm.2016.04.003 http://www.jflmjournal.org/article/S1752-928X(16)30005-1/abstract?cc=y= Accessed January 30, 2017.

35. Lynch, T., Price, A. *The Effect of Cytochrome P450 Metabolism on Drug Response, Interactions, and Adverse Effects.* Eastern Virginia Medical School. The American Family Physician, August 1, 2007 issue. http://www.aafp.org/afp/2007/0801/p391.html Accessed January 23, 2017.

36. National Association of Testing Authorities. Blacktown Molecular Research Laboratory. Blacktown Clinical School. Irina Piatkov. Email: irina.piatkov@health.nsw.gov.au. http://www.nata.com.au/nata/component/jumi/scopeinfo?key=18636 Accessed January 23, 2017.

37. NSW Government, Department of Health, University Clinic and Research Centre, Blacktown & Western Sydney Local Health District. Diversity Health Institute. Transcultural Mental Health Centre. Pharmacogenetic research testing. *Cytochrome P450 2C19 Fact Sheet.* http://www.dhi.health.nsw.gov.au/ArticleDocuments/1720/CYP2C19%20Fact%20Sheet.pdf.aspx Accessed January 30, 2017.

38. Breggin, Peter, MD. *Psychiatric Drugs Are More Dangerous than You Ever Imagined.* YouTube video. November 4, 2014. https://youtu.be/luKsQaj0hzs 9.17 minutes into the video. Accessed February 2, 2017.

39. Ibid.

40. Ibid.

41. BBC News Panorama. *The Secrets of Seroxat.* Aired on BBC One October 13, 2002. https://youtu.be/ZO43efODoug Published September 5, 2014 for the charity website rxisk.org. Accessed February 14, 2017. Full transcript available here: http://news.bbc.co.uk/2/hi/programmes/panorama/2310197.stm Accessed February 13, 2017.

42. Ibid.

43. Ibid.

44. Beyond Blue Website, Australia. *Antidepression Medication Factsheet BL/0125 02/15*, December 2014. http://resources.beyondblue.org.au/prism/file?token=BL%2F0125 Accessed November 18, 2016. Available on request. This factsheet information was updated in December 2016, and uploaded to the website in January or February 2017. The new factsheet was accessed February 11, 2017.

45. *Beyond Blue Website, Australia. Antidepressant Medication Factsheet BL/0125 12/16. December 2016. http://resources.beyondblue.org.au/prism/file?token=BL%2F0125* Accessed May 29, 2017.

46. Ibid.

47. Ibid.

48. Ibid.

49. Healy, D., Le Noury, J., Mangin, D., *Links between serotonin reuptake inhibition during pregnancy and neurodevelopmental delay/spectrum disorders: A systematic review of epidemiological and physiological evidence.* International Journal of Risk & Safety in Medicine 28 (2016) 125-141. DOI 10.3233/JRS-160726. IOS Press. Accepted July 12, 2016. http://rxisk.org/wp-content/uploads/2016/10/2016-SSRIs-ASD-IJRSM.pdf?utm_source=October+2016+News&utm_campaign=October+News&utm_medium=email Accessed October 26, 2016.

50. Healy, David. *Autistic Spectrum Disorder and SSRIs.* Rxisk.org website. http://rxisk.org/autistic-spectrum-disorder-and-ssris/ October 25, 2016. Accessed October 26, 2016.

51. Purcell, Andrew. *Antidepressants: How drugs got into Australia's system.* Sydney Morning Herald. October 11, 2015. 4.49 am. http://www.smh.com.au/national/advance-antidepressants-fair-how-drugs-got-into-australias-system-20151006-gk2jjh.html Accessed January 26, 2017.

52. Healy, David, Le Noury, Jo, Mangin, Dee. *Antidepressants*, Rxisk.org website https://rxisk.org/antidepressants/ Accessed Feb 14, 2017.

53. Urato, Adam, Professor of Obstetrics & Gynecology at Tuft's University. *New Epidemic: Antidepressants During Pregnancy.* July 9, 2012. David Healy website. https://davidhealy.org/a-new-epidemic/ Accessed February 14, 2017.

54. Beyond Blue, The National Depression Initiative. Perinatal Mental Health Consortium. *Perinatal Mental Health. National Action Plan.* 2008-2010 Full Report. September 2008. Intervention for Depression during the Perinatal Period, Page 78. Beyond Blue Website. https://www.beyondblue.org.au/docs/default-source/8.-perinatal-documents/bw0125-report-beyondblues-perinatal-mental-health-(nap)-full-report.pdf?sfvrsn=2 Accessed December 8, 2016.

55. Gøtzsche, Peter. *Overprescribing antidepressants: where's the evidence?* British Medical Journal, June 30, 2014. BMJ 2014;348:g4218 http://www.bmj.com/content/348/bmj.g4218/rr/759524 Accessed November 18, 2016.

56. Whitaker, Robert *Anatomy of an Epidemic. Magic Bullets, Psychiatric Drugs, and the Astonishing Rise of Mental Illness in America.* Broadway Paperbacks, New York. Page 165 referencing a paper written by D. Goldberg "The effect of detection and treatment on the outcome of major depression in primary care," British Journal of General Practice 48 (1998): 1840-44.

57. Ibid. Page 168. Referencing Coryell, W. *Characteristics and significance of untreated major depressive disorder.* American Journal of Psychiatry 152 (1995): 1124-29. My figures approximate, visually estimated from the *NIMH's Study of Untreated Depression* graph on page 168.

58. Ibid. Referring to Rosenbeck, R, *The Growth of Psychopharmacology in the 1990s,* International Journal of Law and Psychiatry 28 (2005): 467-83. Page 168.

59. Breggin, Peter, MD., *Psychiatric Drugs are More Dangerous than you ever Imagined.* Mentioned earlier in this chapter. Youtube video https://youtu.be/luKsQaj0hzs

60. Ibid.

61. Ibid.

62. Purcell, Andrew. *Antidepressants: How drugs got into Australia's system.* Sydney Morning Herald. October 11, 2015. 4.49 am. http://www.smh.com.au/national/advance-antidepressants-fair-how-drugs-got-into-australias-system-20151006-gk2jjh.html Accessed January 26, 2017.

63. Healy, David. *Study 329 Taper Phase.* October 10, 2016. http://davidhealy.org/study-329-taper-phase/ Accessed November 14, 2016.

64. Gøtzsche, Peter. *Deadly Psychiatry and Organised Denial.* 2015. https://books.google.com.au/books/about/Deadly_Psychiatry_and_Organised_Denial.html?id=K99wCgAAQBAJ&redir_esc=y&hl=en Accessed February 27, 2017.

65. Gøtzsche, Peter. *Does long term use of psychiatric drugs cause more harm than good?* BMJ 2015; 350 doi: https://doi.org/10.1136/bmj.h2435 (Published 12 May 2015) BMJ 2015;350:h2435 British Medical Journal. http://www.bmj.com/content/350/bmj.h2435 Accessed June 18, 2017.

66. Australian Government. Australian Institute of Health and Welfare. Mental Health Services in Australia (MHSA). *Mental Health-related prescriptions.* 2015-2016 (and previously 2014-15). https://mhsa.aihw.gov.au/resources/prescriptions/
Accessed August 18, 2017.

67. Ibid.

68. Ibid.

69. Ibid.

70. Ibid.

71. Ibid.

Chapter 11. The Cost of Lack of Sleep and Mental Health to Australia.

1. Wade, M. *Now for the good news: Life got better for Australians in 2016.* The Sydney Morning Herald March 4-5, 2017. Figures from the Fairfax-Lateral Economics wellbeing index 2016. The index's author is Dr Nicholas Gruen who is also the Chair of The Australian Centre for Social Innovation.

2. Wade, M. *The wellbeing cost of mental health hits $ 200 billion.* The Sydney Morning Herald. Published September 9, 2016. http://www. smh.com.au/national/the-wellbeing-cost-of-mental-health-hits-200-billion-20160909-grcxxl.html Accessed March 6, 2017.

3. Swan, Dr Norman and Balendra, Jaya. *Wasted.* Four Corners. September 28, 2015. Presented by Dr Norman Swan. http://www.abc. net.au/4corners/stories/2015/09/28/4318883.htm. Accessed January 14, 2016. Full transcript available on the website.

4. Australian Government, Australian Institute of Health and Welfare, Australia's Welfare 2015, Australian Institute of Health and Welfare 2015. *7.2 How are people with mental illness faring?* Page 2. http:// www.aihw.gov.au/WorkArea/DownloadAsset.aspx?id=60129552309 Accessed April 10, 2017.

5. Ibid.

6. Czeisler, Charles, Baldino Director of Sleep Medicine and Director of the Division of Sleep Medicine, Harvard Medical School and Team Leader of Human Performance Factors at NASA's National Space Biomedical

Research Institute. *Sleep Deficit: The Performance Killer.* YouTube video published November 9, 2012. https://youtu.be/pNHcXmiYsBk. Accessed January 18, 2016.

7. Wood, Patrick. *'Alarming' number of drowsy drivers on Australia's roads, sleep study finds.* February 8, 2017. ABC News Breakfast. http://www. abc.net.au/news/2017-02-08/sleep-study-finds-alarming-number-of-dozy-drivers-on-our-roads/8250780 Accessed May 21, 2017. Full *Report to the Sleep Health Foundation 2016, Sleep Health Survey of Australian Adults* is available at this link.

8. Czeisler, Charles, *Sleep Deficit: The Performance Killer.* YouTube video published November 9, 2012. https://youtu.be/pNHcXmiYsBk. Accessed January 18, 2016.

9. Purcell, Andrew. *Antidepressants: How Drugs Got into Australia's System.* Sydney Morning Herald, October 10, 2015. http://www.smh.com.au/ national/advance-antidepressants-fair-how-drugs-got-into-australias-system-20151006-gk2jjh.html. Accessed May 8, 2017.

10. Australian Government, Department of Health. The Pharmaceutical Benefits Scheme. *Expenditure and Prescriptions Report 2015-16,* Table 12. ATC Level 2 Drug Groups Sorted by Highest Script Volume, 2015-16. Includes subsidized and under co-payment scripts. Section 85 only; incl. Drs Bag. http://www.pbs.gov.au/statistics/expenditure-prescriptions/2015-2016/expenditure-prescriptions-report-2015-16.pdf Accessed May 8, 2017. The new figure accessed August 18, 2017 is 36 million scripts. See the updated figures at the end of Chapter 10.

11. Cha, Ariana Eunjung. *Researchers: Medical errors now third leading cause of death in United States.* Washington Post. May 3, 2016. https:// www.washingtonpost.com/news/to-your-health/wp/2016/05/03/ researchers-medical-errors-now-third-leading-cause-of-death-in-united-states/?utm_term=.3a431b5c2e40 Accessed May 21, 2017.

12. Swan, Dr Norman and Balendra, Jaya. *Wasted*. Four Corners. September 28, 2015. Presented by Dr Norman Swan. This is a quote from Robyn Ward. http://www.abc.net.au/4corners/stories/2015/09/28/4318883. htm. Accessed January 14, 2016. Full transcript available on the website.

13. ABC News, Sydney. *Key Facts: Gambling in Australia*. 8 Jun 2011. http://www.abc.net.au/news/2011-05-25/key-facts-gambling-in-australia/2730414 Accessed May 22, 2017.

14. Australian Government, Department of Employment, *Australian Jobs 2016*. https://australianjobs.employment.gov.au/jobs-industry/health-care-and-social-assistance Accessed March 6, 2017.

15. Mental Health Commission of NSW, *What We Know*, https://nswmentalhealthcommission.com.au/our-work/strategic-plan/what-we-know Accessed March 6, 2017.

16. *The Fairfax Lateral Economics Index of Australia's Wellbeing report of 2014*, Mental Health, page 56. Also known as the HALE index (Herald/Age Lateral Economics Index). http://lateraleconomics.com.au/wp-content/uploads/2014/02/Fairfax-Lateral-Economics-Index-of-Australias-Wellbeing-Final-Report.pdf Accessed March 6, 2017

17. Ibid.

18. Australian Government, Australian Institute of Health and Welfare, Australia's Welfare 2015. Part 7.2, page 2. *How are people with mental illness faring?* http://www.aihw.gov.au/WorkArea/DownloadAsset.aspx?id=60129552309 Accessed April 10, 2017.

19. *Stats and Facts*, Youth Beyond Blue website, quoting figures from the ABS National Survey of Mental Health and Wellbeing: Summary of Results 2007 (2008), p 9 https://www.youthbeyondblue.com/footer/stats-and-facts Accessed April 10, 2017

20. Citizens Committee on Human Rights (CCHR), *Release of Australian Documentary about Psychotic Drug, Selling Australian Children Down the Drain.* http://cchr.org.au/articles/release-of-australian-documentary-about-psychiatric-drugs Accessed April 10, 2017. (Note I am *not* associated in any way with Scientology or CCHR.)

21. Ibid.

22. Ibid.

23. Schizophrenia Research Institute, *About Schizophrenia.* 26 June 2013. http://www.schizophreniaresearch.org.au/schizophrenia/about-schizophrenia/ Accessed April 10, 2017.

24. Ibid.

25. Ibid.

26. Ibid.

27. Hutcheon, Jane, interview with Fay Jackson, Deputy Commissioner with the NSW Mental Health Commission. ABC News television, *One Plus One.* Broadcast April 7, 2017 http://iview.abc.net.au/programs/one-plus-one/NU1741H010S00 Accessed April 10, 2017.

28. Gøtzsche, Peter. *Mental Health: Overdiagnosed and Overmedicated.* YouTube video uploaded May 12, 2015. https://youtu.be/ZMhsPnoIdy4 Accessed April 10, 2017.

29. Ibid. 25 minutes in. Accessed April 10, 2017.

Chapter 12. Why a 10 Minute Quickie with Your Doctor is Never Enough.

1. Gøtzsche, P.C., *Mental Health, Overdiagnosed and Overmedicated.* YouTube video uploaded May 12, 2015. https://youtu.be/ZMhsPnoIdy4 Accessed July 24, 2015.

Chapter 13. Preventative Medicine. Why Bother when the Money is in the Illness?

1. Australian Government, Department of Employment, *Australian Jobs 2016*. https://australianjobs.employment.gov.au/jobs-industry/health-care-and-social-assistance Accessed March 6, 2017.

2. Ibid.

3. SurfacePro4 advertisement. November 6, 2016. https://youtu.be/Yjs2uiKPo2c Accessed March 13, 2017.

Chapter 14. The Medical Profession Created Their Own Terminal Case.

1. Cromie, William J. *Suicide high among female doctors: More than double the rate of general public.* Harvard Gazette, February 3, 2005. http://news.harvard.edu/gazette/2005/02.03/11-suicide.html Accessed June 5, 2017.

2. O'Meara, Cindi. *Pharmageddon is the Story of a Tragedy by Dr David Healy.* November 14, 2012. https://changinghabits.com.au/pharmageddon-is-the-story-of-a-tragedy-by-dr-david-healy/ Accessed March 1 2017

3. Sydney Morning Herald Commentary. *Three of my Colleagues have Killed Themselves: Medicine's Dark Secret can't go on.* February 10, 2017. http://www.smh.com.au/comment/three-of-my-colleagues-have-killed-themselves-medicines-dark-secret-cant-be-allowed-to-go-on-20170209-gu9crd.html Accessed February 12, 2017

Chapter 15. Our Kids at School. Mental Health Care or the New Marketing Frontier?

1. Australian Government, Department of Health, Therapeutic Goods Administration website. *SSRI antidepressants: Actions by the Therapeutic Goods Administration concerning use of antidepressants in children and adolescents.* October 15, 2004. https://www.tga.gov.au/alert/

ssri-antidepressants-actions-therapeutic-goods-administration-concern-ing-use-antidepressants-children-and-adolescents Accessed March 13, 2017.

2. Australian Government, Department of Health, Therapeutic Goods Administration website, Adverse Drug Reactions Advisory Committee, historical document. *Use of SSRI Antidepressants in Children and Adolescents. October 15, 2004* https://www.tga.gov.au/use-ssri-antidepressants-children-and-adolescents-october-2004 Accessed March 6, 2017.

3. Headspace, website of the National Youth Mental Health Foundation. *Headspace Evidence Summary: Using SSRI Antidepressants and Other Newer Antidepressants to Treat Depression in Young People: What are the issues and what is the evidence?* Page 2. Version 2, Updated December 2012. https://headspace.org.au/assets/Uploads/Resource-library/Health-professionals/ssri-v2-pdf.pdf Accessed March 6, 2017.

4. Ibid.

5. Ibid.

6. Ibid.

7. Ibid. Page 1.

8. Le Noury, Joanna, Nardo, John, M., Healy, David, Jureidini, Jon, Raven, Melissa, Tufanaru, Catalin, Abi-Jaoude, Elia. *Restoring Study 329: efficacy and harms of paroxetine and imipramine in treatment of major depression in adolescence.* BMJ 2015; 351 doi: https://doi.org/10.1136/bmj.h4320 (Published 16 September 2015) BMJ 2015;351:h4320 Res. http://www.bmj.com/content/351/bmj.h4320 Accessed March 13, 2017.

9. Australian Antidepressants Class Action, Facebook page. https://www.facebook.com/AustralianAntidepressantClassAction/?pnref=story Accessed March 13, 2017.

10. Le Noury, Joanna, Nardo, John, M., Healy, David, Jureidini, Jon, Raven, Melissa, Tufanaru, Catalin, Abi-Jaoude, Elia. *Restoring Study 329: efficacy and harms of paroxetine and imipramine in treatment of major depression in adolescence*, Open Access. https://study329.org/wp-content/uploads/2015/09/Study-329-Final.pdf (Accessed March 13, 2017) and https://study329.org/bmj-press-release-and-materials/ Accessed March 6, 2017.

11. Australian Government, Department of Health, Therapeutic Goods Administration (TGA), Adverse Drug Reactions Bulletin Volume 23, Number 6, December 2004. https://www.tga.gov.au/publication-issue/australian-adverse-drug-reactions-bulletin-vol-23-no-6 A statement by ADRAC dated 15 October 2004. Mentions increased risk of suicidal ideation amongst other side effects. Accessed March 6, 2017.

12. Harvard Medical School, Division of Sleep Medicine. *Stiffened Penalties for Night-time Teen Driving Associated with Fewer Fatal Crashes. June 17, 2015.* https://sleep.med.harvard.edu/news/547/Stiffened+Penalties+for+Nighttime+Teen+Driving+Associated+With+Fewer+Fatal+Crash. *Accessed October 2, 2017.*

13. The National Institute of Mental Health (USA). *Mental Illness Exacts Heavy Toll, Beginning in Youth.* Press Released June 6, 2005. Based on National Comorbidity Survey Republication (NCS-R) study. http://www.nihmh.nih.gov/news/science-news/2005/mental-illness-exacts-heavy-toll-beginning-in-youth.shtml. Accessed August 22, 2015.

Chapter 16. What has Sleep got to do with Fatigue? And Other Scarily Common Organisational Questions.

1. Shantha M. W. Rajaratnam, PhD; Laura K. Barger, PhD; Steven W. Lockley, PhD; et al *Sleep Disorders, Health, and Safety in Police Officers.* JAMA. 2011;306(23):2567-2578. doi:10.1001/jama.2011.1851. December 21, 2011. Downloadable at: http://jamanetwork.com/journals/jama/fullarticle/1104746 Accessed May 1, 2017.

2. JAMA and Archives Journals. *Sleep disorders common among police officers.* Science Daily, 23 December 2011. https://www.sciencedaily.com/ releases/2011/12/111220172618.htm Accessed May 1, 2017.

3. University at Buffalo. *Night beat, overtime and a disrupted sleep pattern can harm officers' health.* ScienceDaily. ScienceDaily, 17 November 2009. https://www.sciencedaily.com/releases/2009/11/091117161120. htm Accessed May 1, 2017.

Chapter 17. Media Games and the Need for an Overhaul.

1. Robbins, Rebecca. *Drug makers now spend $5 billion a year on advertising. Here's what that buys.* Stat News. March 9, 2016. https://www. statnews.com/2016/03/09/drug-industry-advertising/ Accessed April 3, 2017.

2. Australian Government, Department of Health. Therapeutic Goods Administration. *Regulation of Therapeutic Goods in Australia.* April 8, 2011. https://www.tga.gov.au/regulation-therapeutic-goods-advertising-australia Accessed April 3, 2017.

Chapter 18: Politicians are Not Capable of Doing Their Job.

1. Parliament of Australia website. *The Pharmaceutical Benefits Scheme: A Quick Guide.* 7 April 2016. http://www.aph.gov.au/About_Parliament/ Parliamentary_Departments/Parliamentary_Library/pubs/rp/rp1516/ Quick_Guides/PBS Accessed March 1, 2017

2. McEwan, John. *A History of Therapeutic Goods Regulation in Australia,* September 2007. https://www.tga.gov.au/sites/default/files/history-tg-regulation.pdf Accessed December 12, 2016

3. Ibid., page 29.

4. Ibid., page 32.

5. Ibid., page 40.

6. Williams, MJ, Kevat, Dev A S Kevat, and Loff, B. *Conflict of Interest Guidelines for Clinical Guidelines.* Medical Journal of Australia. Med J Aust 2011; 195 (8): 442-445. doi: 10.5694/mja10.11130 https://www. mja.com.au/journal/2011/195/8/conflict-interest-guidelines-clinical-guidelines Accessed December 8, 2016. Downloadable here: https://www. mja.com.au/system/files/issues/195_08_171011/wil11130_fm.pdf

7. Ibid.

8. Ibid.

9. Ibid.

10. Ibid.

11. Ibid.

12. Ibid.

13. Ibid.

14. Ibid.

Chapter 19. The Seventh Dwarf.
No references cited.

Chapter 20. A Royal Commission with Broad Ranging Terms of Reference.

1. Raymond, Nate and Grzincic, Barbara. *GSK must pay $3 million in generic Paxil suicide lawsuit: U.S. jury.* Reuters Business News. April 20, 2017. http://www.reuters.com/article/us-gsk-lawsuit-idUSKBN17M2SH Accessed May 1, 2017.

2. Fiddaman, Bobby. *Exclusive: Interview with Wendy Dolin.* April 25, 2017. Fiddaman Blog. http://fiddaman.blogspot.com.au/2017/04/exclusive-interview-with-wendy-dolin.html Accessed May 1, 2017.

3. NBC Chicago 5. *Did a Common Prescription Drug Cause a Chicago Attorney's Death?* April 18, 2017. http://www.nbcchicago.com/investigations/paxil-lawsuit-chicago-419775753.html Accessed May 1, 2017.

4. Baum Hedlund Law. Paxil Trial Exhibits, Dolin vs. GSK Trail. *Plaintiff's Exhibit 347:* Each picture depicts a real person who committed suicide while taking Paxil in a GSK-clinical trial. The red "Vs" mean their specific suicides were violent in nature. There were multiple suicides using firearms, including a murder suicide by one patient. There were also two deaths from people jumping in front of trains. https://www.baumhedlundlaw.com/prescription-drugs/paxil-injuries/paxil-trial-exhibits/ Accessed May 1, 2017.

5. Wroe, David. *Criminal Conduct: Confidential Report Reveals Military's Sex Abuse Response was Tainted.* Sydney Morning Herald November 12, 2016. http://www.smh.com.au/federal-politics/political-news/criminal-conduct-confidential-report-reveals-militarys-sex-abuse-response-was-tainted-20161109-gsl6ad.html Ac cessed February 24, 2017.

6. Wroe, David. *Defence rape cases 'cover-up' could be criminal.* Sydney Morning Herald, November 12-13 2016 page 10-11. 7. Parliament of Australia website. *The Pharmaceutical Benefits Scheme: A Quick Guide.* 7 April 2016 http://www.aph.gov.au/About_Parliament/Parliamentary_Departments/Parliamentary_Library/pubs/rp/rp1516/Quick_Guides/PBS Accessed March 1, 2017

Part Three. Sleep Mojo. You've Lost it, Now Get it Back.
Chapter 21. The 10 Insomnia Types.
No references cited.

Chapter 22. Why Natural?
No references cited.

Chapter 23. Natural Solutions for Everyone.

1. Shannon, E., *Five Reasons to Sleep Cool* video, http://compatibilityblanket. com/sleepcool Accessed March 15, 2017

2. Latz, Dr T, *Over Energy Correction Exercise for Anxiety, Sleep and Stress*, YouTube video May 31, 2009. https://youtu.be/FOzjOOiTJ_Q Accessed February 4, 2016

Chapter 24. Type A: Difficulty Falling Asleep.

1. Latz, Dr Tracy. *Over Energy Correction Exercise for Anxiety, Sleep, Stress.* You Tube video. May 31, 2009. https://youtu.be/FOzjOOiTJ_Q Accessed May 15, 2017.

2. Yates, Brad. *Tap O' the Mornin' - EFT.* September 2, 2007. https:// youtu.be/aoSzivsQkVI Accessed June 19, 2017.

Chapter 25. Type B: Difficulty Staying Asleep.

No references cited.

Chapter 26. Type C: Waking Too Early in the Morning.

1. Marano, H. E. *Bedfellows: Insomnia and Depression*, Psychology Today, 1 July 2003, https://www.psychologytoday.com/articles/200307/bed-fellows-insomnia-and-depression. Accessed February 4, 2016.

Chapter 27. Type D: Drugs, Food Additives and Chemicals.

1. Dengate, Sue, as guest presenter with Shannon, E., *Fed Up with Sleep Disturbance, Sleep with the Experts*, July 8, 2009.

2. Dengate, Sue. The Food Intolerance Network website. https://www. FedUp.com.au. Accessed August 5, 2016.

3. Op. cit.

4. Dengate, Sue. The Food Intolerance Network website, factsheets on symptoms. https://fedup.com.au/factsheets/symptom-factsheets. Accessed August 5, 2016.

5. Ibid., *Sleep Disturbance and Insomnia Factsheet*. https://fedup.com. au/factsheets/symptom-factsheets/sleep-disturbance-and-insomnia. Accessed June 4, 2017.

6. Ibid., *ADHD and Diet Factsheet*. https://fedup.com.au/factsheets/ symptom-factsheets/adhd-and-diet Accessed June 4, 2017.

7. Ibid., *Bedwetting Factsheet*. https://fedup.com.au/factsheets/symptom-factsheets/bedwetting Accessed June 4, 2017.

8. Ibid., *Chronic Fatigue Factsheet*. https://www.fedup.com.au/factsheets/ symptom-factsheets/chronic-fatigue Accessed August 5, 2016.

9. Ibid, *Depression Factsheet*. https://www.fedup.com.au/factsheets/symptom-factsheets/depression Accessed August 5, 2016.

10. Ibid, *Joint Pain, Arthritis and Diet Factsheet*. https://www.fedup.com.au/ factsheets/symptom-factsheets/arthritis-joint-pain-and-diet-1 Accessed August 5, 2016.

11. Ibid, *Oppositional Defiance Disorder Factsheet*. https://www.fedup.com. au/factsheets/symptom-factsheets/opposition-defiance-disorder-odd Accessed August 5, 2016.

12. Ibid, *Sleep Apnea Factsheet*. https://www.fedup.com.au/factsheets/ symptom-factsheets/sleep-apnea Accessed August 5, 2016.

13. Ibid, *Teeth Grinding and Diet Factsheet*. https://www.fedup.com.au/ factsheets/symptom-factsheets/teeth-grinding Accessed August 5, 2016.

14. Ibid, *Glutamates Factsheet*. https://www.fedup.com.au/factsheets/additive-and-natural-chemical-factsheets/621-msg-msg-boosters-flavour-enhancers-and-natural-glutamates Accessed June 4, 2017.

15. Ibid, *Propionic Acid and Bread Preservatives Factsheet*. https://www.fedup.com.au/factsheets/additive-and-natural-chemical-factsheets/280-283-propionic-acid-and-its-salts-the-bread-preservative Accessed June 4, 2016.

16. Dengate, S., as guest expert with Shannon, E., *Fed Up with Sleep Disturbance, Sleep with the Experts*, July 8, 2009.

17. The Food Intolerance Network Website, *How to Start FAILSAFE Eating*. https://fedup.com.au/factsheets/support-factsheets/how-to-start-failsafe-eating Accessed August 5, 2016.

18. ibid. *Join Failsafe Newsletter Subscriber List*. https://fedup.com.au/join-failsafe-newsletter-subscriber-list-3 Accessed August 5, 2016.

19. Dengate, S. *Fed Up with Sleep Disturbance, Sleep with the Experts* August 2009. Information not checked recently.

20. The Food Intolerance Network website, *Nasty Food Awards*. https://fedup.com.au/information/fin-campaigns/product-of-the-year Accessed August 11, 2016.

21. Rxisk.org search of Lipitor (the most commonly prescribed drug in this classification). https://rxisk.org/drug/203/atorvastatin/88154/lipitor/ Shows depression and insomnia as reported side-effects. Accessed August 11, 2016.

22. Lucas, Nic, as guest expert with Shannon, E., *Sleep With The Experts, Training Series 2009, Episode 3 Anxiety*.

23. Dengate, S. *Fed Up with Sleep Disturbance, Sleep with the Experts* August 2009. Information not recently checked.

24. Skovlund, Charlotte Wessel, Mørch, Lina Steinrud, Lessing, Lars Vedel, Lidegaard, Øjvind. *Association of Hormonal Contraception With Depression.* British Medical Journal. Downloadable article is at: http://www.bmj.com/sites/default/files/response_attachments/2016/09/23.pdf Accessed June 22, 2017.

25. Medhora, Shalailah. ABC Triple J Hack. *Being on the Pill puts you at Greater Risk of Depression, study finds.* September 29, 2016. http://www.abc.net.au/triplej/programs/hack/pill-can-increase-risk-of-depression/7888306 Accessed June 22, 2017.

26. Ibid.

27. Lidegaard, Øjvind, Skovlund, CW, Morch, LS, et al. *Association of Hormonal Contraception With Depression,* JAMA Psychiatry. 2016;73(11):1154-1162. doi:10.1001/jamapsychiatry.2016.2387 November 2016. http://jamanetwork.com/journals/jamapsychiatry/article-abstract/2552796 Accessed June 22, 2017.

Chapter 28. Type E: Varying Sleep Times, Circadian Rhythm.

1. Macdonald, Kenneth. *Night Shifts Spark Cancer Pay-out.* BBC Scotland Special Correspondent March 15, 2009. http://news.bbc.co.uk/2/hi/uk_news/scotland/7945145.stm Accessed August 17, 2016.

2. ibid.

3. *What's Good for You* television series. Aired on Australian television August 14, 2006.

Chapter 29. Type F: Muscles and Restless Legs Syndrome.
1. American National Sleep Foundation website. *Restless Legs Syndrome (RLS) Treatment.* https://sleepfoundation.org/content/restless-legs-syndrome-rls-treatment Accessed August 17, 2016.

2. ibid.

3. ibid.

Chapter 30. Type G: Illness and Pain.
1. Dengate, Sue. The Food Intolerance Network. *Joint Pain, Arthritis and Diet factsheet.* https://fedup.com.au/factsheets/symptom-factsheets/arthritis-joint-pain-and-diet-1 Accessed September 5, 2016.

2. Everett, Peter. *Survival in a Toxic Soup: Book One of the Broken Planet Trilogy.* Xlibris Corporation LLC, 2013. Page 11. (Quoting naturopath Phillip Alexander's book *It Could be Allergy and it can be Treated.*)

3. Phillips, J.S., McFerran, D. *Tinnitus Retraining Therapy, TRT, for Tinnitus.* Cochrane Evidence Library. http://www.cochrane.org/CD007330/ENT_tinnitus-retraining-therapy-trt-for-tinnitus Accessed September 5, 2016.

4. Martinez-Devesa P, Perera R, Theodoulou M, Waddell A. *Cognitive Behavioural Therapy for Tinnitus.* Cochrane Evidence Library, ENT Group. http://www.cochrane.org/CD005233/ENT_cognitive-behavioural-therapy-for-tinnitus Accessed September 5, 2016.

Chapter 31. Type H: Mind Games.
1. Gøtzsche, Peter, C. *Mental Health, Overdiagnosed and Overmedicated.* https://youtu.be/AMhsPnoldy4. Accessed July 24,

2. Ibid.

3. Whitaker, Robert. *Mad in America*. Cambridge: Perseus Books Group; 2002.

4. Whitaker, Robert. *Anatomy of an Epidemic: Magic Bullets, Psychiatric Drugs and the Astonishing Rise of Mental Illness In America*. Crown Publishing Group. 2010.

5. Gøtzsche, Peter, C. *Forced Admission and Forced Treatment in Psychiatry Causes more Harm than Good* (short version). http://www. deadlymedicines.dk/wp-content/uploads/2016/03/Abolishing-forced-treatment-in-psychiatry-short-version.pdf. Accessed September 5, 2016.

6. Mercola, Joseph and Whitaker, Robert. *Doctor Mercola's Interview with Robert Whitaker on Mental Health*. Uploaded April 29, 2010. https:// youtu.be/OOcJA4Tyw50 (7 part interview) Accessed September 26, 2016.

7. Guskiewicz, Kevin M, et al. *Recurrent Concussion and Risk of Depression in Retired Professional Football Players*. The Indiana Sports Concussion Network. http://indianasportsconcussionnetwork.com/ recurrentriskofdepressionnfl.pdf Accessed September 26, 2016.

8. Hadhazy, Adam. *Concussions Exact Toll on Football Players Long After They Retire*. Scientific American. September 2, 2008. http://www. scientificamerican.com/article/football-concussions-felt-long-after-retirement/ Accessed September 26, 2016.

9. Schwarz, A. *Concussion tied to Depression in ex-NFL Players*. New York Times, May 31, 2007. http://www.nytimes.com/2007/05/31/sports/ football/31concussions.html?_r=3. Accessed September 26, 2016.

10. Shannon, E. *Loss Grief and Shock*. https://www.sleeplessnomore.com/ loss-grief-and-shock/ Accessed September 2016.

11. Karitane Careline Australia. *Depression and Anxiety in Parents.* http://karitane.com.au/mybabyandme/parent-support/peri-and-postnatal-depression-and-anxiety-in-parents/ Accessed September 27, 2016.

12. Shannon, E. *Waking Too Early.* Sleepless No More website. https://www.sleeplessnomore.com/insomnia-type-tm/waking-too-early-c-2/ Accessed September 27, 2016.

13. Shannon, E. *Mind Games, Psychological Health.* Sleepless No More website. https://www.sleeplessnomore.com/insomnia-type-tm/mind-games-psychological-health/ Accessed September 27, 2016.

14. Mercola, Dr Joseph. *Shocking Update – Sunshine Can Actually Decrease Your Vitamin D Levels.* https://www.youtube.com/watch?v=J1sTYuL-QsU Accessed September 27, 2016.

15. Virtual Clinic, Australia – a Cognitive Behavioural Therapy (CBT) research centre, researching CBT and depression, generalized anxiety disorder, social phobia, panic disorder, and others. https://www.virtualclinic.org.au/our-programs.html Accessed September 27, 2016.

16. Omega Brite Website. *Facts on Omega 3 and Brain Health.* This brand of Omega 3 supplement has a high EPA/DHA ratio and has been the preferred Omega 3 supplement in a number of university research studies, including Natalie Parletta (Sinn)'s work in Australia with ADHD children. https://www.omegabrite.com/benefits/brighter-mood/

17. ABC Television Documentary Program *Making Australia Happy.* Aired 2014, 2015. http://www.abc.net.au/tv/programs/making-australia-happy/ Accessed September 27, 2016.

18. www.Rxisk.org. Established to allow individuals to report side effects of medications, independent of the FDA, TGA, pharmaceutical companies, doctors, psychiatrists and practitioners. A new discovery in my quest to find truth in health and medicine.

19. Shannon, E. *Nutrition, Food Additives, Supplements*. Sleepless No More website. https://www.sleeplessnomore.com/nutrition-food-additives-supplements/ Accessed September 27, 2016.

20. Lucas, Nic as guest expert with Shannon, E., *Sleep with the Experts*, Anxiety episode. August 2009.

21. Ibid.

22. . SBS television *Insight*, 2014 Summer Season, *Anxiety* episode. Published November 25, 2014 and available on YouTube https://youtu.be/0-_dVxJi16E Accessed September 27, 2016.

23. Ng, Dr Franzi, *Introduction to Colarbone Breathing*. Published on YouTube May 15, 2009. https://www.youtube.com/watch?v=KAe1zptu_jc Accessed September 27, 2016.

24. Wikipedia, Thought Field Therapy and Roger Callahan. https://en.wikipedia.org/wiki/Thought_Field_Therapy Accessed September 27, 2017.

25. Wikipedia, Meridian. https://en.wikipedia.org/wiki/Meridian_(Chinese_medicine) Accessed September 27, 2017.

26. Shannon, E. *Online Mental Health Treatment – Prof. Gavin Andrews*. June 17, 2010. https://www.sleeplessnomore.com/insomnia-treatments/online-mental-health-treatment-prof-gavin-andrews/ Accessed September 27, 2016. Note that Crufad.org has now become https://thiswayup.org.au/ Accessed September 27, 2016.

27. Birath, J. Brandon et al. *Sleep Disorders in Older Adults*. UT Health Science Centre, San Antonio. http://familymed.uthscsa.edu/geriatrics/reading%20resources/virtual_library/Syndromes/Sleep/Sleep%20Disorders09.pdf Accessed September 27, 2016.

28. Verity, A. *The Innate System Life Insight process. Stress Relief Strategies and Tips Video #1.* http://stressreliefstrategiestips.com/stressreleiftipsvideo1-17.html#comments Accessed September 28, 2016. Think of your stressing problem while you do the exercise described. Clockwise and anti-clockwise with your eyes open, then again with your eyes closed, breathing in each eye position.

29. Gøtzsche, Peter C. *Mental Health: Overdiagnosed and Overmedicated,* Australia 2015. YouTube video uploaded May 12, 2015. https://youtu.be/ZMhsPnoIdy4 Accessed July 24, 2015.

30. Dengate, Sue. The Food Intolerance Network. http://fedup.com.au/factsheets/symptom-factsheets/adhd-and-diet Accessed September 28, 2016.

31. Sinn, Natalie (now Natalie Parletta) *Omega-3, Concentration and Hyperactivity.* Flinders University, Australasian Science, Hawksburn. Jan/Feb 2007. Vol. 28, Iss. 1; pg. 23, 2 pages http://ehlt.flinders.edu.au/education/DLiT/2007/food/Website/Omega%203%20concentration%20and%20hyperactivity.pdf Accessed September 28, 2016.

32. PR News Wire, London, April 17. *New Published Trial Bolsters Evidence that Omega-3 fish Oil can benefit children with ADHD Symptoms.* Source Aquazen UK Ltd. http://www.prnewswire.co.uk/news-releases/new-published-trial-bolsters-evidence-that-omega-3-fish-oil-can-benefit-children-with-adhd-symptoms-154943355.html Accessed September 28, 2016.

33. Sinn, Natalie. An interview by Newshub. *Study: Omega-3 Improves Learning and Behaviour.* Thursday November 13, 2008. http://www.newshub.co.nz/entertainment/study-omega-3-improves-learning-and-behaviour-2008111319 Video previously cited July 2009, now archived (September 28, 2016).

34. Wendee Nicole. US National Library of Medicine. *Secret Ingredients: Who Knows What's In Your Food.* Environmental Health Perspective. V. 121 (4); 2013 Apr. PMC3620743. https://www.ncbi.nlm.nih.gov/pmc/articles/PMC3620743/ Accessed September 28, 2016.

Chapter 32. Type I: Environment.
1. Shannon, E., *Sleep Statistics, Snoring, Adults.* Sleepless No More website. https://www.sleeplessnomore.com/sleep-statistics/ Accessed January 9, 2017.

2. Brew BK, Marks GB, Almqvist C, Cistulli PA, Webb K, Marshall NS. *Breastfeeding and snoring: A birth cohort study.* PloS one. 2014. DOI: 10.1371/journal.pone.0084956. US http://onlinelibrary.wiley.com/o/cochrane/clcentral/articles/512/CN-00984512/frame.html Accessed January 9, 2017.

3. American National Sleep Foundation. *Snoring in Children.* https://sleep-foundation.org/sleep-news/snoring-children. Accessed October 17, 2016.

4. Halbower, Ann C, et al. *Childhood Obstructive Sleep Apnea Associates with Neuropsychological Deficits and Neuronal Brain Injury.* US National Library of Medicine, National Library of Health. https://www.ncbi.nlm.nih.gov/pmc/articles/PMC1551912/ Accessed October 17, 2016.

5. Beebe, Dean, W, et al. *Persistent Snoring in Preschool Children: Predictors and Behavioural and Developmental Correlates.* Pediatrics, September 2012. http://pediatrics.aappublications.org/content/130/3/382. Accessed October 17, 2016.

6. Ibid.

7. The American Academy of Otolaryngology, Patient Health Information. *Snoring and Sleep Apnea.* http://www.entnet.org/content/snoring-and-sleep-apnea. Accessed October 17, 2016.

8. Molloy, H, and Egger, G. *Good Skin: Safe and simple skin care for today's world.* Allen and Unwin, Sydney, 2000.

9. Ibid.

10. Shannon, E. *Wedding Tackle… Yes… Scrotal Temperature.* Sleepless No More website. January 10, 2009. https://www.sleeplessnomore.com/ insomnia-treatments/wedding-tackle-yes-scrotal-temperature/ Accessed January 9, 2017.

11. Teo, Lynne. *Australia's fresh approach to indoor air quality.* 2 July 1999, *ABC Science website.* http://www.abc.net.au/science/ articles/1999/07/02/33084.htm Accessed January 17, 2017.

12. Dengate, Sue. *Home Sick. Failsafe Newsletter 26.* https://www.fedup. com.au/fedup-newsletters/2001/failsaf26-june-july-2001 Accessed January 17, 2017.

13. Dengate, Sue. *Fumes and Perfumes Factsheet.* Food Intolerance Network website. http://www.fedup.com.au/factsheets/support-factsheets/ fumes-and-perfumes Accessed January 17, 2017.

14. *Wolverton, BC; Douglas, WL; Bounds, K. A study of interior landscape plants for indoor air pollution abatement (July 1989, Report). NASA-TM-108061.* https://en.wikipedia.org/wiki/NASA_Clean_Air_ Study Accessed January 17, 2017.

15. Blakeslee, Sandra. *Study Offers Surprise On Working of Body's Clock.* January 16, 1998. New York Times. http://www.nytimes.com/1998/01/16/ us/study-offers-surprise-on-working-of-body-s-clock.html Accessed January 17, 2017.

16. *US Couples Seek Separate Bedrooms.* BBC News. March 12, 2007. http://news.bbc.co.uk/2/hi/americas/6441131.stm Accessed January 17, 2017.

Chapter 33. Type J: Decisions, Decisions.
No references cited.

Chapter 34. Age Related Sleep.
1. Thomson, Helen *The People Who Need Very Little Sleep*. BBC Future. July 7, 2015. http://www.bbc.com/future/story/20150706-the-woman-who-barely-sleeps Accessed January 17, 2017.

2. Kirkup, James. *Margaret Thatcher's Mental Decline Revealed by her Daughter*. August 24, 2008. http://www.telegraph.co.uk/news/politics/conservative/2614020/Margaret-Thatchers-mental-decline-revealed-by-her-daughter.html Accessed January 17, 2017.

3. American National Sleep Foundation. *Sleeping By the Trimesters: 3rd Trimester*. Quoting the study by Dr. Mindell and Barry Jacobson, *Sleep Disturbances During Pregnancy*. https://sleepfoundation.org/sleep-news/sleeping-the-trimesters-3rd-trimester Accessed January 17, 2017

4. Roberts, RE, Roberts CR, Duong HT. *Chronic Insomnia and its negative consequences for health and functioning of adolescents: a 12-month prospective study*. 2008 Mar;42(3):294-302. doi: 10.1016/j.jadohealth.2007.09.016. Epub 2007 Dec 21. https://www.ncbi.nlm.nih.gov/pubmed/18295138 Accessed March 2, 2017.

5. University of Texas Health Science Center at Houston. *Adolescents With Chronic Insomnia Report 'Twofold To Fivefold' Increase in Personal Problems*. March 23, 2008 https://www.sciencedaily.com/releases/2008/03/080320192339.htm Accessed March 2, 2017.

6. Marqueling, et al. *Depression and suicidal behaviour in acne patients treated with isotretinoin: a systematic review.* Seminars in Cutaneous Medicine and Surgery. 2005;24(2):92-102 http://onlinelibrary.wiley.com/o/cochrane/cldare/articles/DARE-12005004733/frame.html Accessed March 2, 2017

7. Joshi, S., Khandwe, R., Bapat, D., Deshmukh, U. *Effect of Yoga on Menopausal Symptom,* Menopause International, Volume 17, 2011. Page 78. http://onlinelibrary.wiley.com/o/cochrane/clcentral/articles/990/CN-00805990/frame.html Accessed March 3, 2017.

8. Newton, KM et al. *Efficacy of yoga for vasomotor symptoms: A randomized controlled trial.* Menopause, New York. 2014, volume 21, issue 4. Pages 339-46. http://onlinelibrary.wiley.com/o/cochrane/clcentral/articles/550/CN-00984550/frame.html Accessed March 3, 2017.

9. Guthrie, KA et al., *Pooled Analysis of Six Pharmacologic and Nonpharmacologic Interventions for Vasomotor Symptoms,* Obstetrics and Gynecology, August 2015. http://onlinelibrary.wiley.com/o/cochrane/clcentral/articles/131/CN-01107131/frame.html Accessed March 3, 2017.

10. Chattha, R., Raghuram, N., Venkatram, P, Hongasandra, NR. *Treating the climacteric symptoms in Indian women with an integrated approach to yoga therapy: a randomized control trial.* Menopause, New York 2008 http://onlinelibrary.wiley.com/o/cochrane/clcentral/articles/813/CN-00664813/frame.html Accessed March 3, 2017.

11. National Sleep Foundation (USA), *Survey of women's sleeping patterns including during pregnancy and after giving birth.* Summary of Findings. https://sleepfoundation.org/sites/default/files/Summary_Of_Findings%20-%20FINAL.pdf Accessed March 3, 2017.

12. Mednick, Sara, Ehrman, Mark. *Take a Nap! Change Your Life.* Workman Publishing, 2006.

13. J. Brandon Birath, MA, Joseph B Kim MD MS, and Jennifer L. Martin PhD *Sleep Disorders in Older Adults,* Pages 1-31. UT Health Science Centre, San Antonia. http://familymed.uthscsa.edu/geriatrics/reading%20resources/virtual_library/Syndromes/Sleep/Sleep%20Disorders09.pdf Accessed March 15, 2017.

14. McCrae CS, Lichstein KL *Secondary Insomnia: Diagnostic challenges and intervention opportunities*. US National Library of Medicine, National Institutes of Health, Sleep Medicine, Feb 5, 2001. Sleep Medicine Reviews, Vol. 5, No. 1, pp 47–61, 2001 doi:10.1053/smrv.2000.0146, downloadable from http://www.med.upenn.edu/cbti/assets/user-content/documents/LichsteinSIreview.pdf Accessed March 22, 2017.

15. Irwin MR, Olmstead R, Motivafa SJ. *Improving sleep quality in older adults with moderate sleep complaints: A randomized controlled trial of Tai Chi Chih*. US National Library of Medicine, National Institutes of Health, Sleep Medicine. July 31, 2008. Sleep 2008, 31:1001-1008. https://www.ncbi.nlm.nih.gov/pubmed/18652095 Accessed March 22, 2017.

16. Birath, JB, Kim, JB, Martin, JL, *Sleep Disorders in Older Adults*, Pages 1-31. UT Health Science Centre, San Antonia. Download this document for Table IV, *Components of Cognitive-Behavioural Therapy for Insomnia: Stimulus-Control Therapy, Sleep-Restriction Therapy, and Sleep Hygiene*, page 28 http://familymed.uthscsa.edu/geriatrics/reading%20resources/virtual_library/Syndromes/Sleep/Sleep%20Disorders09.pdf Accessed March 22, 2017.

17. MacDonald, Fiona. *Can't Sleep? A Weekend of Camping Could Reset Your Circadian Rhythm, Study Suggests*. February 2, 2107. Science Alert. https://www.sciencealert.com/can-t-sleep-a-weekend-of-camping-can-help-reset-your-circadian-rhythm-study-suggests Accessed August 22, 2017.

Chapter 35. More Strategies for Better Sleep and Improved Mental Health.

1. The Association of Systematic Kinesiology. *History of Kinesiology*. http://systematic-kinesiology.co.uk/home/what-is-systematic-kinesiology#history-of-kinesiology Accessed May 15, 2017.

2. Latz, Tracy. *Over Energy Correction Exercise for Anxiety, Sleep, Stress.* You Tube video. May 31, 2009. https://youtu.be/FOzjOOiTJ_Q Accessed May 15, 2017.

3. Gallo, Fred P and Vincenzi, Harry. *Energy Tapping: How to Rapidly Eliminate Anxiety, Depression, Cravings and More Using Energy Psychology.* New Harbinger Publications, Oakland, CA, 2008. https://www.amazon.com/Energy-Tapping-Eliminate-Depression-Psychology/dp/1572245557/ Accessed May 15, 2017.

4. Ng, Franzi. *Introduction to Collarbone Breathing.* Thought Field Therapy. YouTube video, May 15, 2009. https://youtu.be/KAe1zptu_jc Accessed May 15, 2017.

5. *The Music Instinct - Science: Song* https://www.youtube.com/watch?v=m5pwSMDTD4M Accessed May 15, 2017.

6. O'Connor, Sinead and the Chieftains, *Foggy Dew.* YouTube video February 23 2006. https://www.youtube.com/watch?v=13MQFCfCYdQ Accessed May 15, 2017.

7. Kokin Gumi. *Relax Buddhist Meditation Music – Zen Garden.* YouTube video, February 1, 2008. https://youtu.be/CR3dM-GlZK8 Accessed May 15, 2017.

8. Goldman, Jonathan. *Crown of Creation.* June 14, 2007. https://youtu.be/NmA-dWdaI5k Accessed May 15, 2017.

9. Gregorian Chant - "Dies Irae" https://youtu.be/Dlr90NLDp-0 Accessed May 15, 2017.

10. Williams, Vaughn. *O My Brave Soul* A Sea Symphony, Lorna Kelly, audio. https://youtu.be/agC1koZceE0 Accessed May 15, 2017.

11. Ave Maria. April 6, 2007. https://youtu.be/aQVz6vuNq7s Accessed May 15, 2017.

12. Debussy, Claude, *Clair de Lune*. YouTube video uploaded October 2, 2007. https://youtu.be/-LXl4y6D-QI Accessed May 15, 2017.

13. Motzart, Wolfgang Amadeus - *Piano Concerto No. 21* – Andante. Elvira Madigan. YouTube video uploaded January 14 2008. https://youtu.be/df-eLzao63I Accessed May 15, 2017.

14. Goldstein, Barry. *The Most Relaxing Music: Ambiology: A Musical and Visual Journey to Deep Relaxation*. YouTube video uploaded August 19, 2008. https://youtu.be/iQMTH66y60E Accessed May 15, 2017.

15. Valez, Glen. *Frame Drum*. YouTube video uploaded July 26, 2007. https://youtu.be/fB0hE-YlfzQ Accessed May 15, 2017.

16. Kaur, Snatam, *Ek Ong Kaar*, YouTube video uploaded October 7, 2007. https://youtu.be/f3zUYK4YU8M Accessed May 15, 2017.

17. Kaur, Snatam - *Long Time Sun*. YouTube video uploaded March 7, 2008. https://youtu.be/T1D3ejwQiVg Accessed May 15, 2017.

18. Thomson, Jeffrey, *Theta Meditation System: Let Go of Stress, Renew Your Spirit, Gain Insight and Intuition,* Audio CD. https://www.amazon.com/Theta-Meditation-System-Insight-Intuition/dp/1559617578 Accessed May 15, 2017.

19. Appleton, Katherine M, Sallis, Hannah M, Perry, Rachel, et al. *Omega-3 fatty acids for depression in adults*. Cochrane Database of Systematic Reviews 2015. US: http://onlinelibrary.wiley.com/doi/10.1002/14651858.CD004692.pub4/abstract Accessed May 15, 2017.

20. Klaus, L., Berner, Michael M., Levente, K., *St John's Wort for Major Depression*. Cochrane Database of Systematic Reviews 2008. http://onlinelibrary.wiley.com/doi/10.1002/14651858.CD000448.pub3/full Accessed May 15, 2017.

Chapter 36. Survival Skills During a 'Tired Day'.

1. Mednick, Sara C, Ehrman, M. *Take a Nap! Change Your Life.* Workman Publishing, New York, 2006. https://www.amazon.com/ Take-Nap-Change-Your-Life/dp/0761142908 Accessed March 22, 2017.

2. Mednick, Sara C. *Take a Nap! Change Your Life.* Distinctive Voices at the Beckman Centre, Insights on Science Technology and Medicine. Uploaded on Sep 7, 2010 https://www.youtube.com/ watch?v=nG2sJjwO2QQ Accessed March 22, 2017.

3. Ibid.

4. Ibid.

5. Ibid.

6. Ibid.

7. Harold, Glenn. *A Chakra Meditation.* https://www.youtube.com/ watch?v=YOx_uIkZo0c Accessed March 27, 2017.

8. Sheele, Paul R. *10-Minute Supercharger.* Paraliminal audio. Learning Strategies Corporation 2005. https://www.amazon. com/10-Minute-Supercharger-Paraliminal-CD/dp/0925480053 Accessed March 27, 2017.

9. Wild, James. *Songs of the Forest with the Grey Shrike-thrush.* http:// www.quietearth.org/james-wild/music-mp3s/songs-of-the-forest-mp3/ Accessed March 27, 2017.

10. Brown, Chris. *Guided Meditation for Full Body Relaxation.* Published on YouTube December 11, 2013. https://www.youtube.com/ watch?v=m3vXZpSOgcU Accessed March 27, 2017.

Part Four. Where to from Here? Healthy, Happy and Smart.
Chapter 37. Who to Believe, Who to Watch and What to Read.

1. Houghton, Jack, Brennan, Rose and Hennessy, Annabel. News Corp Australia Network. *Dr Sarang Chitale whose identity stolen by conman Shyam Acharya is 'shocked and distressed'*. March 9, 2017 at 10.33 pm.

2. Ibid.

3. Australian Antidepressants Class Action Zoloft and Aropax, Facebook page. A community page raising awareness about the dangers of antidepressants and the inadequacy of the drug warnings and listed side effects in Australia, and portal for the class action being prepared by Drayton Sher lawyers. https://www.facebook.com/AustralianAntidepressantClassAction/ Accessed March 27, 2017.

4. Go Fund Me, Antidepressants Class Action in Australia. https://www.gofundme.com/HelpOurAussieKids Accessed March 27, 2017.

REFERENCES FOR APPENDICES

Appendix 1. Fatigue and Mental Health: Bedroom to Boardroom. Do the Numbers.

References and explanations to accompany the spreadsheet.

Assumptions and Calculations - we have taken a conservative view.

For the purpose of the calculations we are assuming that people work an 8 hour day on average.

1. What is the Average Daily Earnings of an Australian Worker? Australian Bureau of Statistics, Average Weekly Cash Earnings February 2012 Average weekly earnings = 1346.00 (seasonally adjusted), daily = $ 269.20 (assuming 5 days work/week). Released May 17, 2012 http://www.abs.gov.au/AUSSTATS/abs@.nsf/mf/6302.0

2. *Sleeping Pills Linked to Premature Death Published by the Sydney Morning Herald.* February 29, 2012 quoting the British Medical Journal's open journal. February 28, 2012. http://www.smh.com.au/national/health/sleeping-pills-linked-to-premature-death-20120228-1u13o.html "Up to 10 per cent of adults took sleeping pills in 2010, the drugs were associated with 320,000 to 507,000 extra deaths that year." US figures. This figure does not indicate how many times those pill taking adults took a sleeping pill. At the time of print: this article in the Sydney Morning Herald is no longer available. The British Medical Journal's open journal publication of the original study is here: *Kripke DF, Langer RD, Kline LE Hypnotics' association with mortality or cancer: a matched cohort study* BMJ Open 2012;2:e000850. doi: 10.1136/bmjopen-2012-000850 http://bmjopen.bmj.com/content/2/1/e000850 Accessed August 24, 2017. It was reported in the BBC News February 28, 2012 as *Are Sleeping Pills Dangerous?* http://www.bbc.com/news/av/health-17192074/report-suggests-sleeping-pills-linked-to-early-death Watch the video interview. Accessed August 24, 2017. How many of your staff are taking sleeping pills?

3. Ibid. How many times a year do your sleeping-pill-taking staff take a sleeping pill? "Low rates of prescription" are shown in this report to be

fewer than 18 doses a year. Exact figures on how many tablets have been ingested and the loss of production the next day because of the "hangover effect" have not been found by the author of this book. Further research is required to be done. See 2, 21, 33, 39, 40, 41 for further information.

4. As many as 20% of insomniacs report to untested over-the-counter substances or alcohol. http://jama.jamanetwork.com/article.aspx?volume=295&issue=24&page=2851

5. The average worker gets about 6 hours sleep a night. Australian figures. 2010 Galaxy Research independent survey for Virgin Active.

6. MacLean AW, Davies DR, Thiele K. *The Hazards and Prevention of Driving While Sleepy.*

7. The Danish Government has commenced paying compensation to long-term shift workers for their increased occurrences of cancer. BBC News 2009 http://news.bbc.co.uk/2/hi/uk_news/scotland/7945145.stm No payout figures have been disclosed on the internet, that the author can find.

8. The US National Sleep Foundation, *2008 Sleep In America Poll, Summary of Findings.* Washington DC. https://sleepfoundation.org/sites/default/files/2008%20POLL%20SOF.PDF Accessed October 27, 2016

9. Ibid.

10. Ibid. 65% of Americans report having a sleep problem such as difficulty falling asleep, waking during the night, and waking feeling unrefreshed at least a few times each week, with nearly half (44%) of those saying they experience that sleep problem almost every night. The 44% of the 65% equates to 28.6% of the population. Nearly a third of those surveyed (32%) say they only get a good night's sleep a few nights per month. *Longer Work Days Leave Americans Nodding off on the Job.* http://

www.sleepfoundation.org/article/press-release/longer-work-days-leave-americans-nodding-the-job Accessed October 27, 2016.

11. The US National Sleep Foundation, *2009 Sleep in America Poll, Summary of Findings*. Washington DC. https://sleepfoundation.org/sites/default/files/2009%20SLEEP%20IN%20AMERICA%20SOF%20EMBARGOED_0.PDF Accessed October 27, 2016.

12. The US National Sleep Foundation, *2008 Sleep In America Poll, Summary of Findings*. Washington DC. https://sleepfoundation.org/sites/default/files/2008%20POLL%20SOF.PDF Accessed October 27, 2016. 29% of participants admitted being very sleepy or falling asleep at work in the past month. We have assumed this to be 15 minutes per sleepy person/month of lost productivity. 29% of 100 staff x 15 minutes each time x 12 months x daily salary of $ 269.20 = $ 2,927.55/year

13. The Queensland Centre for Mental Health Research, the University of Queensland reports that on average each employee with depression symptoms will cost their employer $ 9,665 per year, of which they estimate $ 7,878 could be recouped if the affected individuals accessed treatment for their symptoms. Calculated at 7.62% of the population who were prescribed antidepressants in Australia in 2006-7.

14. Shields, Margot. *Stress and Depression in the Employed Population*. http://www.statcan.gc.ca/ads-annonces/82-003-x/pdf/4194128-eng.pdf According to the 2002 CCHS, 3% of male workers and 6% of female workers had experienced a major depressive episode in the year before their survey interview. For workers of both sexes, high stress, on and o the job, was associated with depression, a result consistent with othe studies. Men in high strain jobs were 2.5 times more likely and wome 1.6 times more likely than their counterparts in low strain jobs to hav experienced depression.

15. Australian Bureau of Statistics. 1301.0 Year Book Australia 2008 *Feature article 4: Work-Related Injuries*. Shift workers accounted for sixth (16%) of all people who worked at some time in the 12 month

to June 2006. Work related injuries that resulted in death are excluded from this report. Tradespersons and related workers were the only group reported in this report that showed similar incidences of injury between those that work normal hours and shift workers. (108 and 107 per 1000 employed people).

16. Australian Bureau of Statistics, 2006 figures, as above. Almost two-thirds (63%) of injured workers were men. There are more employed men than women, but a higher proportion are still men - 7.4% compared with 5.1% respectively. Men are more likely to work in hazardous occupations and industries than women.

17. Canadian Community Health Survey: *Mental Health and Well-being 2002.* http://www.statcan.gc.ca/daily-quotidien/030903/dq030903a-eng.htm Accessed October 27, 2016. "Any anxiety" is the addition of panic disorder, social anxiety/social phobia and agoraphobia.

18. "Decrements in performance" are not the only side effects of sleeping pills that might affect workers. Side effects include headache, addiction, dizziness, drowsiness, nausea, myalgia, dyspepsia, arthralgia, backpain, halucinations, anxiety, disorientation, drugged feeling, fatigue, lethargy, memory disorders, weird behaviour, and have even been connected to over a four fold risk of death and increased rates of cancer for people taking large amounts of pills per year. See note 2.

19. Fatigue Science. http://www.fatiguescience.com/assets/pdf/Alcohol-Fatigue.pdf

20. Roehrs, T., and Roth, T. *Sleep, Sleepiness and Alcohol Use.* NIH National Institute on Alcohol Abuse and Alcholism. http://pubs.niaaa.nih.gov/publications/arh25-2/101-109.htm Accessed October 27, 2016.

21. Johnson, Lavern C. and Chernik, Doris A. *Sedative-hypnotics and Human Performance.* Naval Health Research Centre, San Diego, California. http://scholar.google.com.au/scholar_url?url=http://www.dtic.mil/cgi-bin/GetTRDoc%3FAD%3DADA108297&hl=en&sa=X&scisig=AA

GBfm3SICiIx7-JiJSvPeZOHMh66VeKCw&nossl=1&oi=scholarr&ve d=0ahUKEwjYxPTL6fnPAhXHppQKHUd_CS0QgAMIHCgAMAA Report No. 81-19. Accessed October 27, 2016. 7.14% of 100 people x 18 times/year x .33 lost productivity x 269.20 = $ 11417.20 per 100 workers "All hypotics, at some doses, produce decrements in performance the next day. Higher doses consistently showed a decrement, and this decrement was usually persistent over the entire day." For my calculations I have assumed that each insomniac in the workplace takes 18 sleeping pills per year (low end of the figures), and that that they perform at 2/3 the productivity for that day after they have taken the sleeping pill. We have also assumed that they have taken only one pill at a time, for one night (not consecutive nights) – not the 'higher doses' or topping up the next night (or subsequent nights).

22. *Re-awakening Australia. The Economic Cost of Sleep Disorders in Australia 2010.* Deloitte Access Economics October 2011, page 56. The Sleep Health Foundation. http://www.sleephealthfoundation.org.au/pdfs/ news/Reawakening%20Australia.pdf Accessed October 27, 2016. Lost performance due to presenteeism equivalent to 7.8 days per annum per individual with insomnia after controlling for comorbid conditions.

23. Ibid. Executive Summary page iii. Prevalence of sleep disorders given as 8.9% of the population - the addition of 3 disorders focused on in this study "since these account for the majority of sleep impacts studied." They are not totals for 'sleep disorders' generally. Obstructive Sleep Apnea (OSA) 4.7% of the population, Primary Insomnia 3%, Restless Legs Syndrome 1.2% total 8.9%. These rates do not overlap. "Costs may be underestimated given the prevalence of people experiencing symptoms of insomnia, RLS or OSA is substantially higher than the proportion of people who are diagnosed with these conditions, and given the exclusion of other sleep disorders" Page iii. These figures are calculated from the 8.9% from these 3 disorders from this report.

24. American Academy of Sleep Medicine (AASM). *Insomnia costing US workforce $ 63.2 billion a year in lost productivity, study shows.* Thursday September 1, 2011. http://www.aasmnet.org/articles.aspx?id=2521

Accessed October 27, 2016. The study estimates the loss of human capital from loss of work performance from insomnia was valued at $ 2,280 per person per year.

25. *Australians in a Depressed State and Antidepressant Prescriptions Skyrocket.* Courier Mail, June 26, 2010. http://www.couriermail.com.au/news/australians-in-a-depressed-state-as-antidepressant-prescriptions-skyrocket/story-e6freon6-1225884636195 Accessed October 27, 2016. In 2008-09 there were 12.3 million prescriptions for antidepressants written in Australia. It shows a 46% rise in the number of prescriptions written for antidepressants and other mental health medications in Australia since it began collecting that series of data 12 years ago. About one in five aged 16 to 85 will have had a mental disorder at some time in a 12-month period. It is worse in people aged 16 to 24, with one in four suffering the effects of a mental illness. Australian Institute of Health and Welfare (AIHW) http://www.aihw.gov.au/publication-detail/?id=6442468376 Accessed October 27, 2010.

26. The US National Sleep Foundation, *2009 Sleep in America Poll, Summary of Findings.* Washington DC. Page 6. See 11 above.

27. Maas, Dr. James B. *Power Sleep: The Revolutionary Program that Prepares Your Mind for Peak Performance.* 1998. Page 129, paraphrased. While the coffee or cola break is seen as a legitimate part of the workday, why isn't there are greater acceptance of a direct response to lack of sleep through a daytime short nap at work?

28. Stephens, D.G. *Midday Naps Get the Nod from Researchers, Workers.* Chicago Tribune. May 8, 1996. Quoting Gerald Celente of the Trends Research Institute, Rhinebeck, NY. "In the future people will understand that naps are a healthy benefit and not a sign of being lazy. Naps are one of the top ten trends for 1996." http://articles.chicagotribune.com/1996-05-08/news/9605080326_1_naps-full-spectrum-fitness-afternoon-craving Accessed October 27, 2016.

29. Maas, Dr James, *Power Sleep* p137. See reference 27. Shift workers average one to two hours less sleep than their daytime counterparts during the week, and three or four hours less on weekends. Sourced from Dr Martin Moore-Ede, Institute for Circadian Physiology, brochure, Human Alertness Research Centre, Cambridge, Mass.

30. Belenky G, Wesensten NJ, Thorne DR, et al. Patterns of performance degradation and restoration during sleep restriction and subsequent recovery: a sleep dose response study. J Sleep Res. 2003;12:1-2. https://www.ncbi.nlm.nih.gov/pubmed/12603781 Accessed October 27, 2016.

    Only 2 hours less sleep per night than optimal over a week can lead to performance decrements equal to 24 hours of consecutive wakefulness.

32. Dr James Maas, *Power Sleep*, Page 137. Sourced from Moore-Ede, see 29 above. 32. In interpreting the information in 33, 34, 35, 36 note that individual prescriptions will vary in the number of doses, the strength of each individual dose and the type of preparation.

33. Australian Institute of Health and Welfare (AIHW). *Mental Health Related Prescriptions.* In 2006-7 over 12 million scripts for antidepressants were written to approximately 1.6 million patients in Australia. This represents 7.62% of the population (understatement, as the total population includes babies and children). www.aihw.gov.au/WorkArea/DownloadAsset.aspx?id=6442456971 Accessed October 27, 2016. (Update: 16.6 percent of Australians are now taking an antidepressant – 2016.)

34. Original data for some tables was sourced from the Pharmaceutical Benefits Scheme and Repatriation, Pharmaceutical Benefits Scheme data (DoHA). See reference 32 above. These figures assume that 100% of depressed people are seeing their medical professional and are 'prescribed', which would actually not be the case, hopefully.

34. In 2006-7 there were 2.77 million scripts for hypnotics and sedatives written to approximately 568,000 patients in Australia. Source: refer 32

and 33 above. This represents 2.71% of the population. Note: the total number of patients is less than the sums of the numbers in the groups as the same patient may obtain prescriptions for medications in more than one group/medicine type. The reductions in the numbers of patients in Table 11.6 was significant. For example, in the general-practioner-prescribed mental health related patient total - the total number of patients added by prescription type amounted to 2,800,165 which was reduced to 2,149,344 total for Australia for the general practitioners. This reduction of 650,821, if it related to the number of patients taking two classes of mental health-related prescriptions would indicate that 30.3% are prescribed medications from, say, 2 groups of the 5. These totals are then reduced for the totals at the bottom of table 11.6 for "All Prescribers". Does this mean that patients are sourcing scripts from different prescriber types? Note (e) talks about 'groups' which is a little ambiguous. See more ambiguous figures at 48. (We are accepting the ones above.)

35. In 2006-7 there were 3.26 million scripts for anxiolytics (anti-panic or anti-anxiety agents) written for approximately 572,000 Australians. Source: see 33 above, notes and 32. This represents 2.72% of the population.

36. Refer 32 and 33 above. In total there were over 20.6 million scripts written in 2006-7 in Australia for mental health related issues. 3.3 million anxiolytics, 2.6 hypnotics and sedatives, 10.6 antidepressants plus other. (Update for 2017 is 36 million scripts.)

37. Refer 32 and 33 above. 20.6 million scripts were written for 2.3 million patients, which represents an average of 8.7 prescriptions per patient for that year. This represents 11.1 percent of the Australian population being prescribed for mental-health-related issues in total in 2006-7. (Update for 2017 is 36 million scripts and 16.6 percent of the population.)

38. The Australian Bureau of Statistics (ABS) 2006-7. *Population Change.* Australia's population in 2006-7 was 21 million. http://www.abs.gov.

au/AUSSTATS/abs@.nsf/Lookup/3218.0Main%20Features32006-07?opendocument Viewed October 27, 2016.

39. Charles, J., Harrison, C., Britt, H., et al. *Bettering the Evaluation and Care of Health* (BEACH). April 2006 – March 2008. Australian GP Statistics and Classification Centre, the University of Sydney. The most commonly prescribed sleeping tablet in Australia, Temazepam (at 1.7 million prescriptions in 2011) has a half life of 8 - 20 hours.

40. Ibid. The most commonly prescribed sleeping pills in Australia were Temazepam 48.1% of scripts, Zolpidem 13.4%, Oxazepam 11.3%, Nitrazepam 11.0%, Diazepam 3.3%. BEACH program, April 2006-March 2008. If 48.1% equated to 1.7 million scripts then the 'real' number of scripts written per year would be 3,541,666. This figure varies significantly to other sources. On July 29, 2015 the RACGP reported nearly 7 million benzodiazepine scripts are written each year in its online media release *New benzodiazepines guide for GPs to improve patient care,* available at *http://www.racgp.org.au/yourracgp/news/media-releases/benzodiazepines-guide/* Accessed April 19, 2017. Has the number of scripts written about doubled between 2006-8 and 2015?

41. Note: The percentages stated for prescriptions/population for hypnotics/sedatives (sleeping pills), anxiety/panic and depression are mutually exclusive - the numbers do NOT overlap.

42. American National Sleep Foundation, March 3, 2008. *Longer Work Days Leave Americans Nodding Off on the Job.* National Sleep Foundation March 3, 2008. See 10 above. https://sleepfoundation.org/media-center/press-release/longer-work-days-leave-americans-nodding-the-job Accessed October 27, 2016.

43. Roehrs, Timothy R and Roth, Thomas. *Sleep, Sleepiness and Alcohol Use.* Vol 25, Number 2, 2001. The US National Institute of Health (NIH), National Institute on Alcohol Abuse and Alcoholism (NIAAA)

publications. http://pubs.niaaa.nih.gov/publications/arh25-2/101-109. pdf Accessed October 27, 2016.

44. Czeisler, C.A. *Sleep Deficit: The Performance Killer, Harvard Business Review. A conversation with Charles A Czeisler, the Baldino Professor of Sleep Medicine at Harvard Medical School.* Harv Bus Rev. 2006 Oct;84(10):53-9, 148. https://www.ncbi.nlm.nih.gov/pubmed/17040040 Accessed October 27, 2016.

45. Ibid. "A company's sleep policy should not permit anyone, under any circumstances, to take an overnight flight and then drive to a business meeting somewhere - period."

46. The US National Sleep Foundation, *2008 Sleep In America Poll, Summary of Findings.* Washington DC. https://sleepfoundation.org/sites/default/files/2008%20POLL%20SOF.PDF Accessed October 27, 2016.
    More than one third of Americans (34%) say their workplace permits napping during breaks at work, with 16% reporting their employer provides a place for them to nap. An additional 26% say they would nap on a break at work if their employer were to allow it.

47. Refer 8 and 89. Caffeine and alcohol disturb sleep.

48. Richardson, David. *Sleeping Pill Safety Test.* Today Tonight television program, May 17, 2008. http://au.news.yahoo.com/today-tonight/health/article/-/3385659/sleeping-pill-safety-test/ The numbers of prescriptions being written for sleeping pills is difficult to ascertain. The Today Tonight show May 17, 2008 quote 2.8 million prescriptions written for Temazepam alone, with an additional 2.1 million for Diazepam, 1.4 million for Serapax and Zolpidem/Stilnox was prescribed to 770,000 Australians. (Some of these figures are similar to those in the UK.)

49. Peetz, Murray, Muurlink. *The Impact of Working Arrangements on the Physical and Psychological Health of Workers and Their Partners.* ACES Mining and Energy Employees Survey. 2012. Page 12 Table 2. Use of sleeping pills was almost twice as high amongst those who wished to

reduce their hours than those content with their hours. 4.1% to 8.0%. And an even higher 11.3% where workers wanted fewer hours and had no say over their hours. Having a say makes a difference to their ability to sleep and they feel safer at work and traveling to and from work. Page 15.

50. Ibid. Pp 6-7.

51. Ibid, page 13.

52. A third of Australians have tried it, but a lack of quantitive evidence around sleep disorders. Overview of Major Drugs, cannabis, Northern Territory Government website. http://www.nt.gov.au/health/healthdev/ health_promotion/bushbook/volume2/chap1/cannabis.htm

53. Rajaratnam, Barger et al. *Sleep Disorders, Health, and Safety in Police Officers.* American Medical Association. JAMA December 2011. A study of 4,957 police officers in US and Canada (2005-7). Positive screening of any sleep disorder was associated with increased risk of self-reported health and safety related outcomes - roughly double the occurrences on having depression, burnout/emotional exhaustion and/or falling asleep while driving. The way this "double" number was arrived at does not allow us to compare these figures with the figures shown for the number of antidepressants prescribed. 10.7% is the figure given here.

54. Moynihan, Ray and Cassels, Alan. *Selling Sickness: How Drug Companies are Turning Us All Into Patients.* This figure varies substantially between sources. Some figures quoted go as high as 30%. See discussion of antidepressants in Chapter 2 of this book. The numbers of prescriptions being written is given to show 'hard figures'.

55. Fahrenkopf, Sectish et al. *Rates of medication errors among depressed and burnt out residents: prospective cohort study.* http://www.ncbi.nlm.nih. gov/pmc/articles/PMC2258399/ Studies have found rates of burnout in residents to be between 41% and 76%, whereas rates of depression range from 7% to 56%. Accessed May 29, 2017.

56. Mednick, Sarah. *Take a Nap! Change Your Life*. Page 16.

57. Ibid. page 13

58. Ibid. page 14. Quoting Dr John A Caldwell, principal research psychologist for the Warfighter Fatigue Countermeasures Program.

59. Ibid. page 18. Quoting from a 2003 report by Circadian Technologies Inc, a leading international consulting firm specializing in extended work hours.

60. The National Sleep Research Project. Www.abc.net.au/science/sleep/default.htm

61. MBF (BUPA) *Healthwatch Survey* - Spring 2007 Specifically - mean hours of sleep per night generally is 6.8 hours. 18-24 age group 7.2 hours, 25-34 6.8, 35-44 6.5, 45-54 6.6, 55-64 6.8 and 65-75 7 hours. The peak mid-career group, 35-44 year olds get the least amount of sleep - 6.4 hours on average.

62. Pfizer Australia and Australasian Sleep Association *National Sleep Study* (sourced from bupa.com.au website June 11, 2012.)

63. MBF (BUPA) *Healthwatch Survey* - Spring 2007. *Australia becoming a sleep deprived nation of 'semi-somniacs'*, media release. www.bupa.com. au. June 11, 2012. The 51% who aren't sleeping enough rate the following as the 'highest' reasons for not sleeping: 11.9% work too much, work related stress, pressure, job insecurity, shift work, and 11.9% too much to do, always busy, not enough hours in the day.

64. MBF (BUPA) *Healthwatch Poll 2009*. One in four Australian adults has taken an action that puts their health at risk as a result of the global financial crisis (GFC). www.bupa.com.au website June 12, 2012.

65. Better Sleep Council. Quoted in Chiropractors' Association of Australia Fact Sheet. *Interesting facts and statistics on sleep. Poor Sleep Affecting*

Accuracy and Attitude On The Job. 2007. www.chiropractors.asn.au Accessed June 11, 2012.

66. *40 Facts About Sleep You Probably Didn't Know,* The National Sleep Research Project. Studies in Canada have shown that reduced sleep during daylight saving adjustments result in 8% more accidents, and having the extra hour during adjustments reduces the number of road accidents. http://www.abc.net.au/science/articles/2002/10/24/689016. htm Accessed June 11, 2012.

67. Sleep Health Foundation, *Re-awakening Australia, The Economic Cost of Sleep Disorders in Australia, 2010.* Oct 2011. Page 30.

68. Ibid., please see calculations.

69. Ibid., please see calculations.

70. Ibid., page 32, please see calculations

71. Ibid. Please note that the report includes costings of other sleep-disorder-related problems such as coronary artery disease, stroke, congestive heart failure and depression. Figures related to the productivity costs of these are included in the *Re-awakening Australia* report in total, based on absenteeism, assumed to be 5.5 days per person employed per year. Calculations and table 4.9 on page 65 of that report.

72. Ibid., page 42 PAF is 'population attributable fraction', the proportion of one health condition, injury or risk factor that can be directly attributed to another. E.g. to a sleep disorder, injury, etc.

73. Ibid., page 42. We have included the base case percentages here.

74. Jason Om reporting: *Higher Suicide Rate Among Doctors.* ABC radio, PM program. August 18, 2010. With Mark Colvin and Michael Paigent. http://www.abc.net.au/pm/content/2010/s2986807.htm Accessed August 24, 2017.

75. Marcus, Carole L, and Loughlin, Gerald M., *Effect of Sleep Deprivation on Driving Safety in Housestaff,* Sleep 19 (1996) 10: 763-766.

76. K. Gamble, A. Motsinger-Reif et al, *Shift Work in Nurses: Contribution of Phenotypes and Genotypes to Adaption.* April 13, 2011. In one study, approximately 14% of night shift workers had symptoms that met the criteria for 'shift work sleep disorder', and nearly a third of the shift work sleep disorder group were depressed. http://www.plosone.org/article/info%3Adoi%2F10.1371%2Fjournal.pone.0018395 Visited June 12, 2012.

77. Lockley, Steven et al. *Effects of Health Care Provider Work Hours and Sleep Deprivation on Safety and Performance.* http://www.ingentaconnect.com/content/jcaho/jcjqs/2007/00000033/a00111s1/art00002 Accessed June 12, 2012

78. Banks, S., and Dinges, D., *Behavioural and Physiological Consequences of Sleep Restriction,* Journal of Clinical Sleep Medicine. Vol 3, No5, 2007. Important to note that this study also demonstrated that sleep deprived people underestimate the effect that the lack of sleep is having on their performance. See graphs of subjective vs. objective sleepiness. http://www.ncbi.nlm.nih.gov/pmc/articles/PMC1978335/pdf/jcsm.3.5.519.pdf Accessed June 12, 2012

79. Refer reference 17. *Canadian Community Health Survey: Mental Health and Well-being 2002.* http://www.statcan.gc.ca/daily-quotidien/030903/dq030903a-eng.htm Only 32% sought help from a health professional (incl. doctor, psychiatrist, specialist, psychologist, nurse)

80. Pidd et al. *Proportion of employed recent drinkers who missed work because of alcohol use or illness/injury, who went to work under the influence of alcohol, and who usually drank at work, by risk category.* Australia, 2001(per cent). 2006. Accessed via "Statistics on Drug Use in Australia 2006" (full publication) Australian Institute of Health and Welfare. Employees, Alcohol in the Workplace. Please note that some industries

we don't normally associate with 'risky and high risk' on this list include education, financial, wholesale, retail, and services.

81. Ohayon and Caulet et al (1997b) *How sleep and mental disorders are related to complaints of daytime sleepiness.* US National Library of Medicine, National Institutes of Health, PubMed. Arch Intern Med. 1997 Dec 8-22;157(22):2645-52. https://www.ncbi.nlm.nih.gov/pubmed/9531234 Accessed June 22, 2017.

82. Maas, James D. *Power Sleep.* Page 10

83. Ibid, page 11

84. Ibid, page 12

85. Ibid, page 54. Original study Stanley Coren, Professor of Psychology at the University of British Columbia. It has been shown that alertness, energy, vigilance, the ability to process information, creativity and critical thinking are affected.

86. Ibid, page 54. Thinking skills are all enhanced with 10 hours sleep, original study by Timothy Roehrs and Thomas Roth.

87. Ibid., pp 59 - 61

88. Hewlett, Sylvia Ann. *Top Talent.* Harvard Business Press, page 24

89. Op. cit., page 90-91. Using alcohol might help you fall asleep more quickly but it supresses both REM (active, dreaming) sleep and non REM (NREM, deep, restorative) sleep. Sleep deprivation greatly magnifies the effects of alcohol, regardless of your physical build. "One drink of alcohol can make you stone cold drunk if you are carrying a large sleep debt." Drinking at bedtime can also start or aggravate sleep apnea, and might prevent the momentary arousals necessary to resume breathing causing you to die in your sleep.

90. Ibid., pages 91 and 117. Sleeping pills, like alcohol, might prevent the necessary momentary arousals necessary to resume breathing in sleep apnea sufferers. "Sleeping pills are respiratory depressants and can exacerbate sleep apnea and related illnesses".

91. Ibid., page 119.

92. Ibid., page 125.

93. Ubell, Earl. *Do You Have Trouble Sleeping?* Parade, September 16, 1984.

94. Moore-Ede, Martin. Institute for Circadian Physiology, brochure, Human Alertness Research Centre, Cambridge, Mass.

95. Stanford Sleep Disorders Centre. *Why Should We Care About Sleep* pamphlet.

96. Irwin, Michael et al. *Partial Night Sleep Deprivation Reduces Natural Killer and Cellular Immune Responses in Humans.* Journal of the Federation of American Sleep Societies for Experimental Biology, 10 (1996): 643-653.

97. Butler, Nancy H. National Forum on Sleeplessness and Crashes Staged in Washington, DC. *The National Sleep Foundation Connection*, Winter 1995.

98. Maas, James D. *Power Sleep* page 154.

99. Chandrasekaran, Rajiv. *Eighteen Wheels and Forty Winks*, The Washington Post, June 22, 1995.

100. Fritz, Roger. *Sleep Disorders: America's Hidden Nightmare*, Nashville: National Sleep Alert, Inc. 1993.

101. Cole, Richard. *Study Finds Sleep Apnea Raises Risk of Car Crash*, Associated Press, 22 May 1997.

102. Maas, James D. *Power Sleep*, page 156.

103. Ibid.

104. National Forum on Sleeplessness and Crashes Staged in Washington, DC.

105. Coven, Stanley, *Sleep Thieves*, Free Press, New York, 1996.

106. Maas, James D, *Power Sleep*, page 164

107. Croucher, John S., *Number Crunch*, Sydney Morning Herald Good Weekend Magazine.

108. Hewlett, Sylvia Ann. *Top Talent*. Harvard Business Press. Page 21. "As employees struggled to cope, negative strategies - such as taking sleeping pills, drinking, smoking, biting one's nails, overeating, and losing one's temper - trumped positive ways of coping".

109. Ibid., page 20. *Hidden Brain Drain* January 2009 survey.

110. Ibid., page 23.

111. Ibid., page 57.

112. Ibid. "Productivity Reduces with Length of Hours Worked" (*General Behaviour and Attitude at Work* section).

113. Rogersa, Peter J and Dernoncourta, Claire. *Regular Caffeine Consumption: A Balance of Adverse and Beneficial Effects for Mood and Psychomotor Performance*. Elsevier. "We conclude that overall there is little unequivocal evidence to show that regular caffeine use is likely to substantially benefit mood or performance. Indeed, one of the significant factors motivating caffeine consumption appears to be "withdrawal relief". http://www.sciencedirect.com/science/article/pii/S0091305797005157

114. Kripke, D., Langer et al. *Hypnotics Associated with Mortality or Cancer: A matched cohort study.* http://bmjopen.bmj.com/content/2/1/e000850.full See reference 3 above.

115. Lakhani, Nina. *Doctors sued for creating 'Valium Addicts'.* The Independent, Thursday 29 December 2011. More than 6.6 million benzodiazepine prescriptions for anxiety were dispensed by England's pharmacies in 2010, a 15 per cent increase in 10 years. Prescriptions for Valium have increased by 20 per cent over the same period. http://www.independent. co.uk/life-style/health-and-families/health-news/doctors-sued-for-creating-valium-addicts-6282542.html# Accessed August 13, 2012.

116. Australian Government, Australian Bureau of Statistics (ABS). The most common mental health problem in Australia, according to an ABS study was anxiety disorder. In fact it affected 14 per cent of all people aged 16 - 85 years in the 12 months prior to the survey. Women were more likely to experience the disorder (18 per cent) than men (11 per cent). http://www.abs.gov.au/AUSSTATS/abs@.nsf/Lookup/4102 .0Main+Features30March%202009 Accessed August 18, 2012

117. Ibid. In the 12 months prior to the ABS Survey 2007 the following showed symptoms of a mental health disorder: 22 per cent of women and 18 per cent of men. What was defined as a mental illness was anxiety, mood or substance use disorder. http://www.abs.gov.au/ AUSSTATS/abs@.nsf/Lookup/4102.0Main+Features30March%20 2009 Accessed August 18, 2012

118. Ibid. Over a lifetime 45 per cent of Australians between the ages of 16 and 85 experienced at least one of the selected mental disorders - of anxiety, mood or substance use disorder. http://www.abs.gov.au/AUSSTATS/ abs@.nsf/Lookup/4102.0Main+Features30March%202009 Accessed August 18, 2012

119. Australian National Prescribing Service Website. *Sleeping Pills and Older People: The Risks.* Published in Medicinewise Living March 31, 2015.. http://www.nps.org.au/publications/consumer/

medicinewise-living/2015/risks-with-taking-sleeping-pills-as-we-get-older Accessed October 24, 2016.

120. Beyond Blue website. Benzodiazepines. *Benzodiazepines and Side Effects.* https://www.beyondblue.org.au/the-facts/anxiety/treatments-for-anxiety/medical-treatments-for-anxiety/benzodiazepines Accessed October 24, 2016.

121. Australian Bureau of Statistics website. *6302.0 - Average Weekly Earnings, Australia, Nov 2016, Table 1: Average Weekly Earnings, Key Figures, Australia, November 2016* Latest issue released at 11:30 am Canberra time. 23/02/2017 http://www.abs.gov.au/ausstats/abs@.nsf/mf/6302.0 Accessed April 18, 2017

122. Shannon, E. *Alarming Sleep Secrets,* chapters 9 and 10.

123. Manousakis, Jessica. Sleep Health Foundation, Sleep Survey Report 2015. *The sleep habits of an Australian adult population: A report on the 2015 online sleep survey from the Sleep Health Foundation.* September 24, 2015. Available for download: https://www.sleephealthfoundation.org.au/pdfs/sleep-week/SHF%20Sleep%20Survey%20Report_2015_final.pdf Accessed April 19, 2017.

124. Charles, J, Harrison, C, Britt, H. et al. *BEACH Bettering the Evaluation and Care of Health. April 2006 – March 2008.* Australian GP Statistics and Classification Centre, the University of Sydney. Available for download here https://www.sleeplessnomore.com/sleeping-pills-prescribed-for-insomnia/ Accessed April 19, 2017.

125. Royal Australian College of General Practitioners (RACGP) *New benzodiazepines guide for GPs to improve patient care.* Media Release 29 July 2015. http://www.racgp.org.au/yourracgp/news/media-releases/benzodiazepines-guide/ Accessed April 19, 2017.

126. The Australian Government, Department of Health, Pharmaceutical Benefits Scheme, *Australian Statistics on Medicine 2014.* Updated 7

March 2016. http://www.pbs.gov.au/info/statistics/asm/asm-2014#_Toc425339262 Accessed April 19, 2017

127. Purcell, Andrew. *Antidepressants: How drugs got into Australia's system.* Sydney Morning Herald. October 11, 2015. 4.49 am. http://www.smh.com.au/national/advance-antidepressants-fair-how-drugs-got-into-australias-system-20151006-gk2jjh.html Accessed January 26, 2017.

128. Britt, H., Miller, C., Henderson, J., Bayram, C., et al. *General Practice Activity in Australia*, BEACH Bettering the Evaluation and Care of Health 2013-14. Family Medicine Research Centre, Sydney University. General Practice Series No. 36. SAND abstract number 212: The prevalence of common chronic conditions in patients at general practice encounters 2012–14. Page 130. https://ses.library.usyd.edu.au/bitstream/2123/11882/4/9781743324226_ONLINE.pdf Accessed April 19, 2017.

129. Gøtzsche, Peter. *Mental Health: Overdiagnosed and Overmedicated.* YouTube video uploaded May 12, 2015. https://youtu.be/ZMhsPnoIdy4 Accessed April 10, 2017.

130. *Half of Australians not getting enough sleep: study.* Sydney Morning Herald (AAP). October 30, 2007. Quoting studies done by MBF. http://www.smh.com.au/news/health/half-of-australians-not-getting-enough-sleep-study/2007/10/30/1193618850766.html Accessed August 24, 2017.

Appendix 2. The Case for Sleep Education.

1. Czeisler, Professor Charles, Baldino Director of Sleep Medicine and Director of the Division of Sleep Medicine, Harvard Medical School and Team Leader of Human Performance Factors at NASA's National Space Biomedical Research Institute. *Sleep Deficit: The Performance Killer.* YouTube Video https://youtu.be/pNHcXmiYsBk. Published November 9, 2012. Accessed January 18, 2016. Also quoted in this

video is that a million people a week nod off and fall asleep on the nation's highways (USA).

2. Swan, Dr N and Balendra, Jaya. *Wasted*. Four Corners. September 28, 2015. Presented by Dr Norman Swan. http://www.abc.net. au/4corners/stories/2015/09/28/4318883.htm. Accessed January 14, 2016. Full transcript available on the website.

3. Ibid.

4. Stephanie Berzinski with Dr Charles Czeisler. *How To Sleep Better. Harvard Sleep Expert Offers Tips and Tricks.* The link between cancer and night shift work. http://www.wpbf.com/health/how-to-sleep-better-harvard-sleep-expert-offers-tips-tricks/30719704. Accessed July 23, 2015.

5. Australian Government Therapeutic Goods Administration (TGA). *Caffeine and Oxedrine Containing Products*, TGA Website. https:// www.tga.gov.au/monitoring-communication/caffeine-and-oxedrine-containing-products Accessed July 23, 2015.

6. Gøtzsche, Professor P.C., *Mental Health, Overdiagnosed and Overmedicated.* YouTube video uploaded May 12, 2015. https://youtu. be/ZMhsPnoIdy4 Accessed July 24, 2015.

7. Whitaker, Robert. *Anatomy of an Epidemic. Magic Bullets, Psychiatric Drugs, and the Astonishing Rise of Mental Illness in America.* Broadway Paperbacks, a division of Random House. New York. 2010. Library of Congress Cataloguing-in-Publication Data.

8. Le Noury, Joanna; Nardo, John M; Healy, David; Jureidini, Jon; Raven, Melissa; Tafanaru, Catalin; Abi-Jaoude, Elia; *Restoring Study 329: efficacy and harms of paroxetine and imipramine in treatment of major depression in adolescence.* British Medical Journal. *BMJ* 2015; 351 doi: http://dx.doi.org/10.1136/bmj.h4320. Published 16 September 2015.

BMJ 2015;351:h4320. http://www.bmj.com/content/351/bmj.h4320 Accessed January 14, 2016.

9. Australian National Prescribing Service (NPS). *Sleep Right, Sleep Tight.* https://www.nps.org.au/__data/assets/pdf_file/0020/84341/ Factsheet__Sleep_Right_Sleep_Tight.pdf Accessed July 24, 2015.

10. Wang PS, Bohn RL et al. *Zolpidem use and hip fractures in older people.* http://www.ncbi.nlm.nih.gov/pubmed/11844004 Accessed July 27, 2012.

11. Gøtzsche, Peter C., *Mental Health, Overdiagnosed and Overmedicated.* YouTube video uploaded May 12, 2015. https://youtu.be/ZMhsPnoIdy4 Accessed July 24, 2015.

12. Charles, J., Harrison, C., Britt, H. et al. *BEACH Bettering the Evaluation and Care of Health. April 2006 – March 2008.* . Australian GP Statistics and Classification Centre, the University of Sydney.

13. Kripke, Daniel F., Langer, Robert D., Kline, Lawrence E. *Hypnotics' association with mortality or cancer: a matched cohort study.* British Medical Journal Open Journal February 28 2012. http://bmjopen.bmj.com/content/2/1/e000850 Accessed July 24, 2015.

14. Swan, Dr N and Balendra, Jaya. *Wasted.* Four Corners. September 28, 2015. Presented by Dr Norman Swan. http://www.abc.net. au/4corners/stories/2015/09/28/4318883.htm. Accessed January 14, 2016. Full transcript available on the website.

15. Saul, Stephanie. *Sleep Drugs Found Only Mildly Effective, but Wildly Popular.* New York Times October 23, 2007. http://www.nytimes. com/2007/10/23/health/23drug.html?pagewanted=all&_r=0 Accessed July 23, 2015.

16. Marcus, Caroline. *Sleeping pill blamed for weird actions.* The Sun-Herald Sunday May 10, 2009. Of 1669 calls made to the Adverse Medicine

Events Line between September 2007 and February 2009, 12 percent related to one sleeping pill.

17. Gøtzsche, Professor P.C., *Mental Health, Overdiagnosed and Overmedicated.* YouTube video published May 12, 2015. https://youtu.be/ZMhsPnoIdy4 Accessed July 24, 2015.

18. Davies, Julie-Anne. *Anxiety Nation.* Sydney Morning Herald Good Weekend Magazine. July 14, 2012.

19. Swan, Dr N and Balendra, Jaya. *Wasted.* Four Corners. September 28, 2015. Presented by Dr Norman Swan. http://www.abc.net.au/4corners/stories/2015/09/28/4318883.htm. Accessed January 14, 2016. Full transcript available on the website.

20. The National Institute of Mental Health (USA). *Mental Illness Extracts Heavy Toll, Beginning in Youth.* Press Release June 6, 2005. Based on National Comorbidity Survey Replication (NCS-R) study. http://www.nimh.nih.gov/health/topics/ncsr-study/nimh-funded-national-comorbidity-survey-replication-ncs-r-study-mental-illness-exacts-heavy-toll-beginning-in-youth.shtml
Accessed August 22, 2015.

21. Harvard Medical School, division of Sleep Medicine. *Stiffened Penalties for Nighttime Teen Driving Associated with Fewer Fatal Crashes.* June 17, 2015. https://sleep.med.harvard.edu/news/547/Stiffened+Penalties+for+Nighttime+Teen+Driving+Associated+With+Fewer+Fatal+Crash
Accessed July 23, 2015.

22. Gøtzsche, Professor P.C., *Mental Health, Overdiagnosed and Overmedicated.* https://youtu.be/ZMhsPnoIdy4 Accessed July 24, 2015.

23. Whitaker, Robert. *Anatomy of an Epidemic. Magic Bullets, Psychiatric Drugs, and the Astonishing Rise of Mental Illness in America.* Broadway Paperbacks, a division of Random House. New York. 2010. Library of Congress Cataloguing-in-Publication Data.

24. Le Noury, Joanna; Nardo, John M; Healy, David; Jureidini, Jon; Raven, Melissa; Tafanaru, Catalin; Abi-Jaoude, Elia; *Restoring Study 329: efficacy and harms of paroxetine and imipramine in treatment of major depression in adolescence.* British Medical Journal. *BMJ* 2015; 351 doi: http://dx.doi.org/10.1136/bmj.h4320. Published 16 September 2015). BMJ 2015;351:h4320. http://www.bmj.com/content/351/bmj.h4320 Accessed January 14, 2016.

25. Ibid.

26. The Australian National Prescribing Service. NPS MedicineWise. *Side effects of paroxetine.* (SSRIs as a group). http://www.nps.org. au/medicines/brain-and-nervous-system/antidepressant-medicines/ paroxetine-antidepressant-medicines/for-individuals/side-effects-of-paroxetine. Accessed January 14, 2016.

27. Harvard Business Review. *Sleep Deficit. The Performance Killer.* A Conversation with Harvard Medical School Professor Charles A. Czeisler. http://www.ncbi.nlm.nih.gov/pubmed/17040040 Accessed July 24, 2015

28. JAMA and Archives Journals. *Sleep disorders common among police officers.* ScienceDaily. ScienceDaily, 23 December 2011. <www.sciencedaily. com/releases/2011/12/111220172618.htm>. Accessed August 24, 2017.

29. Stephanie Berzinski with Dr Charles Czeisler. *How To Sleep Better. Harvard Sleep Expert Offers Tips and Tricks.* (The link between cancer and night shift work.) http://www.wpbf.com/health/how-to-sleep-better-harvard-sleep-expert-offers-tips-tricks/30719704. Accessed July 23, 2015.

30. Dengate, Sue. The Food Intolerance Network http://www.fedup.com. au Accessed July 23, 2015.

31. Oliver, Jamie. *Teach Every Child About Food.* TED Talk. February 2010. https://www.ted.com/talks/jamie_oliver Accessed January 14, 2016.

Appendix 3. Let's Make a Documentary.

1. The United States of America, Substance Abuse and Mental Health Services Administration (SAMHSA), *Update on Emergency Department Visits Involving Energy Drinks: A Continuing Public Health Concern.* January 10, 2013. http://archive.samhsa.gov/data/2k13/DAWN126/sr126-energy-drinks-use.pdf Accessed May 28, 2017.

2. The United States Food and Drug Administration (FDA), *Voluntary Reports on Red Bull Energy Drink. January 1, 2004, through October 23, 2012.* https://www.fda.gov/downloads/AboutFDA/CentersOffices/OfficeofFoods/CFSAN/CFSANFOIAElectronicReadingRoom/UCM328525.pdf Accessed May 28, 2017.

3. Gunja, Naren and Brown, Jared A., *Energy drinks: health risks and toxicity*, The Medical Journal of Australia (MJA) August 2012. Med J Aust 2012; 196 (1): 46-49. doi: 10.5694/mja11.10838 https://www.mja.com.au/journal/2012/196/1/energy-drinks-health-risks-and-toxicity Accessed May 28, 2017.

4. Leahy, Eileen. *Energy drinks can be dangerous for the adolescent heart. Overconsumption poses risks for arrhythmias and other cardiovascular events, per study in Canadian Journal of Cardiology. April 2, 2015.* https://www.elsevier.com/connect/energy-drinks-can-be-dangerous-for-the-adolescent-heart Accessed May 28, 2017.

5. Jensen, Erik. *Watchdog Admits Energy Drinks Dodged State Food Standards.* Sydney Morning Herald, September 4, 2009. http://www.smh.com.au/national/watchdog-admits-energy-drinks-dodged-state-food-standards-20090903-fa17.html Accessed May 28, 2017.

6. *Take high-caffeine energy drinks off the market: NSW minister.* The Sydney Morning Herald (AAP), September 3, 2009. http://www.smh.com.au/national/take-highcaffeine-energy-drinks-off-the-market-nsw-minister-20090903-f9ak.html Accessed May 28, 2017.

7. Environmental Working Group, Washington, USA. http://www.ewg. org/skindeep/ Facebook page https://www.facebook.com/pg/ewg.org/ about/?ref=page_internal

8. Dengate, Sue. The Food Intolerance Network, *Salicylates Factsheet.* https://fedup.com.au/factsheets/additive-and-natural-chemical-factsheets/salicylates Accessed May 28, 2017.

9. *RACP Submission to the Therapeutic Goods Administration (TGA) Advisory Committee on Medicines Scheduling.* Accessed January 29, 2015.

10. AR. Australian Medical Association website July 15, 2013. *Rescheduling of Benzodiazepines.* https://ama.com.au/ausmed/rescheduling-benzodi-azepines Accessed May 28, 2017.

11. *Dolin vs. GSK Dolin v GSK Paxil Trial Transcripts.* Baum Headlund Law website. https://www.baumhedlundlaw.com/prescription-drugs/paxil-injuries/gsk-paxil-trial-transcripts/ Accessed May 28, 2017.

12. Gøtzsche, Peter. C. *Mental Health: Overprescribed and Overmedicated.* Published May 12, 2015. https://youtu.be/ZMhsPnoIdy4 Accessed May 28, 2017.

13. Le Noury, Joanna et al. *Restoring Study 329: efficacy and harms of par-oxetine and imipramine in treatment of major depression in adolescence.* British Medical Journal. BMJ 2015;351:h4320 http://www.bmj.com/ content/351/bmj.h4320 Accessed May 28, 2017.

14. Townsend, Ian. *Fatigue Factor.* ABC Radio National, May 29, 2011. http://www.abc.net.au/radionational/programs/backgroundbriefing/ fatigue-factor/2948418 Accessed January 29, 2015.

15. Fatigue Science, Readiband data. Previously on YouTube at http:// youtu.be/IJqgte7oMf0. Accessed January 30, 2015.

16. Macdonald, Kenneth, *Night Shifts Spark Cancer Payout.* BBC News, March 15, 2009. http://news.bbc.co.uk/2/hi/uk_news/scotland/7945145.stm Accessed January 29, 2015.

17. Shantha M.W. Rajaratnam PhD, Laura K. Barger, PhD, Steven W Lockley PhD, et al. *Sleep Disorders, Health, and Safety in Police Officers.* December 21, 2011.
    JAMA. 2011;306(23):2567-2578. doi:10.1001/jama.2011.1851 http://jama.jamanetwork.com/article.aspx?articleid=1104746 Accessed January 30, 2015.

18. Hall, Ashley. *Lack of sleep ups mental illness risk.* September 1, 2010. ABC Science. http://www.abc.net.au/science/articles/2010/09/01/2999748.htm Accessed January 29, 2015.

19. Armitage, Catherine. *Students Abusing Drugs to Improve Performance.* Sydney Morning Herald, March 10, 2013. http://www.smh.com.au/national/health/students-abusing-drugs-to-improve-performance-20130309-2fsdy.html Accessed January 30, 2015.

20. Faerber, Adrienne E., and Kreling, David H. *Content Analysis of False and Misleading Claims in Television Advertising for Prescription and Nonprescription Drugs.* September 13, 2013. DOI: 10.1007/s11606-013-2604-0. Journal of General Internal Medicine. http://link.springer.com/article/10.1007/s11606-013-2604-0 Accessed May 28, 2017.

21. Krans, Brian. *Truth in Drug Advertising? Not Always.* Healthline website. September 20, 2013. http://www.healthline.com/health-news/policy-tv-drug-ads-often-false-or-misleading-092013 Accessed January 30, 2015.

22. US Food and Drug Administration website. *Prescription Drug Advertising: Questions and Answers.* Guide for Consumers. http://www.fda.gov/Drugs/ResourcesForYou/Consumers/PrescriptionDrugAdvertising/UCM076768.htm Accessed January 30, 2015.

23. Scott, Sophie and Branley, Alison. *Primary Health Care Investigated Again Over Claims of Incentives for GPs to Overservice.* ABC News. December 2, 2014. http://www.abc.net.au/news/2014-12-01/primary-health-care-investigated-for-potential-over-servicing/5930502 Accessed January 28, 2015

Appendix 4. Executive Function Report.
No references cited.

Appendix 5. The Poisons Schedule/Standard.
1. Australian Government, Department of Health, Therapeutic Goods Administration website. *Scheduling of Medicines and Poisons.* 15 July 2016. https://www.tga.gov.au/scheduling-medicines-poisons Accessed November 14, 2016.

2. Australian Government, Department of Health, Therapeutic Goods Administration. *Scheduling Basics.* https://www.tga.gov.au/scheduling-basics Accessed November 14, 2016.

Appendix 6. Sleep Diagnosis Questionnaire.
No references cited.

RECOMMENDED READING

Alphabetical by author.

Ashton, Heather. *The Ashton Manual. Benzodiazepines: How they Work and How to Withdraw. http://www.benzo.org.uk/manual/* Accessed May 29, 2017.

Blake-Tracy, Ann. *Prozac: Panacea or Pandora? Published June 1994. https://www.amazon.com/Prozac-Panacea-Pandora-Antidepressants-Zoloft/dp/0916095592* Accessed May 29, 2017.

Breggin, Peter. *Brain Disabling Treatments in Psychiatry*. Springer Publishing Company. 2007.

Breggin, Peter. *Psychiatric Drug Withdrawal: A guide for Prescribers, Therapists, Patients and Their Families*. Springer Publishing Company. 2012. https://www.amazon.com/Psychiatric-Drug-Withdrawal-Prescribers-Therapists/dp/0826108431

Breggin, Peter. *Toxic Psychiatry: Why Therapy, Empathy and Love must Replace the Drugs, Electroshock and Biochemical Theories of the "New Psychiatry"*. St Martin's Press 2015.

Dengate, Sue. *Fed Up*. Random House, 1998. https://www.booktopia.com.au/fed-up-fully-updated--sue-dengate/prod9781741667257.html

Gøtzsche, Peter C. *Deadly Medicines and Organised Crime. How Big Pharma has Corrupted Medicine*. Radcliffe Publishing London, New York 2013. ISBN-13: 978 184619 884 7 https://www.amazon.com/Deadly-Medicines-Organised-Crime-Healthcare/dp/1846198844

Gøtzsche, Peter, C. *Deadly Psychiatry and Organised Denial*. ISBN 877 159 6240 https://www.amazon.com/Deadly-Psychiatry-Organised-Denial-Gotzsche-ebook/dp/B014SO7GHS

Healy, David. *Pharmageddon.* University of California Press. 2012. ISBN 978-0-520-27098-5 https://www.amazon.com/Pharmageddon-David-Healy/dp/0520275764

Healy, David. *Let Them Eat Prozac.* NYU Press, 2006. ISBN-13: 978-0814736975

Hewlett, Silvia Ann. *Top Talent. Keeping Performance Up When Business Is Down.* Harvard Business Press, Boston, Massachusetts. 2009. ISBN: 978-1-4221-4042-0

Mednick, Sara C. *Take a Nap! Change Your Life.* Workman Publishing Company. New York, 2006. https://www.amazon.com/Take-Nap-Change-Your-Life/dp/0761142908

Moynihan, Ray and Cassels, Alan. *Selling Sickness: How the World's Biggest Pharmaceutical Companies are Turning us All into Patients.* Nation Books. 2005. https://www.amazon.com/Selling-Sickness-Pharmaceutical-Companies-Patients/dp/156025856X

Tye, Larry. *The Father of Spin, Edward L. Bernays and the Birth of Public Relations.* Henry Holt and Company, New York. 1998.

Whitaker, Robert. *Anatomy of an Epidemic. Magic Bullets, Psychiatric Drugs, and the Astonishing Rise of Mental Illness in America.* Broadway Paperbacks. New York. 2010. ISBN: 978-0-307-45242-9 https://www.amazon.com/Anatomy-Epidemic-Bullets-Psychiatric-Astonishing/dp/1491513217

Whitaker, Robert. *Mad In America. Bad Science, Bad Medicine, and the Enduring Mistreatment of the Mentally Ill.* Basic Books, 2001.

Downloadable Articles on the Internet
Alphabetical by author.

Davies, Julie-Anne. *High Anxiety*. The Sydney Morning Herald Good Weekend Magazine July 14, 2012. This article is available, with permission from the Sydney Morning Herald, at http://www.sleeplessnomore.com/anxiety-nation-and-drug-addiction/ Accessed August 8, 2016.

Gøtzsche, Professor Peter C. *Forced Admission and Forced Treatment in Psychiatry Causes More Harm than Good* (short version). March 8, 2016. http://www.deadlymedicines.dk/wp-content/uploads/2016/03/Abolishing-forced-treatment-in-psychiatry-short-version.pdf Accessed August 8, 2016.

Whitaker, Robert. *The Case Against Antipsychotics. A Review of their Long-Term Effects.* http://www.madinamerica.com/wp-content/uploads/2016/07/The-Case-Against-Antipsychotics.pdf Accessed July 28, 2016

Videos, Youtube and TV Shows
Alphabetical order by author.

Blake-Tracy, Ann. International Coalition for Drug Awareness, YouTube Channel. https://www.youtube.com/user/icfda Accessed May 29, 2017.

Breggin, Peter. *Psychiatric Drugs Are More Dangerous than You Ever Imagined.* YouTube video. https://youtu.be/luKsQaj0hzs Accessed May 29, 2017.

Gøtzsche, Peter. C. *Mental Health, Overdiagnosed & Overmedicated.* https://youtu.be/ZMhsPnoIdy4 Accessed August 8, 2016. Don't miss this one, it's a cracker.

Healy, David. Vimeo channel for rxisk.org https://vimeo.com/user11533051 Accessed May 29, 2017.

Healy, David. *04. Secrets of the Drug Trials.* BBC Panorama on suicide and antidepressants: https://vimeo.com/115681494 Accessed June 22, 2017.

Healy, David. *David Healy Lecture – Alcohol.* Excerpt from *The End of Medicine* lecture to medical students in St Bartholomew's Hospital London December 4th, 2012. (Explaining the clinical trial process, using the hypothetical case of alcohol for depression.) From www.rxisk. org and www.davidhealy.org https://vimeo.com/59145379 Accessed June 22, 2017.

Kelly, Shane. *The Benzodiazepine Medical Disaster.* Includes interviews with Emeritus Professors Heather Ashton and Malcolm Lader OBE. https://vimeo.com/188181193 Accessed February 27, 2017.

Shannon E., and Dengate S., *Fed Up with Sleep Disturbance.* Sleep with the Experts webinar 2009. Available in Five Star Sleep Education on Sleepless No More website.

Swan, Dr Norman and Balendra, Jaya. *Wasted.* Four Corners, ABC television. http://www.abc.net.au/4corners/stories/2015/09/28/4318883. htm Full transcript and video available at this link. Accessed August 8, 2016.

Websites with Valuable Information
Alphabetical order by author.

Breggin, Peter. MD. *Violence Caused by Antidepressants: An Update after Munich.* July 25, 2016. http://www.madinamerica.com/2016/07/ violence-caused-by-antidepressants-an-update-after-munich/ Accessed July 28, 2016

Safra, Edmund J, Harvard University, Centre for Ethics. *Institutional Corruption and Pharmaceutical Policy.* https://ethics.harvard.edu/news/ institutional-corruption-and-pharmaceutical-policy Accessed August 11, 2016.

Websites with Reliable Evidence-Based Information
Alphabetical order by website name or topic name.

Akathisia Education - MISSD Akathisia Education. (MISSD: The Medication-Induced Suicide Prevention and Education Foundation in Memory of Stewart Dolin.) Refer Dolin vs. GSK. http://missd.co/

Baum, Hedlund Aristei, Goldman. Dolin vs. GSK case (USA 2017). https://www.baumhedlundlaw.com/prescription-drugs/paxil-injuries/ gsk-paxil-trial-transcripts/

Benzo Organisation and Information. www.Benzo.org.uk Benzodiazepine manual. http://www.benzo.org.uk/manual/ and information by Emeritus Professor Heather Ashton.

British Medical Journal. *Restoring Study 329: efficacy and harms of paroxetine and imipramine in treatment of major depression in adolescence.* Accepted by the British Medical Journal August 3, *2015.* BMJ 2015;351:h4320 doi: 10.1136/bmj.h4320. Open access at: https:// study329.org/wp-content/uploads/2015/09/Study-329-Final.pdf Accessed June 4, 2017.

The Cochrane Library. The Cochrane Database of Systematic Reviews (CDSR) is the leading resource for systematic reviews in health care internationally. http://www.cochranelibrary.com/ Accessed January 26, 2017.

Cytochrome P450 testing. CYP450 enzymes. This test is not routinely recommended, so you will have to find a suitable expert should you want to participate in this testing. If you are in Sydney start with the Blacktown Molecular Research Laboratory, part of the National Association of Testing Authorities. Blacktown Clinical School. http://www.nata.com.au/nata/component/jumi/scopeinfo?key=18636 Accessed June 4, 2017.

Deadly Medicines. Peter Gøtzsche's blog about drugs. http://www.deadly-medicines.dk/category/blog/ Accessed February 27, 2017.

Dolin vs. GSK court case, USA 2017. See Baum, Hedlund Aristei, Goldman (above) which includes court case transcripts.

Food Intolerance Network, Australia. Established by Sue Dengate. For information on food additives, chemicals, and colourings that adversely affect sleeping patterns, behaviours, and mental health. www.Fedup.com.au Accessed January 26, 2017.

International Coalition for Drug Awareness. Ann Blake-Tracy. Online store: https://store.drugawareness.org/ Membership Page: http://members.drugawareness.org/membership/

Mad In America. World leading author of the books *Mad in America* and *Anatomy of an Epidemic* and researcher Robert Whitaker's blog. www.MadInAmerica.com.

MISSD Akathisia Education. MISSD: The Medication-Induced Suicide Prevention and Education Foundation in Memory of Stewart Dolin. http://missd.co/

Preventing Overdiagnosis Conferences. Conferences concerned with over-diagnosis in the medical and mental health disciplines. http://www.preventingoverdiagnosis.net/

Rxisk.org. Register the side effects of prescriptions medications. Established by Professor David Healy. www.Rxisk.org Accessed January 26, 2017.

Selling Sickness, and Selling Sickness Conferences. https://www.facebook.com/sellingsickness/ Accessed June 4, 2017.

Sleepless No More. Elizabeth Shannon's occasional blog. https://www.SleeplessNoMore.com/ *Alarming Sleep Secrets: Your Doctor is Making an ASS out of You, Five Star Sleep Education* and the *Compatibility Blanket.*

SSRI Stories. *Antidepressant Nightmares.* https://www.SSRIStories.org was created by a team of volunteers who wished to build on the legacy of Rosie Meysenburg. Rosie and two colleagues, Ann Blake Tracy and Sara Bostock, compiled the original collection of stories and built the website SSRI stories.com. Rosie maintained it almost singlehandedly from 2006 until her death in March 2012. www.ssristories.net and https://www.ssristories.org. 5000+ Official Database of News Articles documenting antidepressant-induced violence and bizarre behaviour. Index page: http://ssristories.net/archive/indexb6a1.html?sort=date&p

Study 329.org. *Restoring Study 329. Scientific Integrity Through Data Based Medicine.* https://study329.org/ and https://study329.org/bmj-press-release-and-materials/ Accessed June 4, 2017. See British Medical Journal reference above.

Leaders and Truth Tellers

Ashton, Professor C. Heather. www.benzo.org.uk The Benzodiazepine Manual http://www.benzo.org.uk/manual/ and http://www.benzo.org.uk/profash.htm

Blake-Tracy, Dr Ann. International Coalition for Drug Awareness http://www.drugawareness.org/, and Antidepressant Nightmares, Antidepressant Nightmares/SSRI Stories http://www.ssristories.net/, https://ssristories.org/

Dengate, Sue. The Food Intolerance Network. www.FedUp.com.au

Gøtzsche, Professor Peter. Co-founder of the Cochrane Collaboration. Books, papers, BMJ articles, and author of books including *Deadly Medicines and Organised Crime* and *Deadly Psychiatry and Organised Denial*. Peter Gøtzsche's blog. http://www.deadlymedicines.dk/category/blog/

Healy, David, Professor. His blog: https://davidhealy.org/.
Rxisk.org: Making Medicines Safer for All of Us. https://rxisk.org/
https://www.facebook.com/david.healy.7773

Jureidini, Jon, Professor at Adelaide University. One of the authors of Restoring Study 329. http://www.adelaide.edu.au/directory/jon. jureidini And yes, an Aussie.

Le Noury, Joanna, John M Nardo, David Healy, Jon Jureidini, Melissa Raven, Catalin Tufanaru, Elia Abi-Jaoude: The group that reanalysed SmithKline Beecham's Study 329. The work accepted to BMJ August 3, 2015. See references throughout this book. http://www.bmj.com/content/351/bmj.h4320 Accessed June 4, 2017.

Mednick, Dr Sara. *Take a Nap! Change Your Life* author.

Moynihan, Ray and Cassels, Alan. *Selling Sickness* book and Selling Sickness Conference. Ray Moynihan is an Aussie too.

Whitaker, Robert. Author *Mad in America* and *Anatomy of an Epidemic: Magic Bullets, Psychiatric Drugs, and the Astonishing Rise of Mental Illness in America*. https://www.madinamerica.com/
https://www.facebook.com/madinamerica/

Australian Antidepressants' Class Action

http://www.draytonsherlawyers.com.au/class-action-antidepressants/
Accessed July 28, 2016

Australian Antidepressants Class Action and Awareness
https://www.facebook.com/AustralianAntidepressantClassAction/
Accessed June 4, 2017.

Go Fund Me fundraiser for the Antidepressants Class Action https://www.
gofundme.com/HelpOurAussieKids Accessed June 4, 2017.

Sleepless No More Education and Products
Five Star Sleep Education. Downloadable sleep training membership, completed by me in 2013. Book here: https://www.sleeplessnomore.com/
booking-form/

Alarming Sleep Secrets Book: Available from Amazon.com in hard copy
book form, or downloadable Kindle e-book. After publishing I will post
the exact Amazon link on my website at: https://www.sleeplessnomore.
com/alarming-sleep-secrets.

Compatibility Blanket. The bedcovering that solves arguments between
hot and cold bed partners. https://www.SleeplessNoMore.com/
compatibility-blanket. My apologies for the high postage costs overseas,
I'm looking for distributors.

Keynotes. If you would like me to present at your conference, corporate
function, health and wellness event, multi-speaker event, or webinar
please email your proposal to elizabeth@sleeplessnomore.com with
"Speaking Proposal" in the subject line of the email.

Support Groups if you Choose to Come off Medications
Paroxetine (Paxil, Aropax, Seroxat)
https://www.facebook.com/groups/204732929546136/

Life Beyond SSRI Antidepressants - Prozac Effexor and many more https://
www.facebook.com/groups/103788426372995/

Effexor (Venlafaxine) Side Effects, Withdrawal and Discontinuation Syndrome https://www.facebook.com/groups/effexorsupportgroup/

Cymbalta Survivors Support Group https://www.facebook.com/groups/cymbaltasurvivors/

Cymbalta Dangers International https://www.facebook.com/CymbaltaDangersInternational/

Cymbalta Hurts Worse https://www.facebook.com/groups/Cymbaltahurtsworse/

Australian Antidepressants Class Action and Awareness https://www.facebook.com/AustralianAntidepressantClassAction/

Antidepressants Australia Chat https://www.facebook.com/groups/AussieAntidepressantsChat/

Surviving Antidepressants - Antidepressant Withdrawal https://www.facebook.com/survivingantidepressants/

Surviving Antidepressants website http://survivingantidepressants.org/

Letters from Generation RX https://www.facebook.com/LettersFromGenerationRx/

Australia Jons Legacy Prescribed Medications Their Deadly Interactions https://www.facebook.com/JonsLegacy/

International Coalition for Drug Awareness https://www.facebook.com/groups/DRUGAWARENESS/

MISSD Akathisia Education http://missd.co/

Cochrane Research Helper?

If you are impressed by Cochrane's work, you might like to help them in a voluntary capacity.

I think they look for people to do the preliminary screenings of clinical trials, so that the professionals can add the trials to their reviews.

The bonus for this is, if you are into 'alternative medicine' and you can find correctly run clinical trials, you can put natural and alternative trial results forward as well, for consideration.

Cochrane does not only look at drug solutions to health problems.

To find out more go to http://methods.cochrane.org/sdt/welcome, where you might contact Cochrane for more information.

You might be required to do some training, but it will be interesting training whether you end up volunteering or not.

The least that can happen is that you will look at all clinical trials with new and informed eyes.

Jokes

You'll probably need some light relief!

Barker, Arj. *Mattresses and iPods*. The Melbourne Comedy Festival Gala in 2008. Uploaded to YouTube Feb 2, 2009. https://youtu.be/G7aV2KLmsHY Accessed August 8, 2016.

Mayer, Bill. *Anti-Pharma Rant*. Uploaded to YouTube September 30, 2007. https://youtu.be/rHXXTCc-IVg. Accessed August 8, 2016.

Oliver, John. *Last Week Tonight with John Oliver: Marketing to Doctors*, HBO. https://youtu.be/YQZ2UeOTO3I. Accessed August 8, 2016.

Contact Details

Elizabeth Shannon
Sleepless No More
Website: www.SleeplessNoMore.com
Email: elizabeth@sleeplessnomore.com

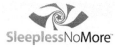

Mobile Phone: + 61 4 58 41 4441 (Sydney, Australia time zone)
Website: https://www.SleeplessNoMore.com
Twitter: @SleeplessNoMore
Facebook: https://www.facebook.com/sleeplessnomore and
https://www.facebook.com/ElizabethMaryShannon
Skype: elizabeth.shannon.

National Television and Media Appearances (Australia and the US): https://www.sleeplessnomore.com/media/

INDEX

CPSIA information can be obtained
at www.ICGtesting.com
Printed in the USA
BVHW041016200619
551532BV00017B/2098/P